Equine Welfare

The Universities Federation for Animal Welfare

UFAW, founded 1926, is an international, independent, scientific and educational animal welfare charity that works to improve high standards of welfare for farm, companion, laboratory and captive wild animals, and for those animals with which we interact in the wild. It works to improve animals' lives by:

- Promoting and supporting developments in the science and technology that underpin advances in animal welfare;
- Promoting education in animal care and welfare;
- Providing information, organising meetings, and publishing books, videos, articles, technical reports and the journal *Animal Welfare*;
- Providing expert advice to government departments and other bodies and helping to draft and amend laws and guidelines;
- Enlisting the energies of animal keepers, scientists, veterinarians, lawyers and others who care about animals.

"Improvements in the care of animals are not now likely to come of their own accord, merely by wishing them: there must be research ... and it is in sponsoring research of this kind, and making its results widely known, that UFAW performs one of its most valuable services."

Sir Peter Medawar CBE FRS, 8th May 1957
Nobel Laureate (1960), Chairman of the UFAW Scientific Advisory Committee (1951–1962)

UFAW relies on the generosity of the public through legacies and donations to carry out its work improving the welfare of animal now and in the future. For further information about UFAW and how you can help promote and support its work, please contact us at the address below.

Universities Federation for Animal Welfare
The Old School, Brewhouse Hill, Wheathampstead, Herts AL4 8AN, UK
Tel: 01582 831818 Fax: 01582 831414 Website: www.ufaw.org.uk
Email: ufaw@ufaw.org.uk

UFAW's aim regarding the UFAW/Wiley-Blackwell Animal Welfare book series is to promote interest and debate in the subject and to disseminate information relevant to improving the welfare of kept animals and of those harmed in the wild through human agency. The books in this series are the works of their authors and the views they express do not necessarily reflect the views of UFAW.

Equine Welfare

Edited by

C. Wayne McIlwraith
University Distinguished Professor,
Barbara Cox Anthony University
Endowed Chair in Orthopaedics,
Director of Orthopaedic Research
Center and Musculoskeletal Program,
Colorado State University, Fort Collins,
Colorado, USA

Bernard E. Rollin
University Distinguished Professor,
Professor of Philosophy,
Professor of Animal Sciences,
Professor of Biomedical Sciences,
University Bioethicist,
Department of Philosophy,
Colorado State University,
Fort Collins, Colorado, USA

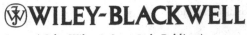

WILEY-BLACKWELL

A John Wiley & Sons, Ltd., Publication

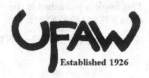

Established 1926

This edition first published 2011 by Blackwell Publishing Ltd.
© 2011 by UFAW

Series Editors
James K. Kirkwood and Robert C. Hubrecht

Blackwell Publishing was acquired by John Wiley & Sons in February 2007. Blackwell's publishing program has been merged with Wiley's global Scientific, Technical and Medical business to form Wiley-Blackwell.

Registered Office
John Wiley & Sons Ltd, The Atrium, Southern Gate, Chichester, West Sussex, PO19 8SQ, UK

Editorial Offices
9600 Garsington Road, Oxford, OX4 2DQ, UK
The Atrium, Southern Gate, Chichester, West Sussex, PO19 8SQ, UK
2121 State Avenue, Ames, Iowa 50014-8300, USA

For details of our global editorial offices, for customer services and for information about how to apply for permission to reuse the copyright material in this book please see our website at www.wiley.com/wiley-blackwell.

The right of the authors to be identified as the authors of this work has been asserted in accordance with the UK Copyright, Designs and Patents Act 1988.

Library of Congress Cataloging-in-Publication Data

Equine welfare / edited by C. Wayne McIlwraith, Bernard E. Rollin.
    p. ; cm.
    Includes bibliographical references and index.
    ISBN 978-1-4051-8763-3 (pbk. : alk. paper)
1. Horses. 2. Animal welfare. I. McIlwraith, C. Wayne. II. Rollin, Bernard E.
[DNLM: 1. Horses. 2. Animal Husbandry. 3. Animal Welfare. 4. Horse Diseases. SF 285.3]
    HV4749.E68 2011
    179'.3–dc22
                                        2010041319

A catalogue record for this book is available from the British Library.

This book is published in the following electronic formats: ePDF 9781444397802; ePub 9781444397819

Set in 10/12.5pt Sabon by SPi Publisher Services, Pondicherry, India

1   2011

Contents

Contributors

Kent Allen, DVM
Virginia Equine Clinic
Middleburg, VA
USA

Rick M. Arthur, DVM
Equine Medical Director
School of Veterinary Medicine
University of California
Davis, CA
USA

Jay Baldwin, DVM
First Equine Horse Health
Services, LLC
Dover, DE
USA

Jerry B. Black, DVM
Director of Equine Sciences
Undergraduate Program
Colorado State University Equine Center
Colorado State University
Fort Collins, CO
USA

Doug Corey, DVM
Associated Veterinary Medical Center
Walla Walla, CA
USA

Andrew F. Fraser, DVM, PhD
Carbonear
Newfoundland
Canada

David Frisbie, DVM, PhD, DACVS
Associate Professor
Gail Holmes Equine Orthopaedic
Research Center
Department of Clinical Sciences
Colorado State University
Fort Collins, CO
USA

Laurie Goodrich, DVM, PhD, DACVS
Assistant Professor
Gail Holmes Equine Orthopaedic
Research Center
Department of Clinical Sciences
Colorado State University
Fort Collins, CO
USA

Kevin K. Haussler, DVM, DC, PhD
Assistant Professor
Gail Holmes Equine Orthopaedic
Research Center
Department of Clinical Sciences
Colorado State University
Fort Collins, CO
USA

Jim Heird, PhD
Executive Professor and Coordinator
College of Veterinary Medicine
and Biomedical Sciences
Texas A & M University
College Station, TX
USA

Albert J. Kane, DVM, MPVM, PhD
Senior Staff Veterinarian
APHIS/BLM Wild Horse and Burro
Partnership
US Department of Agriculture, APHIS,
Veterinary Services
Fort Collins, CO
USA

Marthe Kiley-Worthington, PhD
Centre d'Eco-Etho Recherche et
Education
La Combe, Drome
France

Midge Leitch, VMD, DACVS
Staff Veterinarian in Radiology
University of Pennsylvania
School of Veterinary Medicine
Kennett Square, PA
USA

Tom R. Lenz, DVM, MS, DACT
Senior Director
Equine Veterinary Operations
Pfizer Animal Health
USA

Nancy S. Loving, DVM
Loving Equine Clinic
Boulder, CO
USA

D. Paul Lunn, BVSc, PhD, DACVIM
Department of Clinical Sciences
James L. Voss Veterinary Teaching
Hospital
College of Veterinary Medicine
and Biomedical Sciences
Colorado State University
Fort Collins, CO
USA

Khursheed Mama, DVM, DACVA
Department of Clinical Sciences
James L. Voss Veterinary Teaching
Hospital
College of Veterinary Medicine
and Biomedical Sciences
Colorado State University
Fort Collins, CO
USA

Jay G. Merriam, DVM
Massachusetts Equine Clinic
Uxbridge, MA
USA

Nat T. Messer, IV, DVM, DABVP
Professor
University of Missouri
Columbia, MO
USA

**C. Wayne McIlwraith, BVSc, PhD,
DSc, DACVS, FRCVS, DECVS**
University Distinguished Professor
Barbara Cox Anthony University
Endowed Chair in Orthopaedics
Director, Gail Holmes Equine
Orthopaedic Research Center
Department of Clinical Sciences
Colorado State University
Fort Collins, CO
USA

Richard D. Mitchell, DVM
Fairfield Equine Associates
Newtown, CT
USA

Joe D. Pagan, PhD
Founder and President
Kentucky Equine Research
Versailles, KY
USA

David W. Ramey, DVM
Porter Ranch, CA
USA

Bernard Rollin, PhD
University Distinguished Professor
Professor of Philosophy
Professor of Animal Sciences
Professor of Biomedical Sciences
University Bioethicist
Department of Philosophy
Colorado State University
Fort Collins, CO
USA

Josie L. Traub-Dargatz, DVM, MS,
DACVS
Animal Population Health Institute
College of Veterinary Medicine
and Biomedical Sciences
Colorado State University
Fort Collins, CO
USA

and

US Department of Agriculture, APHIS,
Veterinary Services
Center for Epidemiology and Animal
Health
Fort Collins, CO
USA

Foreword

Having evolved to help us maximize our evolutionary fitness – most recently as we (our ancestors) lived in the trees, descended to the savannahs, and emigrated as hunter–gatherers to the far ends of the Earth – our brains are wired to raise all sorts of 'gut feelings,' 'instincts,' and preferences. Regardless of their relevance to the very different habitats we have since created for ourselves, these default biases – 'Don't touch snakes,' 'Be wary of spiders,' 'Try tasting the red berries,' and many others far less apparent to us – remain subtly powerful and very influential. Unless we take time to stop and consider, using evidence and reason, our brains are inclined to make, and stick to, hasty judgments about what is good or bad, and about what they like and what they don't (to the detriment of the welfare of some species). This can have adverse consequences for animal welfare.

There is something about horses that makes us tend to feel very fondly toward them. Nancy Loving (Chapter 13) captures this very evocatively: 'The whicker of welcome, the soft blow of a horse's sweet breath on one's face, and the velvet touch of a warm muzzle add to the special emotional attachment an owner feels for a horse.' So, too, in more muscular but equally eloquent style, does David Ramey (Chapter 2): 'To ride a horse at speed gives its rider metaphorical wings, freeing man from the constraints of the ground, even if only for a short time. Throughout history, these needs have been celebrated in poetry, writing, sculpture, paintings, and drawings. The horse has been given high marks for honor, intelligence, and wisdom, and has been given a wide and diverse range of symbolic meanings. The horse has been treated with reverence, and man has used the horse as a symbol for his highest aspirations.' As this book shows, such warmth and admiration often foster great concern and effort to provide for the welfare – the quality of life – of horses. Are all animals so fortunate?

Toads, rats, and the very many other species that, in contrast, tend to be judged the other way by our brains are more used to the harsher facets of human behavior. However, they might console themselves by observing that there can be some significant risks in having such close relationships with humans. In the case of horses, as we see in this book, these can include: 'firing' (see Chapter 11), 'soring' to adjust gait and impress show judges (see Chapter 12), suboptimal housing leading to behavioral abnormalities, inappropriate feeding (often reflecting generosity unconstrained by knowledge, or overwhelming it), and being at risk (often for similar reasons) of 'alternative' therapies that have no scientific basis.

UFAW works to improve the welfare of animals by promoting and supporting research aimed at determining animals' needs and how these can be met (both of which can be much more difficult than our hasty, biased, brains often assume) and through education, including publishing information relevant to animal welfare. One way that animal welfare improvements can be brought about is through becoming aware that standards for animal care in some situations fall short of those in others. It is therefore very helpful to look across the range of ways in which animals are kept and used, both between and, as most valuably done in this book, within species. As UFAW's founder, Charles Hume, stated in his foreword to one of the charity's first books, The UFAW Handbook on the Care and Management of Farm Animals (Churchill Livingstone, 1971): 'UFAW does not necessarily support all the procedures that are described, and hopes that as knowledge accumulates some alternative and more humane methods will be developed.' Although horses have been kept for thousands of years, it is only very recently that practices have begun to be scientifically scrutinized from the welfare point of view and there are, no doubt, many improvements to be made, as recognized by the editors in their preface.

We are very grateful to Wayne McIlwraith and Bernie Rollin for their excellent work in drawing together and editing this book (and patiently dealing with all of the editorial comments from UFAW), and to all the authors for their very interesting, informative, valuable, and New- and Old-World flavored chapters on aspects of our interactions with this very appealing animal.

James K. Kirkwood
UFAW

Preface

Western society is in the midst of a major cultural revolution in how animals are viewed and in how they ought to be treated in the course of human use. Despite the fact that rats and mice continue to be viewed by some as vermin, society has nonetheless demanded that the pain and distress they undergo in the process of research be regulated in law. Similar demands are being made regarding the animals used for food. Indeed, in 2004, no fewer than 2100 laws pertaining to animal welfare were proposed in state legislatures across the USA. Inevitably, the ethical searchlight illuminating animal use has focused on the horse, an animal second only to the dog in its iconic stature. Those who view horses as livestock have been outpaced by those who see them as companion animals. Equine uses long taken for granted or ignored by society in general have been thrown into stark relief as emerging animal welfare issues.

The equine industry has often tended to ignore the animal welfare issues following in its wake, and has historically not attracted a great deal of opprobrium. This is even true of the Tennessee Walking Horse show industry, which, despite federal legislation promulgated in the 1970s aimed at correcting welfare abuses, continued to behave as it always had. That this social inattention will not last is patent, given all else that has occurred regarding animal welfare. If society is shocked by a practice, it will act, even if it has not thought through the consequences of its actions – witness what has occurred in regard to horse slaughter. If the industry wishes to retain its autonomy, it must address animal welfare issues in an anticipatory way, even if the issues have not yet reached societal consciousness.

This book is intended to stimulate thought and discussion in the equine industry regarding horse welfare in general and various issues specific to different industries. Toward this end, we have gathered knowledgeable experts in diverse aspects of equine use. Their chapters are not meant to be the final word on the topic, but the first word. They review what has been done regarding equine welfare and where we are going.

The book has grown out of a thirty-year collegial and friendship relationship between the two editors, one of us an equine surgeon and researcher, and the other a philosopher focusing on animal ethics. Our extensive history of watching yesterday's acceptable practices turn into today's social issues, combined with our close tracking of animal welfare concerns, convinced us of the timeliness – indeed exigency – of such a book.

We are grateful to our authors for their willingness to address the issues in their areas of expertise. Virtually no one refused our invitation. We are also grateful to Paula Vanderlinden for her tireless organizational efforts.

Wayne McIlwraith
Bernard Rollin
Fort Collins

Part I
Respecting the Horse's Needs and Nature

Equine Welfare and Ethics

Bernard Rollin

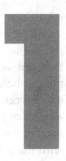

There is an ancient curse that is most appropriate to the society in which we live: 'May you live in interesting times.' From the point of view of our social ethics, we do indeed live in bewildering and rapidly changing times. The traditional, widely shared, social ethical truisms that gave us stability, order, and predictability in society for many generations are being widely challenged by women, ethnic minorities, homosexuals, the handicapped, animal rights advocates, internationalists, environmentalists, and more.

It is very likely that there has been more and deeper social ethical change since the middle of the twentieth century than occurred during centuries of an ethically monolithic period such as the Middle Ages. Anyone over forty has lived through a variety of major ethical changes: the questioning of IQ differentiation, the rise of homosexual militancy, the end of '*in loco parentis*' in universities, the advent of consumer advocacy, the end of mandatory retirement age, the mass acceptance of environmentalism, the growth of a 'sue the bastards' mind-set, the implementation of affirmative action programs, the rise of massive drug use, the designation of alcoholism and child abuse as diseases rather than moral vices, the rise of militant feminism, the emergence of sexual harassment as a major social concern, the demands by the handicapped for equal access, the rise of public suspicion of science and technology, the mass questioning of animal use in science and industry, the end of colonialism, the rise of political correctness – all provide patent examples of the magnitude of ethical change during this brief period.

It is arguable that morally based boycotting of South African business was instrumental in bringing about the end of apartheid, and similar boycotting of some farm products in the USA led to significant improvements in the living situations of farm workers. It is *de rigueur* for major corporations to have reasonable numbers of

Equine Welfare, First Edition. Edited by C. Wayne McIlwraith and Bernard E. Rollin.
© 2011 by UFAW. Published 2011 by Blackwell Publishing Ltd.

minorities visibly peopling their ranks, and for liquor companies to advertise on behalf of moderation in alcohol consumption. Cigarette companies now press upon the public a message that cigarettes kill and extol their involvement in protecting battered women; forestry and oil companies spend millions (even billions) to persuade the public of their environmental commitments. The news station, CNN, reported that 'green' investment funds grew significantly faster than ordinary funds, and reports of child labor or sweatshop working conditions can literally destroy product markets overnight. Monitoring such societal ethical changes and operating in accord with them is essential for all professions, businesses, and governmental agencies.

Not only is success tied to social ethics, but even more fundamentally, freedom and autonomy are as well. Every profession – be it medicine, law, or agriculture – is given freedom by the social ethic to pursue its aims. In return, society basically says to professions it does not understand well enough to regulate: 'You regulate yourselves the way we would regulate you if we understood what you do, which we don't. But we will know if you don't self-regulate properly and then we will regulate you, despite our lack of understanding.' For example, some years ago, the US Congress became concerned about excessive use of antibiotics in animal feeds and concluded that veterinarians were a major source of the problem. As a result, Congress was about to ban extra-label drug use by veterinarians, a move that would have killed veterinary medicine as we know it. However, through extensive efforts to educate legislators, such legislation did not proceed to law. In the same vein, it is much more difficult to be an accountant, post-Enron, because of the proliferation of regulatory restrictions.

One major social ethical concern that has developed over the last three decades is a significant emphasis on the treatment of animals used by society for various purposes. It is easy to demonstrate the degree to which these concerns have seized the public imagination. According to both the US National Cattlemen's Beef Association and the National Institutes of Health (the latter being the source of funding for the majority of biomedical research in the USA), neither group inclined to exaggerate the influence of animal ethics; by the early 1990s, the US Congress had been consistently receiving more letters, phone calls, faxes, emails, and personal contacts on animal-related issues than on any other topic (C. McCarthy, NIH, personal communication; NCBA, 1991).

Whereas twenty years ago, one would have found no bills pending in the US Congress relating to animal welfare, the last decades has witnessed 50 to 60 such bills annually, with even more proliferating at the state level (A. Douglas, American Human Association, Washington, DC, personal communication). The federal bills range from attempts to prevent duplication in animal research, to saving marine mammals from becoming victims of tuna fishermen, to preventing importation of ivory, to curtailing the parrot trade. State laws passed in large numbers have increasingly prevented the use of live or dead shelter animals for biomedical research and training and have focused on myriad other areas of animal welfare. Eight states have abolished the steel-jawed leghold trap (HSUS, 2003). When Colorado's politically appointed Wildlife Commission failed to act on a recommendation from the Division of Wildlife to abolish the spring bear hunt (because hunters were liable to shoot lactating mothers, leaving their orphaned cubs to die of starvation), the general public ended the hunt through a popular referendum. Seventy percent of Colorado's population voted for this as a constitutional amendment (*Denver Post*, 1994). In Ontario, the environmental minister stopped a similar hunt by executive fiat in response to social ethical concern (Animal People, 1999). California abolished the hunting of mountain lions, and state fishery management agencies have been taking a hard look at catch-and-release programs on human grounds (Laitenschloger and Bowyer, 1985).

In fact, wildlife managers have worried, in academic journals, about 'management by referendum.' According to a speech given by the Director of the American Quarter Horse Association, the number of state bills related to horse welfare filled a telephone book-sized volume in 1998 alone (Houston Livestock Show, 1998). Public sentiment for equine welfare in California carried a bill through the state legislature making the slaughter or shipping of horses for slaughter a felony in that state. Municipalities have passed ordinances ranging from the abolition of rodeos, circuses, and zoos to the protection of prairie dogs and, in the case of Cambridge, Massachusetts (a biomedical Mecca), the strictest laws in the world regulating research. There were in fact some 2100 state bills relevant to welfare promulgated in 2004, and everyone in the equine community is aware of how the public forced an end to equine slaughter. Britain has passed a quality-of-life law covering pets that went into effect in 2007. Ever-increasingly, horses are being viewed as companion animals, rather than as livestock.

Perhaps even more dramatic is the worldwide proliferation of laws to protect laboratory animals. In the USA, for example, the US Congress passed two major pieces of legislation (the Animal Welfare Act and the Health Research Extension Act) regulating and constraining the use and treatment of animals in research in 1985, despite vigorous opposition from the powerful biomedical research and medical lobbies. This opposition included well-financed, highly visible advertisements and media promotions indicating that human health and medical progress would be harmed by implementations of such legislation. There was even a less-than-subtle film titled 'Will I Be All Right, Doctor?' with the query coming from a sick child. The response from a pediatrician was, in essence, 'You will be if "they" leave us alone to do as we wish with animals.' With social concern for laboratory animals unmitigated by such threats, research animal protection laws moved easily through the US Congress and have been implemented at considerable cost to taxpayers. In 1986, Britain superseded its pioneering act of 1876 with new laws aimed at strengthening public confidence in the welfare of experimental animals (UK Home Office, 2003). Many other European countries have moved or are moving in a similar direction, despite the fact that some 90% of laboratory animals are rats and mice, which are not often considered the most cuddly and lovable of animals.

Many animal uses seen as frivolous by the public have been abolished without legislation. Toxicological testing of cosmetics on animals has been truncated by public aversion to it driving the science of alternatives (companies such as the Body Shop have been wildly successful internationally by totally disavowing such testing), and free-range egg production is a growth industry across the Western world. Greyhound racing in the USA has declined, in part for animal welfare reasons, with the Indiana veterinary community spearheading the effort to prevent greyhound racing from coming in to the state. Zoos that are little more than prisons for animals (the state of the art during my youth) have all but disappeared, and the very existence of zoos is being increasingly challenged, despite the public's unabashed love of seeing animals. And, as Gaskell and his associates' work has revealed (Gaskell *et al.*, 1997), genetic engineering has been rejected in Europe – not, as commonly believed, for reasons of risk, but for reasons of ethics, in part for reasons of animal ethics. Similar reasons (i.e., fear of harming cattle) have, in part, driven European rejection of bovine somatotropin (BST). Rodeos such as the Houston Livestock Show and the Calgary Stampede have, in essence, banned jerking of calves in roping, despite opposition from the Professional Rodeo Cowboys Association, who themselves never show the actual roping of a calf on national television. Some jurisdictions have banned rodeo altogether.

Agriculture has also felt the force of social concern with animal treatment. Indeed, it is arguable that contemporary concern in society with the treatment of farm animals in modern production systems blazed the trail leading to a new ethic for animals. As early as 1965, British society took notice of what the public saw as an alarming tendency to industrialize animal agriculture by chartering the Brambell Commission, a group of scientists under the leadership of Professor Sir Roger Brambell, who affirmed that any agricultural system failing to meet the needs and natures of animals was morally unacceptable (Brambell, 1965). Though the Brambell Commission recommendations enjoyed no regulatory status, served as a moral lighthouse for European social thought. In 1988, the Swedish Parliament passed, virtually unopposed, what the *New York Times* called a 'Bill of Rights' for farm animals, abolishing in Sweden the confinement systems currently dominating North American agriculture in a series of timed steps (*New York Times*, 1988). Much of northern Europe has followed suit, and the European Union is moving in a similar direction. For example, sow stalls must be eliminated by 2011 (European Union, 2001). Recently, activists in the USA have begun to turn their attention to animal agriculture and have begun to pressure chain restaurants and grocery chains to purchase only 'humanely raised' animal products. In 2007, Smithfield Foods, the largest US pork producer, announced it was phasing out gestation crates, and the US and European veal industries are eliminating confinement veal crates. Key referenda and legislative initiatives have abolished these procedures in a number of states, notably, Colorado, Arizona, and Oregon, with a very major initiative abolishing veal cages, sow stalls, and battery cages for laying hens passed in California in 2008. In a report released in May of 2008, the prestigious Pew

Commission on Industrial Farm Animal Production (www.PCIFAP.org) urged that all high-confinement agricultural systems be abandoned within ten years.

In what follows, I will explain the nature of the ethic informing these activities as well as what implications that ethic has for the equine industry. First, however, it is necessary to explain the concept of animal welfare.

There is one monumental conceptual error that is omnipresent in the animal industries' discussions of animal welfare – an error of such magnitude that it trivializes the industries' responses to the ever-increasing societal concerns about the treatment of agricultural animals. That error is the failure to recognize that the concept of animal welfare contains both empirical and ethical elements.

Societal concerns about animal welfare are emerging as non-negotiable demands by consumers. Failure to respect such concerns can essentially destroy the economic base for animal use. Whether one discusses farm animal welfare or equine welfare with industry groups or with the American Veterinary Medical Association, one finds the same response – animal welfare is solely a matter of 'sound science.'

Those of us serving on the Pew Commission, better known as the National Commission on Industrial Farm Animal Production, encountered this response regularly during our dealings with industry representatives. For example, one representative of the pork producers, testifying before the Commission, answered that, while people in her industry were quite 'nervous' about the Commission, their anxiety would be allayed were we to base all of our conclusions and recommendations on 'sound science.' Hoping to rectify the error in that comment, as well as educate the numerous industry representatives present, I responded to her as follows: 'Madam, if we on the Commission were asking the question of *how* to raise swine in confinement, science could certainly answer that question for us. But that is *not* the question the Commission, or society, is asking. What we are asking is, *ought* we raise swine in confinement? And to this question, science is not relevant.' Judging by her 'Huh?,' I assume I did not make my point.

Questions of animal welfare are at least partly 'ought' questions, questions of ethical obligation. The concept of animal welfare is an ethical concept to which, once understood, science brings relevant data. When we ask about an animal's welfare, or about a person's welfare, we are asking about *what we owe the animal*, and to *what extent*. Thus, when the Council for Agricultural Science and Technology (CAST) report on animal welfare, first published in the early 1980s, discussed animal welfare, it affirmed that the necessary and sufficient conditions for attributing positive welfare to an animal were represented by the animals' productivity (CAST, 1981). A productive animal enjoyed positive welfare; a non-productive animal enjoyed poor welfare.

This notion was fraught with many difficulties. First of all, productivity is an economic notion predicated of a whole operation; welfare is predicated of individual animals. An operation, such as one producing crated veal, can be quite profitable, yet the animals do not enjoy good welfare, since they are inadequately nourished, unable to exercise, and too weak to stand and walk on their own.

Second, as we shall see, equating productivity and welfare is, to some significant extent, legitimate under husbandry conditions, where the producer does well if and only if the animals do well, and square pegs, as it were, are fitted into square holes with as little friction as possible (as when pigs live outside). Under industrial conditions, however, animals do not naturally fit in the niche or environment in which they are kept, and are subjected to 'technological sanders' that allow for producers to force square pegs into round holes – antibiotics, vaccines, hormones, air handling systems – so the animals do not die and produce pounds of meat or milk. Without these technologies, the animals could not be productive. We will return to the contrast between husbandry and industrial approaches to animal agriculture.

The key point to recall here is that, even if the CAST Report definition of animal welfare did not suffer from the difficulties we outlined, it is still an ethical concept. It essentially says 'what we owe animals and to what extent is simply what it takes to get them to create profit.' This in turn would imply that the animals are well if they have only food, water, and shelter, something the industry has sometimes asserted. Even in the early 1980s, however, there were animal advocates and others who would take a very different ethical stance on what we owe farm animals. Indeed, the famous five freedoms articulated in Britain by the Farm Animal Welfare Council (FAWC) during the 1970s (even before the CAST Report) represents quite a different ethical view of what we owe animals, when it affirms the following (see www.fawc.org.uk):

> The welfare of an animal includes its physical and mental state and we consider that good animal welfare implies both fitness and a sense of well-being. Any animal kept by man must at least be protected from unnecessary suffering. We believe that an animal's welfare, whether on farm, in transit, at market or at a place of slaughter, should be considered in terms of 'five freedoms.'
>
> (1) *Freedom from hunger and thirst* – by ready access to fresh water and a diet to maintain full health and vigor.
> (2) *Freedom from discomfort* – by providing an appropriate environment, including shelter and a comfortable resting area.
> (3) *Freedom from pain, injury or disease* – by prevention or rapid diagnosis and treatment.
> (4) *Freedom to express normal behavior* – by providing sufficient space, proper facilities, and company of the animal's own kind.
> (5) *Freedom from fear and distress* – by ensuring conditions and treatment which avoid mental suffering.

Clearly, the two definitions cited contain very different notions of our moral obligation to animals (and there is an indefinite number of other definitions). Which is correct, of course, cannot be decided by gathering facts or doing experiments – indeed, which ethical framework one adopts will in fact determine the shape of science studying animal welfare!

To clarify: suppose you hold the view that an animal is well-off when it is productive, as per the CAST Report. The role of your welfare science in this case will be to study what feed, bedding, temperature, etc. are most efficient at producing the most meat, milk, or eggs for the least money – much what animal science does today. On the other hand, if you take the FAWC view of welfare, your efficiency will be constrained by the need to acknowledge the animal's natural behavior and mental states, and to assure that there is minimal pain, fear, distress, and discomfort – not factors in the CAST view of welfare unless they have a negative impact on economic productivity. Thus, in a real sense, sound science does not determine your concept of welfare; rather, your concept of welfare determines what counts as sound science!

The failure to recognize the inescapable ethical component in the concept of animal welfare leads inexorably to those holding different ethical views talking past each other. Thus, producers ignore questions of animal pain, fear, distress, confinement, truncated mobility, bad air quality, social isolation, and impoverished environment unless any of these factors impact negatively on the 'bottom line.' Animal advocates, on the other hand, give such factors primacy, and are totally unimpressed with how efficient or productive the system may be.

A major question obviously arises here. If the notion of animal welfare is inseparable from ethical components, and people's ethical stance on obligations to farm animals or horses differ markedly across a highly diverse spectrum, whose ethic is to predominate and define, in law or regulation, what counts as 'animal welfare'? This is of great concern to the farm animal industries, worrying as they do about 'animal activists hell-bent on abolishing animal use.' In actual fact, of course, such concern is misplaced, for the chance of such an extremely radical thing happening is vanishingly small regarding food animals, though in all honesty it has happened on occasion – Prohibition is the most notable example. With regard to horses, however, abolitionist concerns should be seen by the industry to be a real and legitimate possibility. US society has witnessed this in a very dramatic way in the area of equine slaughter, which was halted completely in the USA by a groundswell of public opinion.

The differences between horses and food animals as objects of societal moral concern are patent. The vast majority of members of the public consume meat or other products derived from farm animals. On the other hand, a very small percentage is engaged with the equine industry. Of those who own horses, many see them as pets or members of the family – hence, the tension one finds in the legal arena between horses as companion animals and horses as livestock.

To the general public, the horse as an icon is irrevocably associated with the heroic figures of Silver, Trigger, Flicka, Seabiscuit, Black Beauty, Commanche, Mr. Ed, the US Cavalry, the winning of the West, Indian warriors, the wild mustang, Spanish Conquistadors, Genghis Khan, and the Mounties – the list could go on and on. The horse is, as it were, second only to the dog as America's sacred cow. Hence, our revulsion at eating horses or killing them for food, a revulsion not shared by most of Europe.

In the mid-1970s until the mid-1980s, this author was instrumental in drafting what became US laws for protecting laboratory animals, mandating among other things control of pain and distress stemming from their use in research (Rollin, 2006b). The research community opposed the law, and in some advertisements pointed out that 90% of the animals used in research were rats and mice, 'animals people kill in their kitchen.' This argument did not sway the public, nor did the threat that, if constraints were put on animal use, 'the research community would not be able to cure your children.' So strong was public support of this law across bipartisan lines that it was passed within three years of its introduction.

The relevance of this story to the equine industry should be transparent. If society cares enough about the pain of rats and mice to mandate its control, even when the health of children is threatened as a consequence of such legislation, it is easy to imagine the groundswell of concern that would emerge in the face of a well-publicized atrocity emerging from equine use. The public cares a great deal about horses, but very little about the equine industry, much of which is unknown or irrelevant to the average person!

In any case, let us return to societal ethics for animals. By and large, an ethic adopted in society reflects a *societal consensus* – what most people either believe to be right and wrong or are willing to accept upon reflection.

All of us have our own personal ethics, which rule a goodly portion of our lives. In our culture, such fundamental questions as what we read, what we eat, to whom we give charity, what political and religious beliefs we hold, and a myriad of others are answered by our personal ethics. These derive from many sources – parents, religious institutions, friends, reading books, movies, and television. One is certainly entitled to believe ethically, as do some PETA members, that 'meat is murder,' that one should be a vegetarian, that it is immoral to use products derived from animal research, and so on.

Clearly, a society, particularly a free society, contains a bewildering array of such personal ethics, with the potential for significant clashes between them. If my personal ethic is based in radical Islam, and yours is based in celebrating the pleasures of the flesh, we are destined to clash, perhaps violently. For this reason, social life cannot function simply by relying on an individual's personal ethics, except perhaps in singularly monolithic cultures where all members share overwhelmingly the same values. One can find examples of something resembling this in small towns in rural USA, where there is no need to lock one's doors, remove one's keys from the car, or fear for one's personal safety. But of course such places are few, and probably decreasing in number. In larger communities, of course, the extreme case being New York City, one finds a welter of diverse cultures and corresponding personal ethics crammed into a small geographical locus. For this reason alone, as well as to control those whose personal ethic may entail taking advantage of others, a *social consensus ethic* is required, one that transcends personal ethics. This social consensus ethic is invariably articulated in law, with manifest sanctions for its violation.

As societies evolve, different issues emerge, leading to changes in the social ethic. For example, for a long period in the USA, abortion was socially condemned, leading to back-street abortions, and unwanted and abused children. (I am not here taking a position on the morality of abortion; the above statement is factually documentable.) In the 1970s, however, society re-evaluated its position on abortion, relinquishing the decision as to its morality to individual women. Similar actions took place at that time regarding sexual behavior. Whereas, historically, the focus of control of behavior such as homosexuality was believed to reside in the state, the idea that, at least as far as consenting adults were concerned, what one did in the bedroom was paradigmatically up to individual personal ethics, began to rule.

These examples illustrate behaviors once thought to be subject to social ethical control relinquished to personal ethics. The opposite movement may also occur. Historically, to whom one rented or sold one's property was seen as a paradigmatic example of a matter of personal ethical choice. As it became known that this resulted in widespread injustice and unfairness, with people refusing to rent or sell to qualified minorities, society rescinded leaving that behavior to personal ethics. A similar transformation took place with regard to sexual harassment and the enforcement of parental authority over children.

My claim, then, is that, beginning roughly in the late 1960s, the treatment of animals has moved from being a paradigmatic example of personal ethics to ever-increasingly falling within the purview of societal ethics and law. How and why has this occurred, and to what extent?

If one looks to the history of animal use in society back to the beginning of domestication some 11 000 years ago, one finds very little social ethics dictating animal treatment. The one exception to this generalization is the prohibition against deliberate, purposeless cruelty, i.e., needless infliction of pain and suffering. This mandate is well-illustrated in the Old Testament, where many injunctions illustrate its presence. For example, one is told that, when collecting eggs from a bird's nest, one should leave some extant so as not to distress the animal. The requirements of kosher slaughter accomplished by an anatomically trained person using a very sharp knife were clearly intended as a viable alternative to the much more traumatic bludgeoning. (That is not of course to suggest that such slaughter remains welfare-friendly in high-throughput industrialized slaughter houses.) The rule of Kashrut prohibiting the eating of milk and meat – 'do not seethe a calf in its mother's milk' – seems to be aimed at avoiding loss of sensitivity to animal suffering.

In the middle ages, St. Thomas Aquinas provided a more anthropocentric reason for prohibiting cruelty, based in the prescient psychological insight that those who would abuse animals will inexorably progress to abusing humans. Aquinas does not see animals as direct objects of moral concern, but nonetheless strongly prohibits their abuse.

In the late eighteenth century in Britain, and in subsequent years elsewhere, the prohibition against deliberate, sadistic, deviant, willful, malicious cruelty, i.e., inflicting pain and suffering on animals to no reasonable purpose, or outrageous neglect such as not providing food or water, were encoded in the anti-cruelty laws of all civilized societies. While adopted in part out of a moral notion of limiting animal suffering, an equally important reason was the Thomistic one – to ferret out individuals who might graduate to harming humans; case law in the USA and elsewhere make this manifest.

In one revealing case in nineteenth-century Missouri, a man was charged with cruelty after throwing pigeons into the air and shooting them to demonstrate his skill. After killing the birds, he ate them. The court ruled that the pigeons were not 'needlessly or unnecessarily killed,' because the killing was done 'in the indulgence of a healthful recreating during an exercise tending to promote strength, bodily agility and courage' (State v. Bogardus, 1877). In discussing a similar nineteenth-century case of a tame pigeon shoot in Colorado, the court affirmed that 'every act that causes pain and suffering to animals is not prohibited. Where the end or object in view is reasonable and adequate, the act resulting in pain is ... necessary and justifiable, as ... where the act is done to protect life or property, or to minister to the necessities of man' (Waters v. The People, 1896). To the credit of the Colorado Court, it did not find that such tame pigeon shoots met the test of 'worthy motive' or 'reasonable object.' Even today, however, there are jurisdictions where tame pigeon shoots and 'canned hunts' do not violate the anti-cruelty laws.

It is certainly true that cruelty to animals is closely linked to psychopathic behavior – animal cruelty, along with bed-wetting and fire-starting, are the three cardinal signs of future psychopaths. The majority of children who shoot up their schools have early histories of animal abuse, as do 80% of the violent offenders in Leavenworth and most serial killers. Animal abusers often abuse wives and children. Most battered women's shelters must make provisions for keeping the family pet, as the abuser will hurt the animal to hurt the woman. But these laws conceptually provide little protection for animals. Animal cruelty accounts for only a tiny fraction of the suffering that animals undergo at human hands. For example, the USA produces nine billion broiler chickens a year, and many have bruises and fractures or other musculoskeletal injuries. If even 1% of chickens are so injured (a ridiculously low number), then we have 90 000 000 suffering animals there alone – there is nothing like 90 000 000 incidents of cruelty in the USA per year, and those chickens are legally unprotected, not even subject to humane slaughter law!

Upon reflection, it is obvious that growing societal concern with animal treatment would not be content with the anti-cruelty ethic and laws, although society has raised animal cruelty to a felony in more than forty states. These laws are focused on deviant behavior, not on activities that are routinely and widely accepted as, in the word of one court, 'ministering to the necessities of man.' Thus such practices as steel-jawed traps or hot iron branding of cattle are invisible to the anti-cruelty laws.

A 1985 case in New York State vividly pointed out the need for ethical evolution beyond cruelty. A group of attorneys brought suit against the branch of New York

State government charged with administering public lands on the grounds that the agency's permitting the use of steel-jawed traps on public lands without a requirement for regularly checking the traps entailed violation of the cruelty laws, since animals so trapped were deprived of food, water, and medical care for injury. Although sympathetic to the moral point, the judge dismissed the case, reiterating that the cruelty laws did not apply to 'standard' practices such as trapping, which fulfill a legal human purpose – provision of furs and pest control. If the plaintiffs wished to ban steel-jawed traps, said the judge, they needed to go to the legislature, that is, change the social ethic, not to the judiciary, which is bound by the ethic encoded in the anti-cruelty laws (Animal Legal Defense Fund v. The Department of Environment Conservation of the State of New York, 1985).

We will discuss the nature of the emerging ethic shortly, but it is necessary to pause and point out that, while many hurtful practices in animal agriculture do not fall under the anti-cruelty laws, and these require a new ethic and laws following from that ethic, *a goodly number of practices in the equine industry could legitimately be seen as blatant cruelty under the traditional ethic!* These include, but are not limited to, the following:

- The use of severe bits, for example, those made of chain-saw (the so-called mule bit) or bicycle chain.
- The soring of horses (i.e., hurting their feet so they will step high) as done with Tennessee Walkers (this practice evoked federal legislation).
- Excessive whipping.
- Abusive training methods, such as 'tarping' (covering the horse with a tarp and beating him) or use of electroshock.
- Hotshotting (using an electric prod on the horse).
- Abusive cheating at horse shows, including use of firecrackers, whipping, electroshock and anal irritants to excite animals for some show uses, or bleeding, hanging, taping nostrils and even breaking ribs to make the horse appear relaxed.
- Severely cutting tongues in reining horses.
- A general macho attitude toward the horse in some quarters of the industry, often expressed as 'you must beat a horse to establish dominance.'

It is frankly incredible that the industry has escaped public flagellation over the proliferation of such practices. When I have shown a 'mule bit' to my friends not involved with horses, or even to friends who do have horses, but would not have occasion to use such a bit, they are invariably shocked and horrified! Media exposure of these sorts of practices could expose the industry as a whole to adverse publicity it can ill afford.

Let us return to the main thread of our argument. We have thus far argued that the societal ethic for the treatment of animals has moved well beyond a concern for deviant, unnecessary cruelty, which covers only a fraction of annual suffering at human hands, to an ethic that is intended to cover all animal suffering or abuse, even that which is not the result of deliberate cruelty or neglect. We have also indicated that some treatment of horses comes very close to condemnation even by the anti-cruelty ethic. It remains for us to explain the new ethic and look at the applicability to the equine industry.

For the overwhelming majority of human history, until some three decades ago, the anti-cruelty ethic served as the only socially articulated moral principle for animal treatment. Except for a few sporadic voices following in the wake of Darwin's discussion of human–animal continuity, no one spoke of animals' rights, nor did society have moral concepts for animal treatment that went 'beyond cruelty.' The obvious question that presents itself is this: What in the last half-century has led to social disaffection with the venerable ethic of anti-cruelty, which does not cover most sources of animal suffering?

In a study commissioned by USDA to answer this question, I distinguished a variety of social and conceptual reasons (Rollin, 1995).

(1) Changing demographics and consequent changes in the paradigm for animals. Whereas, at the turn of the century, more than half the population was engaged in producing food for the rest, today only some 1.5% of the US public is engaged in production agriculture (AMC, 2003). One hundred years ago, if one were to ask a person in the street, urban or rural, to state the words that come into their mind when one said 'animal,' the answer would doubtless have been 'horse,' 'cow,' 'food,' 'work,' etc. Today, however, for the majority of the population, the answer is 'dog,' 'cat,' or 'pet.' Repeated studies show that some 90% of the pet-owning population view their animals as 'members of the family' (The Acorn, 2002; Harris Poll, 2007), and virtually no one views them as an income source. Divorce lawyers note that custody of the dog can be as thorny an issue as custody of the children!

(2) We have lived through a long period of ethical soul-searching. For almost fifty years, society has turned its 'ethical searchlight' on humans traditionally ignored or even oppressed by the consensus ethic – blacks, women, the handicapped, other minorities. The same ethical imperative has focused attention on our treatment of the non-human world: the environment and animals. Many leaders of the activist animal movement in fact have roots in earlier movements, such as civil rights, feminism, homosexual rights, children's rights, and labor.

(3) The media has discovered that 'animals sell papers'! One cannot channel-surf across normal television service without being bombarded with animal stories, real and fictional. (A *New York Times* reporter recently told me that more time on cable TV in New York City is devoted to animals than to any other subject.) Recall, for example, the extensive media coverage a decade ago of some whales trapped in an ice floe and freed by a Russian icebreaker. It seems someone in the Kremlin realized that liberating the whales was a cheap way to curry favor with US public opinion.

(4) Strong and visible arguments have been advanced in favor of raising the status of animals by philosophers, scientists, and celebrities (Singer, 1975; Rollin, 1981; Regan, 1983; Sapontzis, 1987).
(5) Changes in the nature of animal use have demanded new moral categories.

In my view, although all the reasons listed above are relevant, they are not nearly as important as the precipitous and dramatic changes in animal use that occurred after World War II. These changes include huge conceptual changes in the nature of agriculture and a significant increase in animal research and testing.

For virtually all of human history, animal agriculture was based four-square in animal husbandry. Husbandry, derived from the old Norse word 'hus/band' or bonded to the household, meant taking great pains to put one's animals into the best possible environment one could find to meet their physical and psychological natures – which, following Aristotle, I call *telos* (Rollin, 2006a) – and then augmenting their ability to survive and thrive by providing them with food during famine, protection from predation, water during drought, medical attention, help in birthing, and so on. Thus, traditional agriculture was roughly a fair contract between humans and animals, with both sides being better off in virtue of the relationship. Husbandry agriculture was about placing square pegs into square holes, round pegs into round holes, and creating as little friction as possible in doing so. So powerful is the notion of husbandry, in fact, that when the Psalmist seeks a metaphor for God's ideal relationship to humans, he seizes upon the shepherd in the twenty-third Psalm:

> The Lord is my shepherd; I shall not want. He maketh me to lie down in green pastures; He leadeth me beside the still waters; He restoreth my soul.

We wish no more from God than what the husbandman provides for his sheep. In husbandry, a producer did well if and only if the animals did well, so productivity was tied to welfare. Thus, no social ethic was needed to ensure proper animal treatment; only the anti-cruelty ethic designed to deal with sadists and psychopaths was needed to augment husbandry. Self-interest virtually assured good treatment. The logo of the ASPCA, the first anti-cruelty group in the USA, shows Henry Bergh, its founder, staying the hand of a carter who has beaten his horse to the ground, clearly counter-productive to his own self-interest.

After World War II, this contract was broken by humans. Symbolically, at universities, Departments of Animal Husbandry became Departments of Animal Science, defined not as care, but as 'the application of industrial methods to the production of animals' to increase efficiency and productivity. With technological 'sanders' – hormones, vaccines, antibiotics, air-handling systems, mechanization – we could force square pegs into round holes and place animals into environments where they suffered in ways irrelevant to productivity. If a nineteenth-century agriculturalist had tried to put 100 000 egg-laying hens in cages in a building, they all would have died of disease in a month; today, such systems dominate.

The new approach to animal agriculture was not the result of cruelty, bad character, or even insensitivity. It developed rather out of perfectly decent, *prima facie* plausible motives that were a product of dramatic significant historical and social upheavals that occurred after World War II. At that point in time, agricultural scientists and government officials became extremely concerned with supplying the public with cheap and plentiful food for a variety of reasons. In the first place, after the Dust Bowl and the Great Depression, many people in the USA had soured on farming. Second, reasonable predictions of urban and suburban encroachment on agricultural land were being made, with a resultant diminution of land for food production. Third, many farm people had been sent to both foreign and domestic urban centers during the war, thereby creating a reluctance to return to rural areas that lacked excitement – recall the song popular in the early 20th Century: 'How ya gonna keep 'em down on the farm after they've seen Paree?' (Donaldson *et al.*, 1918). Fourth, having experienced the specter of starvation during the Great Depression, the American consumer was, for the first time in history, fearful of an insufficient food supply. Fifth, projection of major population increases further fueled concern.

When the above considerations of loss of land and diminution of agricultural labor are coupled with the rapid development of a variety of technological modalities relevant to agriculture during and after World War II, and with the burgeoning belief in technology-based economics of scale, it was probably inevitable that animal agriculture would become subject to industrialization. This was a major departure from traditional agriculture and a fundamental change in agricultural values – industrial values of efficiency and productivity replaced and eclipsed the traditional values of 'way of life' and husbandry.

The rise of large amounts of annual research and testing after World War II also superseded the relevance of cruelty-to-animal ethics. People also realized that biomedical and other scientific research, toxicological safety testing, use of animals in teaching, pharmaceutical product extraction from animals, and so on, all produce far more suffering than does overt cruelty. This suffering comes from creating disease, burns, trauma, fractures, and the like in animals in order to study them; production of pain, fear, learned helplessness, aggression, and other states for research; poisoning animals to study toxicity; and performing surgery on animals to develop new operative procedures. In addition, suffering is engendered by the housing of research animals. Indeed, one can argue that the discomfort and suffering that animals used in research experience by virtue of being housed under conditions that are convenient for us, but inimical to their biological natures – for example, keeping rodents, which are nocturnal, burrowing creatures, in polycarbonate crates under artificial, full-time light – far exceed the suffering produced by invasive research protocols.

Thus mid-twentieth-century developments in agriculture and research were a main vector in creating significant sources of animal suffering not captured by the anti-cruelty ethic, and new ethical concepts were called for.

Let us recall that we have argued that the notion of equine welfare must be discussed in terms of societal ethics dictating what we owe animals and to what extent. Thus, once we have described the new ethic, we will be in a position to apply it to the equine industry as a template for what society expects.

Ethical concepts do not arise *ex nihilo*. Plato taught us a valuable lesson about effecting ethical change. If one wishes to change another person's (or society's) ethical beliefs, it is much better to *remind* than to *teach* or, using a martial arts metaphor, it is better to use judo rather than sumo. In other words, if you and I disagree ethically on some matter, it is far better for me to show you that what I am trying to convince you of is already implicit – albeit unnoticed – in what you already believe. Similarly, we cannot force others to believe as we do (sumo). We can, however, show them that their own assumptions, if thought through, lead to a conclusion different from that which they currently entertain (judo). These points are well exemplified in twentieth-century US history. Prohibition was sumo, not judo – an attempt to forcefully impose a new ethic about drinking on the majority by the minority. As such, it was doomed to fail, and, in fact, people drank more during Prohibition. Contrast this with former US President Lyndon Johnson's civil rights legislation. Himself a Southerner, Johnson realized that even Southerners would acquiesce to the following two propositions: (1) all humans should be treated equally; and (2) black people are human. They just had never bothered to draw the relevant conclusion. If Johnson had been wrong about this point, if 'writing this large' in the law had not 'reminded' people, civil rights would have been as ineffective as Prohibition!

So society was faced with the need for new moral categories and laws that reflected those categories in order to deal with animal use in science and agriculture and to limit the animal suffering with which it is increasingly concerned. At the same time, recall that Western society has gone through almost fifty years of extending its moral categories for humans to people who were morally ignored or invisible – women, minorities, the handicapped, children, citizens of the Third World. As we noted earlier, new and viable ethics do not emerge *ex nihilo*. So a plausible and obvious move was for society to continue in its tendency and attempt to extend the moral machinery it has developed for dealing with people, appropriately modified, to animals. And this is precisely what has occurred. Society has taken elements of the moral categories it uses for assessing the treatment of people and is in the process of modifying these concepts to make them appropriate for dealing with new issues in the treatment of animals, especially their use in science and confinement agriculture.

What aspect of our ethic for people is being so extended? One that is applicable to animal use is the fundamental problem of weighing the interests of the individual against those of the general public. Different societies have provided different answers to this problem. Totalitarian societies opt to devote little concern to the individual, favoring instead the state or whatever their version of the general welfare may be. At the other extreme, anarchical groups, such as communes, give primacy to the individual and very little concern to the group – hence they tend to enjoy only transient existence. In our society, however, a balance is struck. Although most of our decisions are made to the benefit of the general welfare, fences are built around individuals to protect their fundamental interests from being sacrificed for the majority. Thus, we protect individuals from being silenced even if the majority disapproves of what they say; we protect individuals from having their property seized without recompense even if such seizure benefits the general welfare; we protect individuals from torture even if they have planted a bomb in an elementary school and refuse to divulge its location. We protect those interests of the individual that we consider essential to being human, to human nature, from being submerged, even by the common good. Those moral/legal fences that so protect the individual human are called *rights* and are based on plausible assumptions regarding what is essential to being human.

It is this notion to which society in general is looking in order to generate the new moral notions necessary to talk about the treatment of animals in today's world, where cruelty is not the major problem, but where such laudable, general human welfare goals as efficiency, productivity, knowledge, medical progress, and product safety are responsible for the vast majority of animal suffering. People in society are seeking to 'build fences' around animals to protect the animals and their interests and natures from being totally submerged for the sake of the general welfare, and are trying to accomplish this goal by going to the legislature. In husbandry, this occurred automatically; in industrialized agriculture, where it is no longer automatic, people wish to see it legislated.

It is necessary to stress here certain things that this ethic, in its mainstream version, is not and does not attempt to be. As a mainstream movement, it does not try to give human rights to animals. Since animals do not have the same natures and interests flowing from these natures as humans do, human rights do not fit animals. Animals do not have basic natures that demand speech, religion, or property; thus, according them these rights would be absurd. On the other hand, animals have natures of their own (*telos*) and interests that flow from these natures, and the thwarting of these interests matter to animals as much as the thwarting of speech matters to humans. The agenda is not, for mainstream society, making animals 'equal' to people. Rather, it is preserving the common-sense insight that 'fish gotta swim and birds gotta fly,' and suffer if they do not.

Nor is this ethic, in the minds of mainstream society, an abolitionist one, dictating that animals cannot be used by humans. Rather, it is an attempt to constrain *how* they can be used, so as to limit their pain and suffering. In this regard, as Suther (1993) points out, the thrust for protection of animal natures is not at all radical; it is very conservative, asking for the same sort of husbandry that characterized the overwhelming majority of animal use during all of human history, save for the last fifty years or so. It is not opposed to animal use; it is opposed to animal use that goes against animals' natures and tries to force square pegs into round holes, leading to friction and suffering. If animals are to be used for food and labor, they should, as they traditionally did, live lives that respect their natures. If animals are to be used to probe nature and cure disease for human benefit, they should not suffer in the process. Thus, this new ethic is *conservative*, not radical, harking back to the animal use that necessitated and thus entailed respect for the animals' natures. It is based on the insight that what we do to animals matters to them, just as what we do to humans matters to us, and consequently, we should respect that in our treatment and use of animals as we do in our treatment and use of humans. And because respect for animal nature is no longer automatic as it was in traditional husbandry agriculture, society is demanding that it be encoded in law.

Strictly speaking, in the eyes of the law, animals have the status of property and thus cannot have rights. But the functional equivalent of rights can be achieved by limiting property use. Thus I own my motorcycle free and clear, but I cannot ride it on the sidewalk, up a one-way street the wrong way, or at any speed I wish. Similarly, the federal laboratory animal laws do not deny that researchers own their animals, but nevertheless restrict how they are used. This explains why we have seen the proliferation of annual protection legislation we mentioned earlier.

It should be clear that I categorically reject the standard dualism rampant in agriculture and veterinary medicine between animal welfare and animal rights. In my view, animal rights, in the mainstream sense I described, is the form that animal welfare has taken in the face of unprecedented animal uses and the social changes described earlier. The notion that animals should have rights, i.e., legalized protections for their basic needs and natures while they are being used, is not the same as saying that animal use should be abolished. In fact, the vast majority of the public would affirm that animals should have rights in this sense.

How does this ethic apply to the equine industry? In varying ways – the industry is far from monolithic. But we can point up some issues which, if not dealt with by the industry, are prone to heavy-handed legislation.

In the first place, despite wishful thinking for some parties, horses are no longer viewed by the public as livestock. In other words, it is not part of their *telos* to be eaten. Hence the massive public sentiment against horse slaughter and shipping for food. This occurred despite the welfare problems inherent in the end of slaughter – slaughter in itself was simply inconceivable. I recently heard a veterinarian lament the waste of protein inherent in stopping equine slaughter in a protein-poor world. This may be true, but it has no more social traction than allowing surplus dogs and cats – a major social problem – to be disposed of as food! In the social mind, horses are akin to large dogs.

It is therefore doubtful that the anti-slaughter movement will be reversed, yet the abandoned, unwanted, horses will continue to proliferate. It is not inconceivable that society could move to stem this tide legislatively – for example, by compelling people to post a bond whenever they acquire a horse, the bond to be forfeited if the owner fails to properly euthanize or place the animal when it is no longer wanted.

Many areas of the equine industry are not in accord with the ethic we have described. Horse racing is an obvious example. Abusive, as opposed to 'natural,' training, is increasingly anathema – revelations of abusive training could do major harm to the industry.

Similarly, drugging, nerving, confining the racehorse for most of the day, will no longer be acceptable to a public with a clear image of how horses should be kept and treated. Nor will trashing them when they can no longer run.

Exactly the same logic applies to horse shows and other equine pursuits. Hurting the horse for the sake of winning could create a groundswell of public opinion banning shows, even as dog-fighting has been societally rejected. Each industry should be courageous enough to address its own abuses and deal with them before that option is removed and the public takes matters into its own hands. As I said in my first talk to the American Association of Equine Practitioners (AAEP) in the early 1990s:

> None of the equine suffering we have mentioned above is necessary – viable alternatives exist to the abusive practices we have mentioned. One can have racing without racing horses who are not biologically ready and without drug abuse; one can have horse training which works with the horse's nature, and not against it, brutally bending it to our will (such training is in any event more beautiful and elegant). One can have horse shows that celebrate and exhibit the horse's *telos*, not our skill at abusive artifice. One can enjoy the horse for what it is, and what we can perfect genetically and environmentally, not for our unfortunate skill in putting square pegs into round holes. In conclusion, I would argue that we should keep as our root metaphor what must surely have informed the ancient vision of the centaur, the symbiotic unity of man and animal, mutually interdependent, rising to heights neither could scale alone.

References

Acorn, The (2002) Survey says pets are members of the family. Available at: http://www.theacorn.com/News/2002/0131/Pets/036.html.

AMC (2003) *18th Annual Agricultural Machinery Conference*, May 5–7, Cedar Rapids, IA. See: http://www.amc-online.org/.

Animal Legal Defense Fund v. The Department of Environment Conservation of the State of New York (1985). Index No. 6670/85.

Animal People (1999) *Animal People*, March. See: http://www.animalpeoplenews.org/.

Brambell, F.W.R. (1965) *Report of the Technical Committee to Stock Husbandry Systems*. Her Majesty's Stationery Office, London.

CAST (1981) *Scientific Aspects of the Welfare of Food Animals*. Council for Agricultural Science and Technology, Report No. 91, November 1981, p. 1.

Denver Post (1994) June 19, 1994, p. D1.

Donaldson, W., Lewis, S.M. and Young, J. (1918) *How ya gonna keep 'em down on the farm?* Waterson, Berlin, and Snyder, New York.

European Union (2001) *Welfare of Dogs*. Health and Consumer Protection Directorate. Luxemburg.

Gaskell, G. *et al.* (1997) Europe ambivalent on biotechnology. *Nature* 387, 845ff.

Harris Poll (2007) Pets are 'members of the family'. No. 120, December 4, 2007. Available at: http://www.harrisinteractive.com/harris_poll/index.asp?PID=840.

Houston Livestock Show (1998) Speech delivered by the Director of the American Quarter Horse Association in Equine Section. See: http://www.hlsr.com/.

HSUS (2003) Fur and trapping. The Humane Society of the United States. Available at: http://www.hsus.org/ace/12031.

Laitenschloger, R.A. and Bowyer, R.T. (1985) Wildlife management by referendum: When professionals fail to communicate. *Wild-Life Society Bulletin* 13, 564–570.

NCBA (1991) National Cattlemen's Beef Association Conference, Denver, CO. See: http://www.beefusa.org/.

New York Times (1988) Swedish farm animals get a bill of rights. October 25, 1988, p. 1.

Regan, T. (1983) *The Case for Animal Rights*. University of California Press, Berkeley, CA.

Rollin, B. (1981) *Animal Rights and Human Morality*, 1st edn. Prometheus Books, Buffalo, NY.

Rollin, B. (1995) *Farm Animal Welfare: Social, Bioethical and Research Issues*. Iowa State University Press, Ames, IA.

Rollin, B. (2006a) *Animal Rights and Human Morality*, 3rd edn. Prometheus Books, Buffalo, NY.

Rollin, B. (2006b) The regulation of animal research and the emergence of animal ethics: a conceptual history. *Theoretical Medicine and Bioethics* 27(4), 285–304.

Sapontzis, S. (1987) *Morals, Reason and Animals*. Temple University Press, Philadelphia, PA.

Singer, P. (1975) *Animal Liberation*. New York Review Press, New York.

State, The v. Bogardus (1877) 4 MO. App 215, 219 (Mo. Ct. App. 1877).

Suther, S. (1993) Are you an animal rightist? *Beef Today*, April.

UK Home Office (2003) Animals in Scientific Procedures Act. Available at: http://www.homeoffice.gov.uk/docs/animallegislation.html.

Waters v. The People (1896) Supreme Court of Colorado, 23 Colo. 33, 46, p. 112.

A Historical Survey of Human–Equine Interactions

David W. Ramey

2

2.1 Introduction

Horse, thou art truly a creature without equal, for thou fliest without wings and conquerest without sword.

The Koran

The structure of human social, economic, artistic, and political life has been long and deeply affected by the relations between human and non-human animals. Horses have almost unquestionably played a larger role in determining the nature of these human interactions than has any other non-human species. The more mundane aspects of horse–human interactions are rather obvious: horses have been served to men as a food source, and have served men in war, for transportation, and at work for millennia, until the Industrial Revolution and the development of the internal combustion engine ultimately rendered them obsolete for such purposes. But horses have met other needs as well: spiritual and esthetic, as well as for excitement and pleasure. To ride a horse at speed gives its rider metaphorical wings, freeing man from the constraints of the ground, even if only for a short time. Throughout history, these needs have been celebrated in poetry, writing, sculpture, paintings, and drawings. The horse has been given high marks for honor, intelligence, and wisdom, and has been given a wide and diverse range of symbolic meanings. The horse has been treated with reverence, and man has used the horse as a symbol for his highest aspirations. With such recognition, and with a litany of accomplishments recorded over time, the horse has been, and is likely to remain, a prominent figure in literature and art for centuries to come. Finally, in modern times, perhaps as a result of such adulation, as well as changes in human ethical considerations, immense changes in human–equine interactions have occurred.

Equine Welfare, First Edition. Edited by C. Wayne McIlwraith and Bernard E. Rollin.
© 2011 by UFAW. Published 2011 by Blackwell Publishing Ltd.

2.2 Early Horse–Human Interactions

... the eating of horsemeat, would remain in the ancient law

Íslendingabók, ch. 7

For all of human history, the horse has inarguably served one important function: as a source of food (Gade, 1976). Horses began to be exploited by modern humans for their meat in many areas of Eurasia during the Pleistocene era (the Ice Age). Bones from Paleolithic horses most likely found a wide variety of uses: in making spears, arrowheads, and harpoon points; for hooks to catch fish; for tools to weave cloth; as implements to assist in the forming of hard stone tools; to scrape hides and make pottery; as hair combs; as musical instruments; and for decorative items such as pendants, rings, and hairpins. Horse skins were probably used for covering human bodies, to help humans ward off the cold. Paleolithic hunters culled herds in Central Europe, as did Paleoindians in North America (Webb and Hemmings, 2006), albeit rarely, when compared to the Central European hunters.

Still, even though horse hunting was widespread, there is a relative lack of large accumulations of horse bones (with the exception of the site of Solutré, in east–central France), which suggests that, for the most part, it was a somewhat haphazard affair, with horses apparently being taken as the opportunity arose, rather than in any sort of systematic hunt. Regardless, especially in the temperate areas of what is now Europe and Asia, horsemeat was a staple of the human diet, at least until the virtual disappearance of wild horses by the sixth millennium BC (Drews, 2004).

Interestingly, while horses served as sustenance in certain areas of the world, in others, where horses were not naturally abundant (most likely due to lack of suitable pasture), horsemeat did not form an important food source. For example, the historical records of Egypt and Mesopotamia fail to record horsemeat as a source of human nutrition. Eating horsemeat was also discouraged by religious edict. Jewish law forbade the consumption of horsemeat; in 732 AD, Pope Gregory III started an effort to ban the practice as 'pagan,' and it has been said that the people of Iceland were reluctant to embrace Christianity largely over the issue of giving up horsemeat. The divergence in the use of the horse as food persists today. Whereas some cultures freely consume horsemeat, e.g., France and Japan, others, especially the USA, revile the practice, and have even enacted laws banning the killing of horses for human consumption. China is actually the world's largest producer of horsemeat.

Nevertheless, while prehistoric man regularly ate horses, there also appears to have been a special relationship between prehistoric man and horses that surpassed the mere use of horses as food. While there is no writing to document such a relationship, horses do appear rather widely in Paleolithic art (Lewin, 2005), for example, in the famous French cave site of Lascaux (discovered in 1940 by four French teenagers). Images of horses far outnumber those of any other species, and the fact that horses were a food source is supported by the inclusion of spears in such drawings (Figure 2.1). Interestingly, the paintings found at Lascaux, as well as other prehistoric

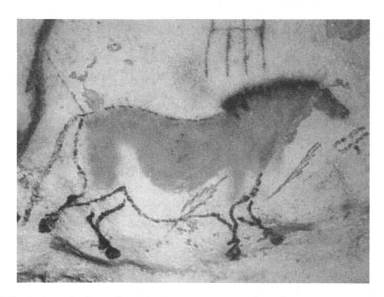

Figure 2.1   Image of a horse from the Lascaux caves. (Wikimedia Commons.)

sites, are usually found in fairly inaccessible and uncomfortable places. This leads to speculation that the paintings themselves were symbolic, and possibly part of some human ritual, rather than decorative. Prehistoric images of horses appear at several sites in Europe, and prehistoric man carved horses on bone, antler, and stone.

2.3 Domesticating Horses

We would not always be soothing and taming nature, breaking the horse and the ox, but sometimes ride the horse wild and chase the buffalo.

Henry David Thoreau

At the end of the Pleistocene period, around 10 000 BC, equids in the New World became extinct. These equids were a distinct species from those in Western and Central Europe (Weinstock *et al.*, 2005). At the same time, in Western and Central Europe, the numbers of the tarpan (*Equus ferus*), the progenitor of the modern horse, became greatly reduced.[1] Small populations of horses likely existed across the northern part of Europe, and perhaps the Near East. Had horses not been domesticated, it is not inconceivable that they would have ultimately become extinct (Budiansky, 1997).

---

[1]The tarpan died out when their natural range was destroyed to make room for people. In addition, farmers killed the wild tarpans to keep them from eating crops or from cross-breeding with domesticated horses. The last tarpan died in captivity, in Russia, in 1876.

However, at some point, horses were domesticated, to the benefit of both horses and humans. Exactly when and where horses were first domesticated is the subject of considerable mystery and controversy. Various sources have concluded that horses were first domesticated during the Neolithic period (New Stone Age), Eneolithic period (Copper Age) or Early Bronze Age; in the Pontic Steppe (the semi-arid grasslands stretching from north of the Black Sea, across Ukraine and southern Russia, to western Kazakhstan), other parts of Eastern Europe, Western Europe, or the Near East; at one or more places; and more or less simultaneously (*Science Daily*, 2006).

A question arises as to what is meant by the word 'domestication.' If the term is used in the more general sense[2] of 'adaptation of an animal or plant through breeding in captivity to a life intimately associated with and advantageous to humans,' then it can be fairly asserted that the horse was kept, almost certainly for its meat, and even perhaps for occasional riding, in the fifth to third millennia BC (indeed, until the later second millennium BC in parts of Europe).

To date, the oldest archeological indicator of an intimate relationship between horses and humans are horse bones, and carved horse images, from Copper Age grave sites of the Khyalynsk culture near the Caspian Sea, in Russia, from about 4800–4400 BC. Here, horse bones and carved horse images have been excavated from over 150 grave sites; other sacrifices occurred on the ground above the graves (Mallory, 1997). Whether the horses had been domesticated or not is unknown – and perhaps unknowable. That horses were sacrificed at least attests to their importance to the people of this time.

Other famous (and still evolving) archeological sites reveal indirect, tantalizing hints as to the earliest horse–human interactions that would ultimately lead to a long, and successful, relationship. Excavations of sites of the Botai culture, in the Agmola Province of Kazakhstan, in Central Asia, offer clues about the domestication of horses. The Botai people lived in houses dug into the ground (Figure 2.2). During their nine-month winter, they dressed in the furs of horses and ate horsemeat. These houses are full of bones, 90% of them from horses, and there are hints that some of these horses may have been domesticated:

(1) The bones of fully grown stallions slightly outnumber those of female horses. If all of these bones were from wild horses, one might imagine that there would be more females, since females tend to form the larger percentage of wild horse bands.

(2) Full horse skeletons are found at the Botai site. Hunters tend to carve up the meaty portions of their kill and take only what they need home, leaving the rest to scavengers.

(3) Large chunks of rock from distant sites suggest that the Botai must have used animals – possibly horses – to pack the rocks (Weed, 2002).

---

[2] See http://www.answers.com/topic/domestication-3.

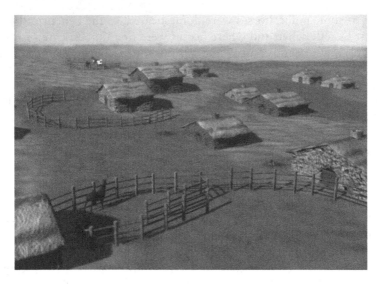

Figure 2.2 Reconstruction of the Botai culture village of Krasnyi Yar (3300 BC), in north–central Kazakhstan. (Artist: Ashley Brickman. Reproduced with permission from Sandra Olsen.)

(4) Geochemical evidence of high ratios of potassium to phosphorus in circular areas, defined by posts, near the pit houses also suggests that horses were living, confined, in close proximity to humans (Stiff *et al.*, 2006).
(5) Radioisotope analysis of milk proteins in pottery shards found at one of the Botai sites suggests that horses were kept for their milk. It is unlikely that anyone would have attempted to milk a wild mare (*Science*, 2008).

Wherever it developed, there is, as yet, no *direct* evidence for the origins of horse domestication. That is, there is no art, no written material, nor any material obtained from grave sites that confirms when horses were first domesticated. There are no saddles nor metal bits that were left behind by early societies – the earliest pieces of horse handling equipment, such as bridles, leads, saddles, or hobbles, would have been made from organic material (e.g., leather), and have long since rotted away. The earliest written and artistic evidence for horse domestication dates back only to the end of the third millennium BC. These domesticated horses were most likely kept for meat or milk. Once horses were domesticated, mare's milk became a welcome addition to the human diet; fermented mare's milk is still consumed in central Asia, e.g., in Kazakhstan as 'koumiss,' and in Mongolia as 'airak' (Figure 2.3).

The use of horses for riding or traction can be documented only to the beginning of the second millennium BC (Littaeur and Crouwel, 1996; Piggott, 1992; Renfrew, 1987). Representations of people riding equids in the Near East appear earlier. However, it is not possible to tell from these drawings if the riders were astride

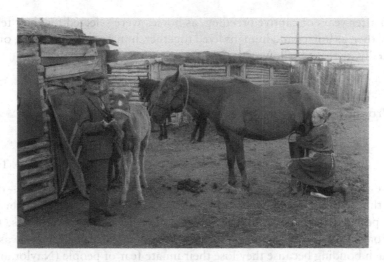

Figure 2.3 Kazakh woman milking a mare at Kenetkul village, in northern Kazakhstan. (Reproduced with permission from Sandra Olsen.)

Equus caballus or if they were riding other Near Eastern equids, such as onagers (also known as the Asian wild ass) and asses.[3]

It is also not possible to tell when horses were domesticated based on changes in their body size. Unlike other species, such as dogs or cattle, where changes in size and other physical characteristics are reliable indicators of domestication and captive breeding, changes in horse bones are not as easily identified. Thus, in general, there are no obvious distinctions between feral and domesticated horses that might indicate the selective breeding that often accompanies domestication. Still, investigators at the Botai sites assert that the lower leg bones of the horses from the site were more slender than those of wild horses and similar in size to those of later domesticated horses. They note that slender bones were a trait later selected by breeders for speed (Maugh, 2009). Further confusing the issue is the fact that domesticated horses could have easily become feral if they escaped captivity, and that all feral horses were similar to those that might have been domesticated, leading to a population of horses of roughly the same size.

Wherever and whenever it developed, horse domestication probably evolved over a period of centuries. Throughout the world, in every culture, aboriginal hunter–gatherers and horticulturists have tamed animals to keep as pets. As horses were tamed, and accompanied humans, it is also possible that slight genetic changes

---

[3] The terms 'donkey' and 'ass' both refer to *Equus assinus*. The animal was first domesticated around 3000 BC, and was widely used as a beast of burden; riding donkeys pre-dates the riding of horses by several centuries. The term 'donkey' has largely replaced the term 'ass' when referring to *E. assinus*, due to the use of the latter term in reference to the human buttocks.

occurred after years of captive breeding, as horses were selected for their temperament. Further, as horses and humans lived together, human understanding of horses
undoubtedly increased, allowing ultimately for horses to be trained.

2.4 Training and Controlling Horses

If horses knew their strength we should not ride anymore.

Mark Twain

While the precise date of domestication is unknown – probably forever – one can
imagine that, if adult horses were kept for meat, their foals would have been handled, or perhaps even made into pets. Certainly, foals bond to humans. Indeed,
orphan foals, if raised by humans, may be notoriously difficult to handle as adults
due to such bonding because they lose their innate fear of people (Naylor and Bell,
1985). On the other hand, humans readily establish emotional connections with
their horses; indeed, evidence exists for people keeping animals as pets from 8000
BC. If foals were kept as pets, over time, it might have been found that horses could
be put to work, or ultimately even ridden. Alternatively, perhaps early hunters
hand-reared foals whose parents had been killed.

Once horses were tamed, they had to be controlled in order to be used as effective human resources. Some of the earliest attempts at horse control may have been
through the use of thongs or straps made of organic materials such as leather or
cord; such artifacts decompose, and so there is no direct evidence for their existence. Nose rings are one of the first documented attempts at controlling horses.
Indeed, a Mesopotamian terracotta plaque from the second millennium that is on
display at the British Museum in London shows a small horse being ridden with a
nose ring. Nose rings were used to control oxen and onagers; if used in a similar
fashion in horses, riders would have held a rein from the nose ring in one hand, and
a whip in the other. If they followed such control methods, early riders were probably also mounted over the horse's rump, as per other species: so-called 'donkey
seat' riding (Figure 2.4). Leg pressure, rider balance changes, whips, or voice commands would have been methods of giving the horse commands. Of course, as
anyone who rides horses might imagine, such a position and method of control
would have been almost totally ineffective for spirited horses, and nose rings for
horses disappeared, at least from the Near East, by 2000 BC.

In order for humans to ride horses, more effective methods of control had to be
developed. Perhaps the first great innovation was the bridle and the bit. The first
use of bridles are unrecorded, and will likely never be dated accurately, since they
were undoubtedly made of organic material, and have long since rotted away.
There is much controversy regarding the date of the first use of bits in horses, with
some scholars suggesting that perforated pieces of antler show evidence of bits
being used as early as 4000 BC. However, antler pieces discovered in association

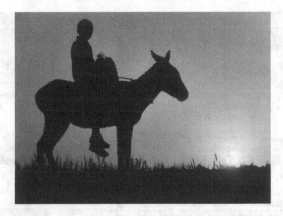

Figure 2.4   Silhouette of boy riding donkey, in 'donkey seat' style. (Istockphoto.com.)

with horse remains – that would more strongly suggest an association between the artifacts and horses – do not occur until approximately 2000 years later. The earliest dating of metal bits is rather more established. Metal bits first appear in the Near East, and were used on Syrian donkeys as early as 2300 BC. Bit wear on horse teeth has been documented in horses from southern Iran during approximately the same time period, and from Egypt in roughly 1700 BC. Control via iron bits enabled riders to be positioned behind the horse's withers, instead of over the hindquarters (where they could more easily dismount if in trouble), and modern riding began.

Humans also recognized fairly early that controlling male horses could be made easier by gelding them. In the frozen tombs of Pazyryk, in the Altai Mountains of Siberian Russia, near the Chinese, Mongolian, and Kazakh borders, are horse mummies, all of which are geldings (Rudenko, 1970). These tombs, first excavated in the 1920s, date to the Iron Age (about 400 BC). How early horses were actually gelded will likely never be known, but Scythian and Sarmatian riders from this part of the world apparently preferred riding geldings. Still, even though ancient commentaries noted that geldings were easier to manage than stallions (Hyland, 1990), essentially all of the classical art and textual material from ancient Greece, Rome, and Egypt show that stallions were the horse of choice for warring and hunting.

2.5 Carts and Chariots

… suddenly a chariot of fire and horses of fire appeared.

The Bible, 2 Kings 2:11

The earliest use of equids was for traction. In most parts of the ancient world, once humans were able to train horses to pull, their value as beasts of burden eventually

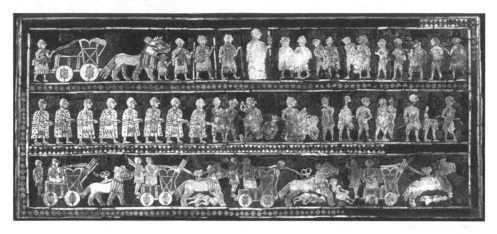

Figure 2.5 Early wagons from the Standard of Ur, c. 2600–2400 BC. (Wikimedia Commons.)

superseded their value as food. Initially, horses and asses were most likely used for pulling, and as pack animals, but apparently not generally for riding. Though occasionally horses were probably ridden as sport for young men (as practiced today in American rodeos), horses were initially trained to pull. Once the practice of using horses for transport and war was adopted, it spread explosively throughout the civilized world. The practice roared across Europe, and by the middle of the second millennium BC horses were being used to pull chariots all over the world, from Greece to Egypt, in Mesopotamia and Anatolia, and on the Eurasian steppe – in China and India, chariots were common by the middle of the first millennium BC. Once harnessed, no other animal had such a tremendous impact on the course of world political developments as has the horse; no other animal served humans in so many different capacities.

The earliest direct evidence of equids used for pulling comes from the Standard of Ur, a hollow wooden box excavated in the 1920s, in the city of Ur, in modern-day Iraq (Figure 2.5). Scenes on the box show humans in four-wheeled vehicles drawn by equids, most likely asses or onagers (Clutton-Brock, 1992); however, it is not clear from the box if the vehicles were used for warfare or transport. Nevertheless, it is felt that contemporaneous Sumerian warriors used solid-wheeled chariots drawn by wild asses.

With the development of the spoked wheel, and the domestication of horses, the age of chariots arose, thrived, and spread like wildfire. The earliest chariots date from around 2000 BC, found in excavations of the timber-grave sites of the Sintashta–Petrovka culture (modern Russia and Kazakhstan). Once horses were hitched to chariots, the innovation spread rapidly – examples have been found in contemporaneous sites throughout the ancient world. In China, the earliest chariots date from the rule of Wu Ding (Shang Dynasty, c. 1200 BC).

The great age of chariot warfare in the early West peaked about 1300 BC, at the Battle of Kadesh, between Egyptian and Hittite forces in what is now modern Syria. Still, in spite of its worldwide spread, the chariot was of minor importance in ancient Greece. Greek topography is unsuitable for chariot warfare; perhaps that is why the chariot was used primarily for ceremonial purposes, for games, and for processions.

Over time, chariots waned in importance, due to the rise of armed horsemen, who were more maneuverable, and especially mounted archers, for whom chariots were an easy target. Gradually, the chariot was relegated to activities such as funeral processions and races, such as the spectacles that were conducted at the Roman Coliseum (Littauer and Crouwel, 2002). Such events have been recorded for posterity on wine vessels and mosaics. Ultimately, chariot racing lost its prestige, although it was still practiced into the Middle Ages.

2.6 Riding Horses in the Ancient World

When I bestride him, I soar, I am a hawk: he trots the air; the earth sings when he touches it; the basest horn of his hoof is more musical than the pipe of Hermes.

William Shakespeare, Henry V

The riding horse was a revolutionary development in horse–human relations. Suddenly, men took flight. Long journeys became possible. Contacts between human societies, previously limited because of distance, became easier. Without horses, humans were sedentary, fixed, and largely unable to explore. Without humans, horses were another large animal: another food source on the plains. Together, they became the most overpowering force in most of recorded history.

There is still some considerable historical dispute as to when riding first began. Some assert that riding was being practiced on the steppe as early as the fourth millennium BC. However, one would think that, if horse riding were being regularly practiced by *any* culture, it would have been rapidly adapted by *all* of them. Examples of such rapid assimilation of horse-related innovations into human culture include when the horse was used for traction: within a few hundred years of horses being trained to pull, horses were being used for such purposes throughout the ancient world. Or, for another example, when the Native Americans of North America saw Spanish explorers riding horses – an animal that was previously unknown to them – they rapidly adopted the practice themselves as soon as they could get their own horses.

In fact, there is no direct evidence for riding in any culture as early as the fourth millennium BC. It is certainly possible that young men jumped on the backs of horses for sport, as young men are wont to do, but there is no evidence of such activity. Further, as previously noted, it would not have been possible to control horses effectively using nose rings, while sitting across the horse's loins. Even during the age of chariot warfare (roughly 1700–1200 BC), when writing and artistic representations of horses and humans became commonplace, there is little evidence of good riding.

It is not until the ninth century BC that evidence for effective horseback riding in the Near East and on the steppe can be found. This might also be in part because to ride horses comfortably, other inventions besides bits were required. Controlling horses is one thing; being able to sit on them for long periods of time without significant discomfort is quite another. One innovation, the saddle, is perhaps obvious; the other, trousers, perhaps less so.

Ancient riders did not use saddles. They undoubtedly rode bareback, or sat on a piece of cloth or hide. As such, it surely must have been difficult controlling horses using only bits, even once metal bits were developed. Early classical art shows riders seated on top of blankets that were unsecured by a girth; one can hardly imagine that this was a secure riding arrangement. Still, the ancient Greeks rode bareback – Alexander the Great's Macedonian cavalry charged their enemies without the benefit of saddles or stirrups, which, if nothing else, makes one admire their riding abilities.

The first use of saddles is generally attributed to the North African Moors. Early saddles were simply pads, but as horse use increased, and horse owning became associated with power and prestige, and saddles became effective control devices, they also became works of art. Assyrian warriors from about 700 BC rode on decorative cloths which were strapped to the horse's back. A saddle from an Iron Age tomb in the Pazyryk Valley of the eastern Altai region of Siberia, from the fifth century BC, is ornately decorated with leather, felt, hair, and gold (Figure 2.6). Saddle trees, which allowed for an even more secure fit for the saddle on the back of the horse, first appeared in Asia in about 200 BC.

Even once a seat on the horse's back could be secured, there was still the problem of rider comfort. Riding horses for long distances chafes human legs; humans developed protection for their legs, accordingly. Mounted Scythian raiders, most likely from what is modern-day Iran, appear to be among the first to wear trousers (Drews, 2004). Such attire was a symbol of status; in ancient China, trousers were only worn by soldiers. Once control of the horse and comfort of the rider were assured, mounted raiding and warfare began in earnest.

Raiding and mounted warfare was undoubtedly a traumatic development for ancient societies. Suddenly, strangers could appear on the horizon and destroy lives and properties within hours. Such an escalation of war power was recorded by ancient artists and historians; the horse also began to appear prominently in the ancient world in art, as well as in histories and literature.

In the late eighth and seventh centuries BC, the Kimmerians and Scythians, (most likely from north of the Black Sea, to northwestern Iran) were able to launch expeditions into Assyria, Lydia, and the Levant (along the western Mediterranean, eastward). These expeditions were documented, albeit somewhat inaccurately, by

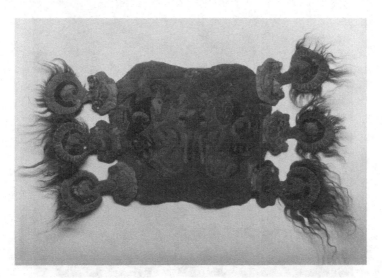

Figure 2.6 Saddle cover, eastern Altai, Pazyryk burial mound 1; felt, leather, horsehair; fifth century BC; length 119 cm, width 60 cm. This cover of thin red felt trimmed along the edges with strips of leather is decorated with appliqué designs in colored felt. On the sides of the cover are two identical compositions: a winged griffin, standing on the ibex he has overwhelmed, holds in his beak one of the victim's horns; the ibex's forefeet are bent under him, while his hind legs, together with the hindquarters, also twisted around, turn upwards; the head faces backward. According to the traditions of ancient Altai art, the animals' bodies are emphasized by appliqué designs in the form of a dot, triangle and drop. On either side the saddle cover has three pendants of yellow felt trimmed with red horsehair and lined with leather. The outer side of each pendant shows an appliqué design in colored felt of a moufflon between two horned tiger's heads. The cover is highly decorative. (Reprinted with permission of The State Hermitage Museum, St. Petersburg, Russia. Photograph © The State Hermitage Museum. Photo by Vladimir Terebenin, Leonard Kheifets, and Yuri Molodkovets.)

the Greek 'Father of History,' Herodotus (*c.* 484–425 BC).[4] Horses gave the Kimmerians and Scythians the elements of speed and surprise, which allowed them to pillage unfortified towns and religious complexes without warning, and to escape pursuers. Armed with bows and swords, these raiders were effective both in hit-and-run battles, as well as in hand-to-hand combat against infantry (Figure 2.7). Mounted soldiers became powerful features of ancient armies (Drews, 2004).

Horses, and their newly mounted riders, rapidly spread throughout the ancient world. Horse remains have been found in burial sites in modern Pakistan, from the early Swat culture (*c.* 1600 BC), as well as at Surkotada (*c.* 2000 BC), and a few other sites. Horses may have been introduced into India by Indo-Aryan people

---

[4]*Herodotus* (transl. A.D. Godley), vol. 4, book 8, verse 98, pp. 96–97. Loeb, 1924.

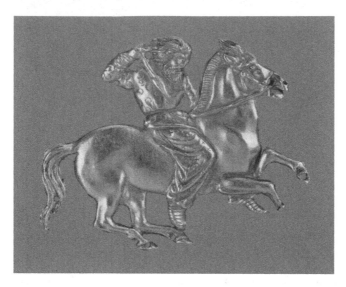

Figure 2.7 Scythian horseman; chased gold plaque; 400–350 BC; Kul-Oba burial mound, Bosporan kingdom, Kerch, eastern Crimea, Ukraine. (Reprinted with permission of The State Hermitage Museum, St. Petersburg, Russia. Photograph © The State Hermitage Museum. Photo by Vladimir Terebenin, Leonard Kheifets, and Yuri Molodkovets.)

from the area around the Caspian Sea (Allchin, 1969). Central Asian raiders invaded ancient India on horseback in the sixteenth century BC and dethroned its king; the cavalry force was called the five hordes (*pañca.ganan*). It was said that the horses of the Sindhu and Kamboja regions were the finest breed; the Kamboja region, and the Ashvaka culture therein, was known as the 'Home of the Horses.' Ancient references to Kambojas as cavalry mercenaries, employed by outside nations, abound. These great horsemen also fought fiercely against Alexander the Great (*c.* 326 BC).

The horse was important throughout most of India's history, but India always depended on western and central Asia for its supply of horses (Bryant, 2001). Some credit Indian riders with the invention of the toe stirrup (a loop of rope that held the big toe), perhaps as early as 500 BC, which is nearly 1000 years before they were employed by Attila the Hun (406–453 AD, leader of the Hunnic Empire of central Asian invaders), who is commonly credited for their invention (Chamberlain, 2006). Like most useful human innovations, the use of stirrups was rapidly adopted by others.

The gratitude and wonder that humans developed for the power and beauty of horses was also recorded in magic and myth. The relationship between horses and humans has commonly moved into the area of the spiritual, and throughout human history, horses have been represented as being favored by the gods. Horses were certainly deemed worthy of sacrifice to human gods; the Ashvamedha

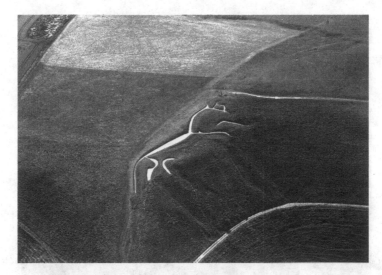

Figure 2.8   The Uffington White Horse. (Copyright David Collier, Faringdon, Oxfordshire, UK.)

(horse sacrifice) is one of the rituals of the Yajurveda (*c.* 1400–1000 BC), one of the four canonical texts of the Hindu religion. The Romans, too, sacrificed horses; every October they would present a horse to the god Mars, and keep the horse's tail through the winter, as a symbol of fertility and renewal. Horses have even been more or less directly consulted, much in the way that ancient humans consulted soothsayers. For example, humans in northern Europe and England kept some favored horses in sacred places, where their activities could be observed, unhindered by human contact, and interpreted as indications of, and omens for, the future. The Uffington White Horse (Figure 2.8), a prehistoric hill figure dating from the Bronze Age, was cut into the slope of White Horse Hill in the English county of Oxfordshire, and may have had religious or magical significance.

The sites of earliest horse concentrations also lie close to the northern border of modern China. As was the case in other cultures, horses were symbols of power and wealth in China; as early as the Shang Dynasty (*c.* 1600–1100 BC), horses and carts were buried with their owners so that all could be together in the afterlife. Horses were even supposed to protect Chinese emperors after death; for example, the 'Terracotta Army' of Chinese Emperor Qin Shi Huang, dating from 210 BC, is perhaps the most spectacular example of funerary statues in the world, with approximately 130 chariots with 520 horses, and another 150 cavalry horses, intended to help rule another empire in the afterlife (Figure 2.9).

During the time of the Western Zhou Dynasty (*c.* 1100–771 BC), a kingdom's military might was measured by the number of its war chariots. With the growth of Chinese empires, horses were necessary for internal communication, control of remote areas, and transportation of goods and supplies throughout the country.

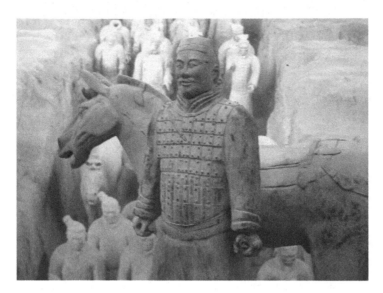

Figure 2.9 Cavalryman of the Terracotta Army of Emperor Qin Shi Huang. (Wikimedia Commons.)

In 307 BC, military commanders and troops were ordered to wear trousers, and practice mounted archery; these adaptations soon spread to other states. Cavalry rapidly replaced the chariot in China; cavalry soon became essential as support for massed ground troops (Ebrey, 1999).

The Chinese are credited with developing other inventions critical to the control of horses. While the toe stirrup may have been developed in India, an illustration of a rider with stirrups attached to the saddle appears in a Jin Dynasty tomb from 322 AD. Breast straps, effective harnessing systems, and horse collars, which allowed horses to haul greater weights more easily than with the breast harness, were also Chinese contributions to advancing man's use of the horse (Cooke, 2001). Unfortunately, the Chinese have, for much of their history, lacked adequate horse pasture to keep their horses, no matter how esteemed, healthy, and active. Alfalfa, a hay crop in much of the world, and the most ancient recorded crop grown solely as forage,[5] was an early introduction, but it was never grown widely enough nor was it suitable for cultivation everywhere. Other feeds were even rarer. Oats, for example, often the feed of choice for war horses in Medieval and Early Modern Europe, were completely unavailable in old China (Smith, 1991).

---

[5] Alfalfa appears to have originated in present-day Iran, or in mountainous regions of adjacent countries east of the Mediterranean Sea in southwestern Asia. The name 'alfalfa' comes from the Arabic *al-fisfisa*, meaning 'fresh fodder.'

As was the case in many cultures, the ancient Chinese celebrated horses for their intelligence. For example, in the 'Spring and Autumn Annals,' the official chronicle of the State of Lu, documenting the period 722–481 BC, Han Fei Zi (c. 280–233 BC) wrote:[6] 'Guan Zhong accompanied Load Huan of Qi in attacking Guzhu. Spring passed and winter returned, and they became lost on the wrong road. Guan Zhong said: "We can use the wisdom of an old horse. Release the old horses and follow them, and thereby reach the right road."'

Indian traditions also celebrate the horse for its wisdom. Hayagriva, a horse-headed god with a human body, is worshipped as the god of knowledge and wisdom in the Vaishnava tradition; Hayagriva also appears in Buddhist traditions. The combination of man and horse was not unique to India, of course; the Centaurs of Greek mythology were half horse and half man. While, in general, the Centaurs were thought of as being wild as untamed horses, Chiron, considered the most superior of his race, was intelligent, civilized, and kind, and had knowledge of, and skill with, medicine. Chiron was a teacher, as well; among his many pupils were Greek cultural icons such as Heracles, Achilles, and Jason. Centaurs have appeared in literature ever since, including most recently in books such as *The Chronicles of Narnia* by C.S. Lewis or the *Harry Potter* series by J.K. Rowling.

Winged horses are common in the mythology of various ancient cultures. A white horse with two wings emerged from the primal ocean of Indian mythology, named Uchchaihshravas [sic]. Indra, one of the Hindu gods, took the horse to Heaven, but later cut off his wings, and gave the horse – now unable to fly back to Heaven – to man as a gift. Pegasus, the great winged horse of Greek mythology, went on many adventures, and ultimately became a servant of Zeus, the king of the gods. On the last day of Pegasus' life, Zeus transformed him into a constellation, where he can still be viewed today. Images of Pegasus adorn company logos and magazines; the horse even has a Turkish airline named after him.

Of course, wings were not the only unique features of mythological horses. Unicorns (Figure 2.10) have been extolled in stories, songs, and poems for centuries. Despite widespread and long-standing beliefs in their existence (during the Renaissance, Leonardo da Vinci even gave details on how they could be captured), and general consensus on their good nature and magical powers, they have never been seen. Unicorns appear to have originated in Chinese folklore, and have taken many forms, from that of a beautiful horse, to combinations such as the body and head of a horse, the beard of a goat, and the tail of a lion; the only consistent feature is a single horn. Unicorns were at least somewhat familiar in form; Sleipnir, the horse of Odin, the king of the Norse gods, had eight legs.

Even the color of horses has also been used as a literary symbol since antiquity. White horses are usually seen as good, representing light, sun, resurrection, and birth, among others. The white horse has been central to world literature since at

---

[6] Han Fei Zi, 'Spring and Autumn Annals,' Discourse on 'Ling Shang,' ch. 22.

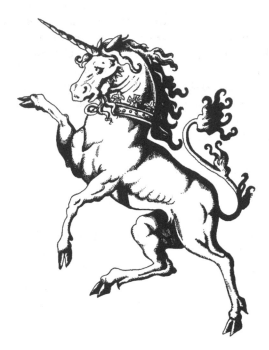

Figure 2.10 Antique illustration of a unicorn. (Published in *Systematischer Bilder-Atlas zum Conversations-Lexikon, Ikonographische Encyklopaedie der Wissenschaften und Kuenste*, Brockhaus, Leipzig, 1844. Istockphoto.com.)

least the Biblical Book of Revelations; St. George, the Patron Saint of England, also rode a white horse. During the Middle Ages, artists portrayed virgins, heroes, saints, and even Jesus Christ riding upon white horses. Conversely, black horses may be feared, representing mystery, night, or death. The third horseman of the Biblical apocalypse rode a black horse, as did the Nazgûl of J.R.R. Tolkein's *Lord of the Rings* trilogy; these fearsome steeds had been specially trained to endure terror.

While horses, and horse cavalry, spread rapidly throughout the ancient world, horses apparently played a relatively minor role in ancient Greece. Still, the Thessalonians were known to produce expert riders, and the Greco-Persian wars showed the Greeks the value of mounted warriors. Xenophon (*c.* 430–354 BC), the Athenian author, soldier, historian and philosopher, wrote several manuals on horsemanship and cavalry (see later footnote), and advocated the maintenance of a small cavalry force. While the value of cavalry was acknowledged, perhaps the mountainous terrain of Greece made keeping horses difficult, posing the same sorts of problems that prevented the ancient Chinese from developing large horse populations; the mountainous terrain of Japan probably limited the development of horse populations there, as well; almost certainly the terrain prevented the adoption of the chariot for Japanese warfare.

On the other hand, the Macedonians (north of Greece) developed a strong cavalry force. Ultimately, this led to the Hetairoi, the heavy companion cavalry of Philip II and Alexander the Great, equipped with metal helmets and various types of body armor, the Prodromoi (literally 'pre-cursors,' in the sense of moving before the rest of the army), light horsemen used for scouting, as well as screening, and the Ippiko (horse rider), the medium cavalry, armed with lances and swords, and covered with leather armor or chain mail (Gabriel, 1990). Thus accompanied, Alexander, astride his great horse Bucephalus, conquered Persia, Bactria, and northwestern India in the third century BC.

The early Roman cavalry was the bailiwick of wealthy men who could afford horses, as well as the necessary arms and armor. The cavalry grew with the addition of foreigners from Gaul, Iberia, and North Africa (Numidia). Whereas initially the Romans used cavalry primarily for scouting, skirmishing, and duties on the outposts of the Empire (see Figure 2.11), ultimately the Romans increased both the numbers and training standards of their cavalry (McCall, 2002).

But horses were not mere war engines in ancient times. Following victory, conquerors needed to maintain contact with their newly acquired land. The Persian Empire (c. fifth century BC) was the largest of its time, and sent messages and gathered information using a network of mounted riders; bas relief carvings of Persian horses adorn the stairways of the great audience hall (the Apadana) of the ancient Persian capitol of Persepolis. In reference to the Persian horses, Herodotus (see earlier footnote) noted, 'It is said that as many days as there are in the whole journey, so many are the men and horses that stand along the road, each horse and man at the interval of a day's journey; and these are stayed neither by snow nor rain nor heat nor darkness from accomplishing their appointed course with all speed'. The motto was eventually adapted by the US Post Office. This system allowed King Xerxes to inform his court at home in Persia that the Greeks had destroyed his fleet off Salamis in 480 BC. Genghis Khan used a similar system to maintain control of what was arguably the greatest empire in world history. The Pony Express, memorialized in story and film, was another famous example. The horse was the fastest method of communication available to man for centuries, not surpassed until the nineteenth century, with the development of the steam engine and the telegraph; it is no stretch to assert that, without the horse, cultures would not have easily encountered each other, travel and trade would not have been as easily accomplished, and ancient empires would not have been as easily built. Indeed, civilization was built on the back of the horse.

Ancient horsemen also found horses to be great sources of entertainment. When horses became domesticated, it is likely that people soon tried to sit on them; one can easily imagine how trying to stay on a wild horse would have been a great source of amusement for both participants and onlookers, as per rodeo today. Both Persians and Greeks raced horses; Roman chariot races were popular then, and have been celebrated in modern film, in movies such as *Ben Hur* and *Gladiator*. As riding became more developed – and, with the development of saddles, bits, stirrups, etc., safer – horsemanship became something to be studied, taught, and developed.

The oldest surviving treatise on horsemanship, written by Xenophon, is *The Art of Horsemanship*; the information in the book is still useful today.[7]

Horses in art also became prominent in the ancient world. The ancient Greeks developed a style of sculpture that was devoted to the perfection of the sculpted form. Greek works, such as the frieze from the interior of the Parthenon from the middle of the fifth century BC, represent horses three-dimensionally, with attention paid to anatomical features such as veins and muscles.

Beginning in ancient times, horses have also been used in innumerable stories, as allegories for human behavior. Aesop (*c.* 620–560 BC), a slave and teller of stories who lived in ancient Greece, often used horses to illustrate morals appropriate for his listeners in his fables.[8] For example, in 'The Horse and the Ass,' the ass professes the wish that he could be dressed in the finery of the warhorse, as opposed to having to carry his heavy weights. However, the next day, the horse was fatally wounded in battle. The ass found the horse, at the point of death, and told him that he had been wrong. The ass concluded that it was better to be secure and humble than ostentatious and in danger.

In the ancient Chinese folktale, 'The Lost Horse,' Sai, a wise man, tells of how good fortune can turn to bad, and vice versa. When Sai's horse runs away, he tells the people who have come to give him comfort that the horse's loss may not be a bad thing; he is proven right when the horse comes back accompanied by a beautiful white mare. But Sai is also reluctant to join the people when they rejoice at his new-found good fortune; his son is later injured in a fall from the mare. But this unfortunate event became a blessing; only because the son was lame from his injury was he unable to go to war against invading nomads; only because the son was lame did father and son survive to take care of each other. The changes in life have no end, and the mystery of life cannot be comprehended (Roberts, 1979).

2.7 Horses and Empires

They say princes learn no art truly but the art of horsemanship. The reason is the brave beast is no flatterer. He will throw a prince as soon as his groom.
Ben Jonson, Discoveries Made Upon Men and Matter and Some Poems,
'Illiteratus princeps'

As man learned to control the horse, horse-mounted soldiers became a feared and potent armed force for nearly two millennia. Cavalry was first used for scouting, for outflanking massed infantry, and for pursuit of a defeated enemy. However, by the beginning of the Common Era, the most powerful cavalry in the world belonged

[7]Xenophon, *The Art of Horsemanship* (transl. M.H. Morgan), Dover, Mineola, NY, 2006.
[8]Aesop's Fables are available at: http://aesop.classicauthors.net/AesopsFables/AesopsFables79.html.

to the Parthian empire of northern Iran, and, later, the Sassanids. While the majority of Persian cavalry comprised light archers, their cataphract – heavy cavalry, fully armored, and armed with lances – was greatly feared by the Romans, with whom the Persians warred for centuries. Eventually, the Romans adapted the Persian heavy armor, as well as their cavalry tactics, as their own.

These ancient warriors idealized and idolized their horses; when horses went to war, they were not mere vehicles for their riders. In cultures from China to Europe, in the Middle East, Greece, and Rome, horses (as well as other equids) were partners, who were considered to participate in various encounters with understanding, wisdom, compassion, and even sadness for his human counterpart (who often lacked those characteristics). So, for example, in the Greek classic, *Iliad* (Homer, *c.* eighth century BC),[9] Xanthus, one of the two great horses of Achilles, speaks back to Achilles when the horse is chastised for leaving the body of Patroclus on the field of battle. The horse not only speaks, but cries, as he has been given the knowledge that Fate had also mandated the death of Achilles.

As Rome declined, in the fourth and fifth centuries AD, it became harder to support large forces of armed men, and armed cavalry took on increasing importance. Better riding equipment, in particular stirrups, pommels, and cantels (adapted from the Persians), meant that riders could be more secure on horseback and cavalry became a more important, and dominant, force. Even though Roman saddles had no stirrups, their saddles did have horns, so riders were fairly secure. Ultimately, the armored Roman cavalry was the predecessor of the medieval knight (Figure 2.11).

However, in other parts of the world, potent cavalry forces developed without armor. Light, fast-moving cavalry was a feature of the Arabs during the Islamic conquests of the seventh century AD. During the period of the Rashidun, under the rule of the first four caliphs after the death of the prophet Muhammed, light cavalry was used to rapidly attack, retreat, and change the point of attack during battle. Such rapid tactics allowed the caliphate to easily conquer Syria; they could easily outmaneuver the Byzantine (late Roman) armies against which they were deployed (Armstrong, 2000). In 751 AD, the Islamic armies defeated the infantry of the Chinese Tang Dynasty at the Battle of Talas, helping the Islamic world to gain control over central Asia, and helped start the decline of the Tang Dynasty (Hoberman, 1982).

The early Islamic dynasties also trained slave soldiers to serve them. The Mamluks were taken as children from parts of central Asia, and then trained within the Islamic world to serve their masters. Mamluks were often trained as cavalrymen; their code of conduct (*al-furusiyya*) valued courage and generosity, but also a knowledge of horsemanship and cavalry tactics. Over decades, the Mamluks became powerful; on several occasions they triumphed over the invading armies of the Crusaders. The Mamluks ruled Egypt from 1250 to 1517; they served even into the nineteenth century as a unit of Napoleon's army (Waterson, 2007). The names

---

[9] Homer, *Iliad*, XVI, 149, 467; XIX, 400.

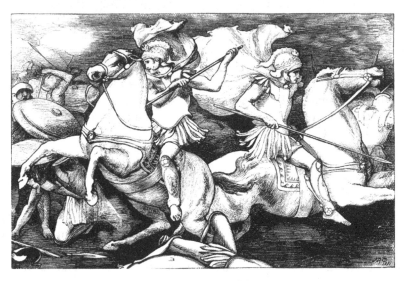

Figure 2.11 Roman knights. A vintage engraving of the Roman heroes Castor and Pollux at the ancient Roman battle of Lake Regillus, a legendary early Roman victory won over the Latin League led by the expelled Etruscan former king of Rome, c. 499 BC. (Istockphoto.com.)

of other cultures with expertise in horsemanship have also become legend; cultures such as the Huns, Avars, Kipchaks, Mongols, and Cossacks were among the most feared of their times, due to their armed might and rapid mobility.

Eastern cultures used the horse to further their empires, as well. Korean kingdoms had cavalry since at least the third century BC, and King Gwanggaeto the Great (c. 374–413 AD) led cavalry expeditions of as many as 50 000 horses against Japanese invaders. The Japanese horsemen of the Kofun period (c. 250–538 AD) wore armor, carried weapons, and used advanced military methods; much of this culture can barely be distinguished from that which occurred on the southern Korean peninsula. Tibetan horsemen also were cavalry warriors, and fought several battles against the Chinese Tang Dynasty (618–907 AD). Indian cavalry was a potent force from the period of the Gupta Dynasty (320–600 AD) forwards.

The horse has had great impact on Chinese history. Han Dynasty rulers made great efforts to import horses; the Tang Dynasty (618–907 AD) saw improvements in breeding practices, as well as stock, through the importation of Arab and Turkish horses. However, during the subsequent Song Dynasty, the Tang breeding programs fell into shambles, leaving a shortage of horses. Thus, ironically, during the period of the Mongols (Yuan Dynasty, 1279–1368 AD, led by Genghis Khan), a period where the largest empire the world has ever known was achieved on the back of the horse, while Chinese influence increased, the quality of Chinese horses declined. Subsequently, horses declined in importance in China. Still, in 1995, it was estimated that China's horse population exceeded 11 million animals, and at least 26 breeds (Cooke, 2001).

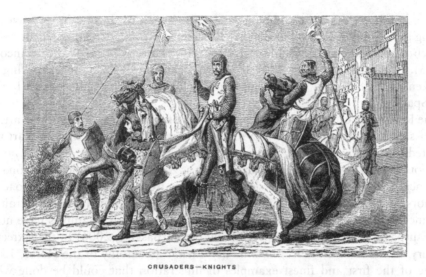

CRUSADERS—KNIGHTS

Figure 2.12 Vintage engraving, from the 1880s, of Crusader knights. (Istockphoto.com.)

After the fall of the Roman Empire, a new horse soldier emerged in Europe, carrying the banner of Christianity. These horsemen combined fighting skill with their faith, and tempered their power with courtesy and politeness. Saddles that wrapped around the horse's barrel provided mounted warriors with ever greater security in combat, stirrups reduced the likelihood of a rider being dismounted while fighting, and spurs added to the rider's control over his charger. As such, the armed charge became a powerful innovation in battle. Ultimately, this led to the 'knight in shining armor,' the ultimate in mounted cavalry force; it was an exchange of flexibility for power. These knights followed the code of Chivalry (from the Old French, *cheval*, meaning horse). Christian holy warriors battled the Moors in Spain, the Turks at the gates of Vienna, and went on Crusades to Jerusalem to battle 'infidels.'[10] By the end of the Middle Ages, Christendom had been firmly established in Europe on the back of the horse.

Armed knights were a political, as well as a military, force; a landowner's social position was measured by how many armored and mounted men he could supply his lord. In exchange for his lord's protection, the vassal pledged himself, or money or land sufficient to support a mounted fighting man. Thus, the feudal system was born (Bloch, 1961). Even so, foot soldiers and bowmen, with cheap, easy-to-use weapons, were the basis of armed warfare in the Middle Ages, and sieges and wars of attrition were the primary method of bringing foes to their knees; mounted knights charging to victory are more the purview of romance than reality (Figure 2.12).

---

[10]It is commonly thought that the Crusades also served as the first introduction of European riders to lighter, faster Middle Eastern horses.

As a combat weapon, the mounted warrior began to decline in effectiveness during the Hundred Years War. English bowmen were able to slaughter the heavy French cavalry at battles such as Crécy (1346), Poitiers (1356), and Agincourt (1415). Even so, by the early sixteenth century, during the flowering of the Renaissance, cavalry made up as much as 50% of the armed forces of France and Spain.

The Renaissance also brought about a revival of the horse as a subject for art. To Renaissance artists, the horse was a relatively new subject; most Medieval art was devoted to religious subjects, and ancient sculptures and mosaics depicting horses had not yet been uncovered. Thus, artists such as Antonio Polliaiuolo and Leonardo da Vinci began looking at the horse with relatively fresh eyes, and they approached the horse with an interest not only in art, but also in anatomy. Formal portraiture that included horses appeared in the fifteenth century; early examples have never been surpassed in terms of perspective and detail (Baskett, 2006) In the sixteenth century, Carlo Ruini's book *Anatomia del Cavallo* (Anatomy of the Horse, 1598) is one of the first and finest examples of illustration that could be done when animals were studied for their own sake (and not as a branch of human anatomy) (Figure 2.13).

From at least the mid-sixteenth century onwards, the use of cavalry began to wane, albeit with notable exceptions, for example, the Polish winged hussars, who were the primary component of the Polish Army between the sixteenth and eighteenth centuries. Several reasons likely led to the decline of the mounted warrior as a primary weapon of battle, including the development of gunpowder in the fifteenth and sixteenth centuries, which allowed infantry to inflict casualties at long range, the expense of maintaining mounted fighters, and the fact that highly trained cavalrymen were much more difficult to replace than foot soldiers, who could be trained in weeks. Thus, the role of cavalry primarily returned to its earliest functions of charging flanks, reconnaissance, attacks on specific targets (e.g., the general of the opposing army), or counter-attack (e.g., by Napoleon's cavalry at the Battle of Marengo in 1800), rather than massed attack. And horses found other uses at war; the development of field artillery made horses important for hauling arms and ammunition to and from the field of battle.

The fifteenth century also brought about the return of the horse to the New World. Columbus brought horses with him on his second voyage, in 1493, and the Spanish explorers of the early sixteenth century conquered much of the New World on horseback. However, contrary to popular belief, horses that escaped from these early expeditions did not become the root of the wild horse herds in North America. Instead, the Spanish mission system was responsible; both escaped horses, as well as horses captured by Native American raiders, made up the foundation animals for the current herds. Thus, the 'wild mustang' of the American plains is actually a bit of a mutt, having come from a cross-section of various breed types (Sponenberg, 1992).

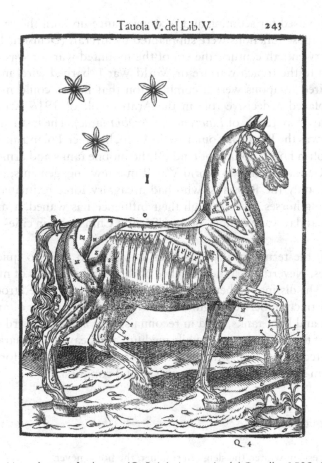

Tauola V. del Lib. V.   243

Q. 4

Figure 2.13 Musculature of a horse. (C. Ruini, *Anatomia del Cavallo*, 1598, 243.)

In the eighteenth century, cavalry forces on both sides of a conflict regularly confronted each other, but cavalry charges against infantry most commonly met with failure. However, cavalry was often used to help chase down infantrymen that had been scattered by artillery, at least until firearms became more accurate. The Charge of the Light Brigade, immortalized in poetry by Alfred Lord Tennyson, was a disastrous charge of British cavalry against Russian forces in 1854 during the Crimean War through artillery and armed infantry; the charge mostly highlighted the futility of charging men with guns on horseback.

Cavalry was still employed by British Empire commanders during the nineteenth-century Imperial expansion; horses were still effective against poorly armed foes. Still, cavalry was indispensable for scouting, harassing supply lines, and screening troop movements, such as in the US Civil War; mounted soldiers battled mounted Native Americans in the late nineteenth century in the Indian wars. Men on horseback were used for scouting and reconnaissance up until the early twentieth century, when those functions were supplanted by aircraft (Denison, 1913).

By the mid-twentieth century, the era of the mounted warrior was over. Horses were ill-suited to the trench warfare of World War I; barbed wire, machine guns, and rapidly fired weapons were a combination that horses could not overcome. Still, horses played a decisive role in the Arab revolt of 1916 (which included Thomas Edward Lawrence, of *Lawrence of Arabia* fame). The last major recorded cavalry battle was the Battle of Komarów, in 1920, between Poland and the Russian Bolsheviks. Polish horses could not fend off the mobile tanks and armored units of the invading German armies in World War II in a few engagements; by the end of World War II, only the Russians, who had a cavalry force estimated at 300 000 men, were using horses. Even though their influence has waned, armed men still patrol borders today, for example, in the USA and China, and in cities (as mounted police).

In addition, the term 'cavalry' has been co-apted to refer to quickly moving armored forces. Nevertheless, the influence of thousands of years of mounted warfare remains. The distinction between the light and heavy armored troops of today mirrors the distinction between light and heavy mounted cavalry of ancient times. Armored cars and light tanks, used in reconnaissance and quick strikes, recall the light cavalry of the Muslim world, while medium and heavy tanks hark back to the heavily protected battle cavalry that was the Byzantine cataphract. Horses, it seems, still have a firm hold on man's designs of war and conquest.

2.8 Horses at Work

The wagon rests in winter, the sleigh in summer, the horse never.

Yiddish Proverb

Even though horses were used for war almost as soon as they were trained to carry riders, horses were not immediately adapted to become working animals. Up until early Medieval times, the primary work animals were the ox and the donkey. Oxen could pull heavier loads than the light horses of the time, and horses were more expensive to keep than either oxen or the smaller donkey. The widespread adaptation of the working horse required the development of larger horses.

As the age of Medieval knights drew to a close, and farming techniques improved, the larger horses that were bred to carry the weight of the knights were put to other uses. Draft horses were developed from the horses of the northern Germanic tribes, horses that were heavier than those in the Mediterranean or Middle East. The horse collar, developed in China, but adapted by Europeans at some unknown date, allowed for much more efficient harnessing of these larger horses to carts and wagons. Horse collars allowed farmers to put the horse's speed and strength to use, allowing for cultivation of larger areas, and pulling of heavier loads.

As stable governments were formed throughout Europe, resources were organized to construct and maintain roads. Larger working horses became commonplace, and they were used to pull plows, carts, coaches, and wagons, as well as turning grindstones to make flour. In Germany, roads of wooden rails, called wagonways, were constructed as early as 1550. Horses pulled wagons or carts over these railways (the progenitor of the modern railroad) more easily than over dirt roads. Wooden rails were replaced with iron rails; wagonways evolved into tramways; railed transport spread throughout Europe, with horses still providing all the pulling power (Lewis, 1970). However, by the early nineteenth century, steam engines had replaced horses as engines of locomotion.

Legend states that the first Japanese horse was born from the head of the dead Uke-mochi, the food goddess. Stones with markings are considered sacred in Japan, and, according to legend, they are the hoof prints of Amida and the other first legendary horses. Japanese emperors used horses to pull carts, as well as to maintain communications in areas under their dominion. However, horses were not used as plow animals; Japanese agriculture centered on the rice harvest, and moist rice paddies are typically seeded by water buffalo, the only beast of burden adapted for life in the wetlands. As in other parts of the world, horses brought a cachet of power and prestige. Curiously, holding a horse's reins was the purview of soldiers in Japan; thus, wealthy merchants could ride, but only if their horse was being led on foot. This, of course, limited the horse's usefulness for individual transport (Kenrick, 1964). The mix of agricultural and social factors probably combined to limit the influence of the horse on economic and political developments in Japan, as well as in other Asian countries.

2.9 Breeding Horses

This most noble beast is the most beautiful, the swiftest and of the highest courage of domesticated animals. His long mane and tail adorn and beautify him. He is of a fiery temperament, but good tempered, obedient, docile and well-mannered.

Pedro Garcia Conde, 1685

The history of planned breeding is blurry, at least in its earliest days. While people undoubtedly bred horses, records of such breeding do not exist until relatively late in history. One of the earliest known horse breeds was the Ferghana horses, which originated in Bactria, an area of modern Afghanistan (Figure 2.14).

Ferghana horses were demanded by the Chinese rulers of the Han Dynasty (c. 200 BC–200 AD), so much so that the Bactrian rulers closed their borders to horse trade, resulting in war (China won). The Chinese demanded at least 100 of the finest Ferghana horses for breeding, and another 3000 ordinary Ferghana horses in tribute (Christian, 1998). According to tradition, Ferghana horses sweated blood; blood-sucking parasites that are endemic to the area may have caused a mixture of sweat and blood that became evident when the horses were worked.

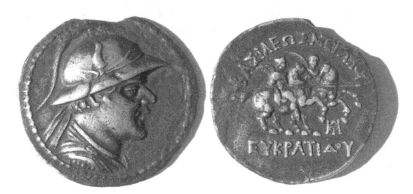

Figure 2.14 Coin showing Eucratides, King of Bactria, and his horse, c. 170–140 BC. (Wikimedia Commons.)

Horses such as the Akhal-Teke have been bred since ancient times, and the Mongol Empire also had an active horse-breeding program. However, the Bedouins, breeders of Arabian horses in the Middle East, appear to be the earliest peoples to document horse breeding. Written pedigrees of Arabian horses date from 1330 AD (Amirsadeghi, 2005).

Different cultures bred different types of horses, depending on their needs. So, for example, light, fast horses were preferred in the Middle East by Muslim warriors, whereas large war horses – called destriers – were bred in Medieval Europe. The heavy European horses later became the foundation animals for a variety of draft horse breeds. Still, Europeans admired the horses of the Middle East, which they encountered in battle during the Crusades, and captured Arabian and Barb horses were crossed with heavier horses to create breeds such as the Percheron, as well as horses used to carry messages, called Coursers, which pre-dated the Thoroughbred horse of today. Horses were subsequently bred for desirable qualities – for example, speedy horses were desirable for communication, heavy horses for work, small ponies for pulling ore out of mines, large horses for pulling carriages, etc.

The sixteenth century marked the beginning of the specialized breeding of horses for purposes other than war. Federico Grison's *The Rules of Horsemanship* initiated *haute école* riding, which became popular among European nobility. The Lippizan horse, named for where it was first bred, from Spanish horse stock in 1580, at the Imperial stud at Lippiza, near Trieste, Italy, became the horse of choice for this purpose, as well as for cavalry officers; the Lippizaners are still the only horses used by the Spanish riding school, in Vienna, Austria.

In England, new breeds were developed, beginning with the reign of King Henry VIII. Foreign horse breeds such as the Barb, Turkoman, and Neapolitan were bred with native English stock to change the make-up of the English horse from being

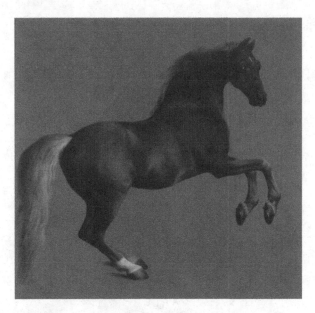

Figure 2.15 *Whistlejacket*, by George Stubbs. (Wikimedia Commons.)

one of mostly 14 hands and below to being one of larger horses. As English horses became bigger, their symbolic value increased as well. While horses have certainly always been prized as symbols of power, horses increasingly became associated with the ruling elite. Young English noblemen were encouraged to learn the art of horse riding; in some ways, mastery of the horse was a metaphor for mastery of the people (Edwards, 2007). As a symbol of power, horses themselves became so important that they were the subjects of portraits *without* their owners; the works of the eighteenth-century English painter George Stubbs are prominent examples (Figure 2.15). The first French *haras* (the National Studs or breeding farms) were created under the reign of Louis XIV in 1665 in Saint-Léger, and developed in the eighteenth century, only to be destroyed during the French Revolution, and re-established by Napoleon in 1806.

The horse's increasing status as a social symbol was accompanied by its other alleged attributes being celebrated as well. For example, the horse's alleged wisdom was the basis for an entire race of wise horses in the famous eighteenth-century satirical novel *Gulliver's Travels*, by Jonathan Swift.[11] The Houyhnhnms [*sic*] were an idealized race, graced with reason and noble qualities; they ruled over the Yahoos, a brutish race that possessed all of men's worst vices. They were a race governed by reason, not emotion; they did not use force, only reasoned persuasion. They did not

---

[11] Officially, the book is titled *Travels into Several Remote Nations of the World, in Four Parts. By Lemuel Gulliver, First a Surgeon, and then a Captain of several Ships.*

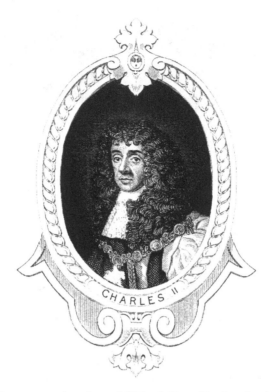

Figure 2.16 Vintage engraving from 1857 of King Charles II of England (May 29, 1630–February 6, 1685). He was popularly known as the Merrie Monarch, in reference to both the liveliness and hedonism of his court and the general relief at the return to normality after over a decade of rule by Oliver Cromwell and the Puritans. (Istockphoto.com.)

lie; they did not have a word for lying in their language. For Swift, horses symbolized an idealized standard of rational existence to which man could aspire.

Horses have probably been informally raced for as long as they have ridden. While the earliest references to horse racing in England date to 1512, breeding specialized horses for racing can be traced to the rule of King Charles II of England. Oliver Cromwell, Lord Protector of England from 1653, until his death in 1658, banned horse racing; in 1660, Charles II restored it (Figure 2.16).

Forty years later, the Thoroughbred horse lineage developed, spurred by the English fascination with Middle Eastern racing horses; the Thoroughbred breed was founded by three horses of Arabian lineage, the Godolphin Arabian, the Byerly Turk, and the Darley Arabian. Horse racing became wildly popular in England, and by 1740 there were so many horse races that government regulation was needed. The popularity of horse racing also led to a change from it being an all-male preserve to part of the social scene of eighteenth-century England. In the late eighteenth century, James Burnett, Lord Monboddo, one of the initial thinkers in the development of the theory of evolution, and also a horse breeder, applied his selective breeding theories to the horse. The multi-billion-dollar modern horse breeding industry still strives to cross particular mares and stallions in an effort to produce champions (Mackay-Smith, 2000).

Or course, the celebrated horses of the ruling elite were not representative of the lives of the majority of horses. The economies of nations were powered on the backs of horses, but life for them was, as seventeenth-century writer Thomas Hobbes described it, 'nasty, brutish, and short' (Hobbes, 1660). English books recording horse sales rarely record horses over ten years old; contemporary accounts routinely recount tales of abused, starved, and neglected horses. As a result, horse care manuals began to be published – for example, by the Englishman Thomas Blundeville, or the Frenchman Jacques de Solleysel – urging readers not to mistreat or overwork their horses, and giving advice on how to care for them; unfortunately, the evidence suggests that such advice was often ignored. While such information may not have been widely distributed, and the advice widely ignored, it almost certainly served as the foundation for the formal development of a new field of study that improved the welfare of the horse: veterinary medicine.

The need for carriage horses in the seventeenth and eighteenth centuries fueled the development of warmblood breeds. Mary Tudor (Queen Mary I, the queen who briefly restored Catholicism to England) first imported Hungarian coaches for herself and her peers. While such transportation initially met with scorn from men who were reluctant to travel in such an 'unmanly' manner, such comfortable transportation soon became fashionable, and a means for the elite to further demonstrate their privileged status. England developed an integrated system of stage coaches in the eighteenth century; the stage coaches of the nineteenth-century American West were the frequent targets of outlaws in legend and film.

The Industrial Revolution started the demise of heavy horses for work; while horses were initially needed to help move the swelling populations of large cities, they ultimately could not compete with automobiles and tractors. Still, lighter riding horses have stayed popular as a means of leisure, sport, and recreation. Draft horses are still used on some small farms, but mostly compete in pulling and plowing competitions.

Quarter Horse racing is a largely American phenomenon. The first recorded match races between two horses – down city streets and country lanes – are from Enrico County, Virginia, dating from 1674. Crowds grew, and large purses were given to the winners; some reports even say that large plantations changed hands based on race outcomes. A Thoroughbred horse named Janus, imported to America in 1756, is the foundation stallion of the Quarter Horse breed; mares of many different breeds were crossed with Janus to foal some of the greatest racing horses in Colonial America. Quarter Horses moved west as the USA expanded, and they found a new use in herding cattle on the American plains. Today, there are distinct types of Quarter Horses: sleek, racing Quarter Horses may be virtually indistinguishable from racing Thoroughbreds, while stock horse types recall the cattle horses of the

American West. The American Quarter Horse Association was founded in 1940, with the aim of registering and preserving the breed (Denhardt, 1991).

2.10 The Modern Horse

I can make a General in five minutes but a good horse is hard to replace.

Abraham Lincoln

There has been an immense shift in human–equine interactions in modern times. Whereas horses initially were prized mostly for their nutritional value, and later as an instrument of war and a beast of burden, the modern horse is mostly a vehicle to be used for sport, leisure, and companionship. Even so, vestiges of the military importance of the horse remain; some monarchies continue to have mounted cavalry as part of their royal guards, for example, the Spanish Royal Guard Escort group.

The evolution of the modern horse was a long time in development. Early horse training could not have been sophisticated, and most likely relied on brute force. However, Xenophon's *The Art of Horsemanship* (see earlier footnote) broke with such tradition, instead emphasizing training the horse through kindness and reward. Equestrian sports were initially viewed mostly as analogues for warfare, and the participants were viewed as practicing skills that would be needed on the battlefield. For example, jousting was designed to simulate horse-mounted combat, but changes in military tactics and equipment quickly destined jousting to ceremony. The artistry of riding that is celebrated today did not being until the Renaissance, as part of a general cultivation of the arts.

As the importance of the horse declined as a weapon of war, horses were trained in any number of airs and schools, and indoor riding became commonplace. The book *Ecole de Cavalerie*, published by the Frenchman François Robichon de la Gueriniere (1688–1751), was one of the most influential and important books on training the horse ever written. Friedrich Wilhelm, Baron Rais d'Eisenberg (*c.* 1700–1770), a member of the aristocracy of the Holy Roman Empire, was one of the most famous horse-lovers of his time, and wrote several important and also lavishly illustrated books on horsemanship, including *La Perfezione e i Difetti del Cavallo* (The Perfection and the Defects of the Horse, 1753). Numerous Portuguese works on the equestrian art were published in the sixteenth and seventeenth centuries, the most famous of which is *Luz da Liberal e Nobre Arte da Cavallaria* (Light of the Noble and Liberal Art of Horsemanship, 1790) published by Manoel Carlos de Andrade. By the Victorian Age (*c.* 1837–1901), equestrianship and indoor horseback riding had become a sophisticated art.

Jumping horses for sport has its roots in French cross-country races, where horses were run literally to their deaths for sport. However, such events were not popular, probably because they could not easily be observed. The 1801 British Enclosures Act, which enclosed common fields in that country in fences, radically

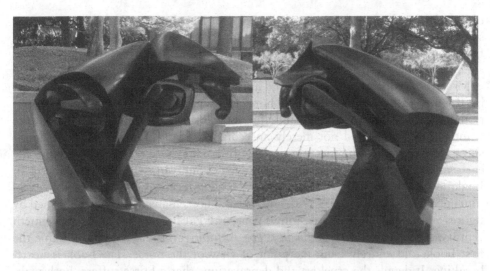

Figure 2.17 Two views of 'Le Grand Cheval,' a bronze sculpture by Raymond Duchamp-Villon, 1914, in the Museum of Fine Arts, Houston, Texas. (Wikimedia Commons.)

altered the sport of hunting in England. Horses and hounds in England were previously used to hunt large game, such as deer and wild boar; fences, and the resulting decline of habitat, reduced the availability of these animals for sport, and resulted in the substitution of the fox for hunting (now banned), with the jumping of fences as an entertaining obstacle. Grand Prix show jumping began in Paris, France, in 1866. In order to facilitate spectators, fences were moved indoors; 'lepping' became a popular competition at the Dublin, Ireland, horse show in 1869. Jumping was introduced as a competitive sport in England in 1907, and recognized as an Olympic sport in 1912. Today, Olympic competitions continue, as well as a lucrative worldwide Grand Prix circuit.

Three-day eventing was originally a race between Berlin and Vienna. The French created the 'Militarie' as an extended training event for cavalry horses in the 1800s. Eventing competitions were first held in Europe in 1902, although the sport did not gain modern Olympic status until 1912, and then only for military men competing on military horses. Numerous other equestrian sports are enjoyed by people around the world, including, but certainly not limited to, the Portuguese *cavaleiro*, where bulls are fought on horseback, combined driving, rodeo, polo, vaulting, cutting, reining, and endurance riding.

While horses have found myriad uses, horses have also taken on different perspectives, especially in modern art. French cubist sculptor Raymond Duchamps-Villon, an expert horseman, who served as an auxiliary doctor in a cavalry regiment during World War I, created his 'Large Horse,' an abstract representation of energy and power (Figure 2.17). Pablo Picasso painted horses as abstract linear objects in his famous painting of the Spanish Revolution, *Guernica*. American sculptor Deborah Butterfield builds popular three-dimensional images of horses from wood pieces or found scraps of metal; her sculptures suggest an almost radiographic view.

Modern developments in ethics and animal welfare have had significant impact on the horse. In many cultures, the horse is now idealized. The undeniable emotional appeal of the horse has resulted in its transformation into the ethos of the companion animal, and not merely an economic entity. Horse–human relationships have moved to the metaphysical, with 'horse whisperers' – dating from the early nineteenth-century Irish horseman, Daniel Sullivan, who became famous in England by rehabilitating vicious horses – having received enormous publicity in film (*The Horse Whisperer*, 1998), and 'natural horsemanship' books published by figures such as Monty Roberts, John Lyons, and Pat Parelli. In the early twentieth century, Anna Sewell's *Black Beauty, The Autobiography of a Horse* became the first book told entirely from the point of view of the horse. The book is heartbreaking. It details the cruelties and depravations that a horse suffers, both malicious and unintentional, at the hand of man. In its time, *Black Beauty* helped bring about the abolition of the 'bearing rein,' a check rein that was used to keep horses' heads high, and was fashionable in late nineteenth-century England, but that was also painful to the horse, and damaging to its neck. The book also helped force more humane treatment of the human cabbies of London. *Black Beauty* also played a part in starting the animal-rights movement – a movement that continues with ever greater influence to this day (Figure 2.18).

More recently, *Sweet William: A Memoir of an Old Horse*, by John Hawke (1996), tells the stories of adversities that are typical of those that torment, and sometimes eventually overcome, most humans. In this, as in other, anthropomorphic books, the horse is able to assert its own good nature in the face of physical and cultural exploitation, and the sympathy evoked for the horse in such books has almost undoubtedly contributed to modern attitudes toward the horse.

Horses have historically existed on the fringes of peoples' moral concepts; as a result, some people accord horses a strong moral status, equivalent to human beings, while others deny them any kind of moral status at all. There have been philosophical discussions regarding the status of animals since the Greek philosopher Aristotle; support can be found for any side of a debate over the place of the horse from such discussions. While a full discussion of the philosophy of animals and ethics is beyond the scope of this chapter, it is indisputable that various philosophies have shaped, and are shaping, the status of the horse in the modern world. Laws exist regarding animal cruelty; no longer can people treat their horses in any manner of their choosing. Philosophical leanings have influenced the passage of laws banning the slaughter of horses in the USA; the 'wild mustang' of the western USA is protected by government legislation, as well. While perhaps wellintended, it remains to be seen if these laws will ultimately benefit horses, as the unwanted horse becomes a problem of increasing concern.

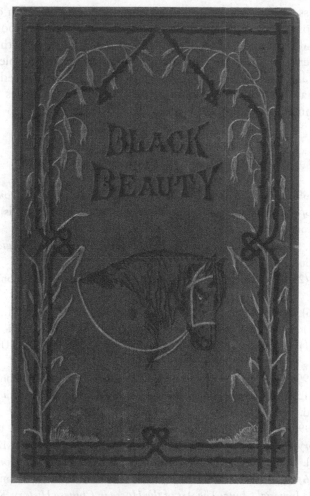

Figure 2.18 The cover of the first edition, 1877, of *Black Beauty*, by Anna Sewell. (Wikimedia Commons.)

2.11 Conclusion

Bless the hoss from hoof to head,
From head to hoof, and tale to mane!
I bless the hoss, as I have said,
From head to hoof, and back again!

James Whitcomb Riley

The history of human–horse interactions has been diverse, complex, long, and mutually beneficial. People likely saved the horse; in turn, horses served man.

For their selfless service, horses were given command of the realm of the mystic. Physically imposing and graceful, they seemed divine. As people look back to the past for spiritual roots and a sense of identity in the modern world, the horse seems again to be a perfect vehicle. It seems that there will always be people who identify with the spirit and power of horses, and see in them a sense of freedom, strength, and nobility that they may not feel in themselves. What that means for the future of horses and humans remains to be seen.

References

Allchin, F.R. (1969) Early domestic animals in India and Pakistan. In *The Domestication and Exploitation of Plants and Animals*, Ucko, P.J. and Dimbleby, G.W. (eds), pp. 317–322. Duckworth, London.

Amirsadeghi, H. (2005) *The Arabian Horse: History, Mystery and Magic.* Thames and Hudson, London.

Armstrong, K. (2000) *Islam: A Short History.* Modern Library/Random House, New York.

Baskett, J. (2006) *The Horse in Art.* Yale University Press, New Haven, CT.

Bloch, M. (1961) *Feudal Society.* University of Chicago Press, Chicago, IL.

Bryant, E. (2001) *The Quest for the Origins of Vedic Culture.* Oxford University Press, Oxford.

Budiansky, S. (1997) *The Nature of Horses.* Weidenfeld and Nicholson, London.

Chamberlain, J.E. (2006) *Horse: How the Horse has Shaped Civilization*, p. 80. Signal Books, Oxford.

Christian, D. (1998) *A History of Russia, Central Asia, and Mongolia*, vol. 1: *Inner Eurasia from Prehistory to the Mongol Empire.* Blackwell Publishing, Malden, MA.

Clutton-Brock, J. (1992) *Horse Power: A History of the Horse and the Donkey in Human Societies*, p. 66, Fig. 4.13. Natural History Museum Publications, London.

Cooke, B. (2001) *Imperial China: The Art of the Horse in Chinese History.* Kentucky Horse Park/Harmony House Publishers. See: http://www.ket.org/artofthehorse/ed/.

Denhardt, R. (1991) *Quarter Horses: A Story of Two Centuries.* University of Oklahoma Press, Stillwater, OK.

Denison, G. (1913) *A History of Cavalry from the Earliest Times: With Lessons for the Future.* Macmillan, London.

Drews, R. (2004) *Early Riders: The Beginnings of Mounted Warfare in Asia and Europe.* Routledge, New York.

Ebrey, P.B. (1999) *The Cambridge Illustrated History of China.* Cambridge University Press, Cambridge.

Edwards, P. (2007) *Horse and Man in Early Modern England.* Hambleton Continuum, London.

Gabriel, R.A. (1990) *The Culture of War: Invention and Early Development.* Greenwood Press, Westport, CT.

Gade, D.W. (1976) Horsemeat as human food in France. *Ecology of Food and Nutrition* 5, 1–11.

Hobbes, T. (1660) *The Leviathan.*

Hoberman, B. (1982) The Battle of Talas. *Saudi/Aramco World* 26–31. See: http://www.saudiaramcoworld.com/issue/198205/the.battle.of.talas.htm.

Hyland, A. (1990) *Equus: The Horse in the Roman World.* Batsford, London.

Kenrick, V. (1964) *Horses in Japan.* J. Allen and Co., London.

Lewin, R. (2005) Art in prehistory. In *Human Evolution: An Introduction*, 5th edn, pp. 229–236. Blackwell Publishing, Malden, MA.

Lewis, M.J.T. (1970) *Early Wooden Railways.* Routledge and Kegan Paul, London.

Littauer, M.A. and Crouwel, J.H. (1996) The origin of the true chariot. *Antiquity* 934–939.

Littauer, M.A. and Crouwel, J.H. (2002) In *Selected Writings on Chariots, Other Early Vehicles, Riding, and Harnesses*, Raulwing, P. (ed.). Brill Publishing, Leiden.

Mackay-Smith, A. (2000) *Speed and the Thoroughbred: The Complete History.* Derrydale Press, New York.

Mallory, J.P. (1997) Yamna culture. In *Encyclopedia of Indo-European Culture.* Fitzroy Dearborn, London.

Maugh, T.H. (2009) Horses were tamed a millennium earlier than previously thought. *Los Angeles Times*, March 6, 2009. Available at: http://www.latimes.com/technology/la-sci-horses6-2009mar06,0,879584.story.

McCall, J.B. (2002) *The Cavalry of the Roman Republic: Cavalry Combat and Elite Reputations in the Middle and Late Republic.* Routledge. New York.

Naylor, J.M. and Bell, R. (1985) Raising the orphan foal. *Veterinary Clinics of North America: Equine Practice* 1(1), 169–178.

Piggott, S. (1992) *Wagon, Chariot and Carriage.* Thames and Hudson, London.

Renfrew, C. (1987) *Archaeology and Language: the Puzzle of Indo-European Origins.* Jonathan Cape, London.

Roberts, M. (1979) *Chinese Fairy Tales and Fantasies.* Pantheon Books, New York.

Rudenko, S.I. (1970) *Frozen Tombs of Siberia: the Pazyryk Burials of Iron Age Horsemen*, Thompson, M.W. (transl.). Dent, London.

Science (2008) Trail of mare's milk leads to first tamed horses. *Science* 332, 368.

Science Daily (2006) New evidence of early horse domestication. Science News. *Science Daily.* Available at: http://www.sciencedaily.com/releases/2006/10/061023192518.htm.

Smith, P. (1991) *Taxing Heaven's Storehouse: Horses, Bureaucrats, and the Destruction of the Sichuan Tea Industry, 1074–1224.* Harvard University Press, Cambridge, MA.

Sponenberg, D.P. (1992) The colonial Spanish horse in the USA: history and current status. *Archivos de Zootecnia* 41(154/extra), 335–348.

Stiff, A.R., Capo, R.C., Gardiner, J.B. *et al.* (2006) Geochemical evidence of possible horse domestication at the Copper Age Botai Settlement of Krasnyi Yar, Kazakhstan. In *Proceedings of the Geological Society of America*, Philadelphia, PA, 2006. Available at: http://gsa.confex.com/gsa/2006AM/finalprogram/abstract_116407.htm.

Waterson, J. (2007) *The Knights of Islam: The Wars of the Mamluks.* Greenhill Books, London.

Webb, S.D. and Hemmings, C.A. (2006) Last horses and first humans in North America. In *Horse and Humans: The Evolution of Human–Equine Relationships*, Olsen, S.L., Grant, S., Choke, A.M. *et al.* (eds), pp. 11–23. Archaeopress, Oxford.

Weed, W.S. (2002) First to ride. *Discover Magazine*, online March 1, 2002. Available at: http://discovermagazine.com/2002/mar/featride.

Weinstock, J., Willerslev, E., Sher, A. *et al.* (2005) Evolution, systematics, and phylogeography of Pleistocene horses in the New World: a molecular perspective. *PLoS Biology* 3(8), e241.

Equine Health and Disease – General Welfare Aspects

3

D. Paul Lunn and C. Wayne McIlwraith

3.1 Introduction

Horse owners or caretakers have a moral, and in some countries a legal, obligation to ensure that the welfare needs of horses are met. In the context of equine health, this means protecting the horse from pain, suffering, injury, and disease. There are any number of components to this responsibility. Protection can best be accomplished by prevention of the occurrence of disease. However, given that no preventive measures are foolproof, protection also requires employing strategies to detect the occurrence of disease in individual horses and populations. When signs of disease are detected, appropriate care will include diagnosis of the disease, followed by treatment and appropriate recuperation. Importantly, for many conditions, and particularly for musculoskeletal injury, or life-threatening diseases such as colic, proper care of the horse demands timely and effective provision of emergency care.

Prevention of the occurrence of injury is less predictable than preventing the occurrence of disease. Different equine athletic activities are associated with different risk of injury and the specifics of those injuries vary. While many injuries are accidents, our concern for the welfare of the horse suggests that attention should be paid to any diseases that might predispose to injury and to early diagnosis of microdamage that can lead to severe (and sometimes catastrophic) injuries. Practices or 'traditions' particular to an individual sport that inflict pain on the horse or place the horse at risk are unacceptable. Specific issues as well as ethics related to individual activities will be documented in the various chapters about those disciplines.

Standards of care in terms of protection from disease may vary significantly for different equine populations, and in different human societies and cultures. Typically, we consider that the responsibility for prevention of disease rests with

---

Equine Welfare, First Edition. Edited by C. Wayne McIlwraith and Bernard E. Rollin.
© 2011 by UFAW. Published 2011 by Blackwell Publishing Ltd.

the owner or caretaker of the horse. However, if the owner ignores or fails to fulfill their responsibility, then society has the responsibility to intervene for the welfare of the horse. Determination of what the standard of care may be is frequently accomplished through legislation. When the horses in question have no owner, as is the case for feral horse populations, then society alone bears responsibility for the welfare of these animals, particularly if society has contributed to the problem (including allowing horses to become feral). Typically, acceptable standards for equine health in feral horse populations may be very different from acceptable standards for privately owned and managed horses. In their natural state, feral horses are subject, for example, to a greater risk of predation, parasitism, and injury than would be acceptable in privately owned horses. Nevertheless, civilized society should and must intervene in the best interests of these animals when health problems develop that are outside the typical range of circumstances affecting these animals. More specifics on feral horses are provided in a separate chapter (see Chapter 24).

Determining acceptable standards for protection of horses from disease is inherently subjective, given the wide range of equine health-care standards practiced by different human societies. The establishment of Codes of Practice for equine health care, which is typically done on a national level, can address this.

3.2 Codes of Practice

In the United Kingdom, the Animal Welfare Act 2006 led to the issuing of a Code of Practice for Welfare of Equines in November, 2008 (www.defra.gov.uk). This document addressed the impact of health on equine welfare, and identified a series of responsibilities for horse owners, which included the need to be able to recognize signs indicating the presence of illness (changes in appetite, droppings, behavior, body condition, or signs of pain), a responsibility to respond appropriately through determining the cause of illness, and offering a treatment, typically achieved through veterinary consultation. Horse owners also have a responsibility to provide routine health care, including parasite control programs, dental and hoof care, and prevention of infectious and contagious disease through hygiene, isolation procedures, and vaccination. Additional health-care responsibilities relate to the use of saddlery and harness, and safety and care during transport. Special responsibilities relating to geriatric or ill horses include consideration of humane euthanasia to avoid unnecessary pain and distress.

Another British organization, the National Equine Welfare Council (NEWC), which is an association of several equine welfare organizations, published the Equine Industry Welfare Guidelines Compendium for Horses, Ponies and Donkeys (second edition) in 2005 (see http://www.newc.co.uk/codes/industry.php), and this provides some additional guidance on appropriate health care in order to maintain equine welfare.

As has been pointed out by Rollin in his introductory chapter (see Chapter 1), the last two decades have witnessed 50–60 bills relating to animal welfare annually being presented to the US Congress. The American Association of Equine Practitioners (AAEP) Mission Statement is: 'To improve the health and welfare of the horse, to further the professional development of its members, and to provide resources and leadership for the benefit of the equine industry' (AAEP, 2009a). All decisions made within this 10 000 member organization have the focus of the health and welfare of the horse in its decision-making.

The AAEP also uses the American Veterinary Medical Association (AVMA) Animal Welfare Principles (AVMA, 2006). The AVMA is a medical authority for the health and welfare of animals, and it offers eight integrative principles for developing and evaluating animal welfare policies, resolutions, and actions:

(1) The responsible use of animals for human purposes such as companionship, food, fiber, recreation, work, education, exhibition, and research conducted for both the benefit of humans and animals is consistent with the Veterinarians' Oath.
(2) Decisions regarding the animal care, use, and welfare shall be made by balancing scientific knowledge and professional judgment with consideration of ethical and societal values.
(3) Animals must be provided with water, food, proper handling, health care, and an environment appropriate for their care and use, with thoughtful consideration for their species-typical biology and behavior.
(4) Animals should be cared for in ways that minimize fear, pain, stress, and suffering.
(5) Procedures related to animal housing, management, care, and use should be continually evaluated, when indicated, refined or replaced.
(6) Conservation and management of the animal population should be humane, socially responsible, and scientifically prudent.
(7) Animals shall be treated with respect and dignity throughout their lives and, when necessary, provided a humane death.
(8) The veterinary profession shall continually strive to improve animal health and welfare through scientific research, education, collaboration, advocacy, and the development of legislation and regulations.

The AAEP also adopts the AVMA's Guidelines on Animal Abuse and Animal Neglect (2002), Animals used in Entertainment, Shows and Exhibition (2007), and Policy on the Humane Transport of Equines (2008). The AAEP also has additional Position Statements on the Stewardship of the Horse (2002), Management of Mares Utilized in the Pregnant Mare Urine (PMU) Collection Industry (1996), the Use of Horses in Urban Environments (2003), the Use of Vesicants (2003), the Practice of Soaring (2002), the Practice of Tail Docking (2003), and Thermocautery (or Pin Firing) (2006) (AAEP, 2009b).

3.3 Monitoring Health and Detecting Disease

Horse owners and caretakers have a responsibility for appropriate monitoring of horses in their charge for signs of illness. Typically, this monitoring should occur at least once daily in horses turned out at pasture, and twice daily for stabled horses, or horses in late pregnancy. It is proposed in the NEWC Guidelines that semi-feral horses, grazed in natural habitats, should be monitored at least once a week. This monitoring must be done by someone capable of identifying signs of disease, such as changes in body or hoof condition, changes in behavior, appetite, droppings, the presence of an injury, other more specific disease signs, and particularly signs of pain. With regards to signs of equine pain, a good source of reference is the International Veterinary Academy of Pain Management website (www.ivapm.org). Recognition and management of pain will also be discussed in detail in Chapter 7. Because of the frequently violent equine response to pain, such as in the case of colic pain, it is vital to address pain management quickly and effectively in order to limit further injury.

Monitoring will require adequate opportunity for proper observation of each horse, which may require individual restraint and handling. Clearly, in populations such as feral horses, opportunities for observation may be limited. There are alternative strategies available for a more global observation of signs of disease. For example, the strategies of syndromic surveillance can be powerfully applied to large horse populations on a regional or national basis. On a national basis, many governments of countries with significant equine populations and industries practice health monitoring, as is in the case in the USA through the National Animal Health Monitoring Service (www.aphis.usda.gov).

Clinical disease, by definition, results in detectable signs. Subclinical, or occult, disease results in no detectable signs, but may still have significant health and welfare implications for horses. Examples include the subclinical spread of equine parasite infection in groups of juvenile horses. For these reasons, physical observation alone does not provide adequate opportunity for detection of disease before significant equine suffering and morbidity result, as with parasitism, and certain infectious and contagious diseases. For these reasons, acceptable welfare standards may often require periodic examination of fecal samples for internal parasites, and serological or microbial isolation techniques to identify, and control the occurrence and spread of, infectious disease. In the USA, a good example is the legal requirement for periodic testing for the presence of antibodies to equine infectious anemia virus. Monitoring of lameness conditions will be discussed separately below.

3.4 Treatment of Disease

Detection of the occurrence of disease brings a responsibility for appropriate specific diagnosis and treatment. Standard veterinary texts detail appropriate diagnostic and therapeutic strategies. It is important to recognize that the value of individual horses may significantly affect which treatments are feasible. Just because a preferred therapy may not be financially practical, does not render treatment impossible in most instances, or excuse the horse owner or caregiver from the responsibility to mitigate the effects of disease. Similarly, incurable disease can still be made tolerable, for example, through use of analgesics in the case of chronic lameness.

A critical component of therapy is provision of adequate circumstances and time for recuperation. In working horses, financial pressures and the pressures of competition can limit this essential component of treatment unless the veterinary advice is carefully followed.

3.5 Disease, Work and Welfare

When disease cannot be eliminated by treatment, a chronic disease state results. This can be mitigated by changes in management and long-term therapy, such as is the case when non-steroidal anti-inflammatory drugs (NSAIDs) are administered for lameness. The decision as to whether to continue to treat chronic disease, or to consider euthanasia, is made after considering the degree to which suffering can be alleviated in the horse. Veterinary advice is critical to this decision-making process, as are issues such as the cost of continued care, and the ability of the horse to complete any work that may be an essential part of its value. The question of whether horses should continue to be used in work when disease cannot be eliminated, and may progress because of the work, is complex and ultimately depends on subjective judgment.

When it is clear that continuing in work will lead to deterioration in the horse's condition, or unreasonable pain and suffering, then clearly the work must end. This can be a vexing issue in performance horses, where use of medication to allow for continued performance in competition is a highly controversial area. There may be circumstances when treatment and continued competition are consistent with the welfare of the horse. For example, mitigation of joint inflammation by intermittent treatment, to allow competition if it does not ultimately accelerate the further progression of the disease, may be acceptable. However, it can also be argued that, in competition, horses should be judged solely on their ability as an athlete to perform. Other competitors expect to compete with the horse, not the combination of the horse and medication. This is not necessarily a welfare issue, and such decisions should be made by appropriate regulatory authorities with oversight of the competition in question. The welfare implications of horses suffering from disease continuing to be involved in competition through the use of medications must focus solely on the well-being of the equine athlete.

3.6 Euthanasia

Euthanasia is a necessary and appropriate component of managing horses that are entrusted to our care. Horse owners and caretakers, and veterinarians, share the important responsibility for making decisions with regard to euthanasia of horses that are suffering from untreatable disease, or have reached the end of their useful lives through reason of age, or lack of resources for their care. In some circumstances, the decision to euthanize a horse is simple and driven by a catastrophic disease or injury. In the case of chronic disease, the decision may be complex and emotionally devastating for the horse owner. Consultation with veterinarians can ease this burden, as can counseling for the decision-maker (Lagoni *et al.*, 1994). When euthanasia has been elected, a variety of methods exist for carrying it out, and they are discussed in Chapter 8. The critical factors in selecting a euthanasia method are clearly to minimize suffering in the horse, and assure the safety of the individuals carrying out the procedure.

3.7 Preventive Health Programs

A wide variety of preventive health programs can be designed for horses. The sophistication of these programs will depend upon the complexity of the health threat the horse faces, and the resources of the caregivers in charge of management of the horse. Generally, preventive health programs focus on parasite control, vaccination, dental care, and foot care. The primary source of information for horse owners and caretakers in designing preventive health programs must be veterinarians. However, horse owners are bombarded with advertisements and numerous other sources of information promoting individual products, such as wormers and vaccines. Similarly, a variety of laypersons offer services such as dental care. The role of the veterinarian is central to making evidenced-based decisions about preventive health programs. Nevertheless, it should be acknowledged that there is an important and valuable role for non-veterinarians when appropriately regulated. Increasingly, farriers and equine dentists are regulated by governmentally recognized associations and work effectively in collaboration with veterinarians.

Parasite control is essential for almost all horses managed under typical agricultural circumstances. Grazing management can significantly impact the prevalence of internal parasites, but anthelmintic treatment is typically essential to manage this form of parasitism effectively. Many factors influence the design of parasite control programs, and standard veterinary texts provide primary resources for this material.

Vaccination is a vitally important strategy for control of infectious and contagious disease. While standard veterinary texts are a valuable source of information for design of vaccination programs, the rapid evolution of available products, and disease behaviors, has led to the use of web-based resources for provision of the most contemporary guidelines, such as those produced in 2007 by the American Association of Equine Practitioners (www.aaep.org).

An annual dental examination should be performed in all healthy horses. Generally, only veterinary surgeons should conduct the evaluation and any required treatment. However, in some jurisdictions, appropriately qualified equine dentists may provide some of the necessary services in collaboration with veterinarians. Foot care requires that hooves be trimmed as often as is necessary to maintain the health of the foot. Depending on the condition of the horse, this can be as frequently as every month, or as infrequently as every 3–6 months. For horses that are shod, foot care will be required every 4–8 weeks.

3.8 Infectious and Contagious Disease

Infectious and contagious diseases represent perhaps the greatest threat to animal health, and the horse is as subject to this concern as is any species. A vital component of equine welfare is paying adequate attention to hygiene and isolation protocols that limit the risk of spread of infectious and contagious microbial disease. Extensive guidelines on this subject were provided by the American Association of Equine Practitioners in 2006 (www.aaep.org). In addition to following best practices, horse owners, caretakers, and veterinarians must also be compliant with governmental regulation. This is of particular importance in regards to movement of forces within and between countries.

3.9 Lameness as a Welfare Issue

There are two broad areas where lameness can potentially be a significant welfare issue: (1) minimum standards of care for the non-athletic horse; and (2) management of lameness in the athletic horse.

As mentioned previously, there are a series of responsibilities for horse owners that have been addressed, and these include recognition of the presence of lameness as well as basic foot care to prevent the development of certain conditions. Under section 3.3 on health and monitoring disease, it was stated that horses should be monitored at least once daily when in pasture and twice daily when stabled; this monitoring should involve assessment of lameness. Lameness at the walk needs to have immediate veterinary assessment. Laminitis is as much an emergency as acute abdominal symptoms, and veterinary expertise is required for assessment of this stage of this disease and recommendations for treatment. Non-weight-bearing is typically associated with fracture but can also be associated with an infected synovial structure. While it is the owner's prerogative to choose treatment options (which may include euthanasia), daily monitoring of the horse for problems and consultation with a veterinarian in obvious cases of lameness is not optional. As discussed previously with disease prevention, there are a number of preventive measures, including regular trimming to prevent overgrowth of hooves and development of obvious disparity in foot balance, and cleaning out the feet to prevent thrush, particularly when horses are confined. Nutritional maintenance, particularly in ponies and older horses, is important to lessen the chances of laminitis.

Horses that are competing athletically typically have closer attention paid with regard to lameness and the various musculoskeletal disorders that lead to lameness. Because of training and competition, lameness conditions are usually recognized at an earlier stage, particularly when there is an astute horseman training or owning the horse. Poor performance is often the first sign of a lameness condition. On the other hand, issues of 'selective vision' also occur when important competitions are occurring. The welfare of the athletic horse is predicated on a good working relationship between trainer and veterinarian. In addition to clinical examination, improvements in imaging – particularly with digital radiographs, ultrasonography, and nuclear scintigraphy – have greatly enhanced diagnostic capabilities and recognition of subtle problems. There is much information on advances in diagnosis and treatment available (McIlwraith, 2005a). Certainly there is individual variation in favorite treatments by clinicians, but the standard of treatment is generally high.

A more controversial issue is the use of medication during competition or in close proximity to it, and the issues of the beneficial and potentially harmful effects of anti-inflammatory and analgesic drugs allowed in competition when there is tissue fragility or risk of more severe injury. This will be discussed separately below.

3.10 Prevention of Injury and Early Diagnosis

As mentioned before, there are a number of means of prevention of disease, such as vaccination. However, there is no prophylaxis for musculoskeletal injury in the horse. It is known that most fractures in athletic horses are pathologic fractures (occurring in previously diseased bone) and a key to prevention of many injuries is early detection of the microdamage in the subchondral bone that leads to these problems (Kawcak et al., 2000, 2001; Norrdin et al., 1998). The need for more aggressive research regarding early diagnosis of pre-fracture disease, as well as the roles of track surface, medication, and conformation, have been highlighted after the tragedy of Eight Belles in the Kentucky Derby in 2008.

The Eight Belles tragedy led to a Congressional Subcommittee Hearing on the welfare of the racehorse. Unfortunately, this hearing focused on two main aspects: (1) the lack of national regulations in racing; and (2) the overuse of medication by equine veterinarians – when there are certainly other issues involved if we are attempting to decrease musculoskeletal injury in the racehorse. It has, however, led to the formation of a number of committees, taskforces, and national organizations, and if meaningful changes happen (and, more importantly, are mandated), there will be considerable benefit to the welfare of the racehorse. Of particular relevance to this chapter was the formation of a Racing Task Force by the American Association of Equine Practitioners, which resulted in a White Paper with veterinary recommendations for the safety and welfare of the Thoroughbred racehorse (AAEP, 2009a). The essential elements were: (1) the adoption of uniform rules on medication usage, testing, security, and enforcement by all industry participants;

(2) increased funding for regulatory functions, including state-of-the-art testing and racetrack security; and (3) continued identification and implementation of procedures and strategies that will significantly reduce the injury rate of horses, such as the recent recommendations to eliminate the use of toe grabs, other than wear plates with a height no greater than 2 mm. The White Paper then made recommendations in four keys areas: (1) societal change and the public perception of horse racing; (2) the racing business model; (3) veterinarian–owner–trainer relationships; and (4) medication. Welfare issues associated with horse racing will also be discussed in a separate chapter by Arthur (Chapter 11).

Because of our knowledge that bone disease precedes fracture, considerable effort has been paid to possible means of early diagnosis. From the demonstration that catastrophic fractures in the humerus were preceded by stress fractures and callus formation (Stover *et al.*, 1992), nuclear imaging became a common procedure when vague lameness was present in racing Thoroughbreds, and has led to the prevention of catastrophic injuries, not only in the humerus, but also in the pelvis, vertebrae, femur, and tibia. Nuclear imaging is also capable of detecting early subchondral bone disease, and this subchondral bone disease can be further defined with computed tomography (CT) and magnetic resonance imaging (MRI) (Kawcak *et al.*, 2000, 2008). The problem is, if the horse is not lame, it is impractical to be routinely screening all horses for presence of this microdamage. One of the best hopes we have for significant decrease in catastrophic injury in racehorses is the validation of serum biomarkers. As just acknowledged, newer imaging modalities such as CT and MRI can pick up early microdamage in musculoskeletal tissues, but the practicality of these modalities as screening devices is an issue. Considerable work has been done in the horse with serum biomarkers and the early detection of disease (McIlwraith, 2005b; Billinghurst *et al.*, 2004; Frisbie *et al.*, 1999, 2005, 2008, 2009), and the hope for the near future is that serum biomarkers can be used as a screening device to identify a horse at risk, and then sophisticated imaging techniques used to confirm the location and extent of injury.

Other factors are involved in contributing to injury and need attention, including track surface (Peterson and McIlwraith, 2008a, b) and conformation (Anderson *et al.*, 2004). More recently, there has been work on conditioning the young musculoskeletal system to prevent injury (Rogers *et al.*, 2008).

3.11 The Ethics of the Equine Veterinarian Working with the Athletic Horse

The equine veterinarian commonly addresses ethical issues when dealing with competition horses. An important ethical equation is whether the horse can compete after treatment without further risk.

As recently pointed out in an article on ethics in human sports medicine (Bernstein *et al.*, 2004), the authors stated that, in most human medicine, several assumptions hold true: (1) the physician works exclusively on behalf of the patient; (2) the patient and doctor are assumed to share the common goal of improving the patient's health; and (3) the doctor–patient relationship is private. However, they pointed out that these assumptions may not apply in human sports medicine, where sports medicine physicians often do not work exclusively on behalf of the patient, but rather report to the team or organization that hires them. The common goal of improved health is therefore subject to skewing factors when the patient is an athlete (Bernstein *et al.*, 2004). The veterinarian working in equine sports medicine is challenged with the first two points on a regular basis. The priority is the patient and, as the equine patient cannot have a discussion with the veterinarian, the trainer and owner have to take part in the decision. It has also been pointed out in human sports medicine that conflicts of interests need to be clarified and corrected, such as, for example, an athletic trainer or team physician being answerable to the coach or the team itself rather than to the player or patient (Spindler, 2009).

In equine sports medicine, the trainer is the agent for the owner and has responsibility for all decisions. The veterinarian makes recommendations to the trainer and in most situations the recommendations are heeded. The importance of open and consistent communication between the owner, trainer, and veterinarian to develop the relationship of trust and shared philosophy is emphasized in the recent White Paper from the AAEP. The current reality of racetrack operations is that the owner is often excluded from the communication chain, and change is necessary. Many owners do not recognize that veterinary care is not given to any racehorse without the trainer's direct or implicit approval, and that their trainer is acting as their legal agent when requesting veterinary services for their horses. Owners as well as trainers need a thorough understanding of the medication and training philosophy of their trainers, and education in these aspects will help. In other equine athletic disciplines, it is equally important for transparency in medication use and understanding of risk (or lack of).

If a horse has an injury that with or without medication poses a risk if training and racing is continued, then the horse needs to be taken out of the race or out of training, as the case may be. With some conditions, the inability of the horse to compete because of the severity of it makes the situation easy. However, if there is subclinical disease or predisposing factors that are known to the veterinarian but are not obvious, the trainer needs to understand (if they don't appreciate it already) that there is risk. In the same lecture by the second author mentioned above (McIlwraith, 2005a), it was interesting that examples were given, such as that a patient with a cruciate injury cannot go back into the game whereas a more minor injury can, with or without the use of acutely placed analgesia.

The use of analgesic agents at the time of racing is illegal. On the other hand, other industries such as cutting have no drug testing. Veterinarians are obligated to recommend the withdrawal of a horse from competition if there is a lack of response to treatment and/or the horse is at risk by continuing training or competing. Much of this can be controlled in racing, but there is still controversy over how close to competition it is appropriate to give NSAIDs and intra-articular medication, and there is considerable disparity in these practices between the USA and elsewhere in the world. The problem goes beyond the control of veterinarians in that, in certain industries, medication is administered by non-veterinarians and, while not illegal, it is certainly not in the best interest of the welfare of the horse.

References

AAEP (2009a) *Putting the Horse First: Veterinary Recommendations for the Safety and Welfare of the Thoroughbred Racehorse.* American Association of Equine Practitioners. White Paper.

AAEP (2009b) *Resource Guide and Membership Directory.* American Association of Equine Practitioners, pp. 34–38.

Anderson, T.A., McIlwraith, C.W. and Douay, P. (2004) The role of conformation in musculoskeletal problems in the racing Thoroughbred. *Equine Veterinary Journal* 36, 571–575.

AVMA (2006) *Animal Welfare Principles.* The American Veterinary Medical Association.

Bernstein, J., Perlis, C. and Bartolozzi, A.R. (2004) Normative ethics in sports medicine. *Clinical Orthopaedics and Related Research* 420, 309–318.

Billinghurst, R.C., Brama, P.A.J., Van Weeran, R. and McIlwraith, C.W. (2004) Evaluation of serum concentrations of biomarkers of skeletal metabolism and results of radiography as indicators of severity of osteochondrosis in foals. *American Journal of Veterinary Research* 65, 143–150.

Frisbie, D.D., Ray, C.S., Ionescu, M., Poole, A.R., Chapman, D.L. and McIlwraith, C.W. (1999) Measurement of synovial fluid and serum concentrations of the 846 epitope of chondroitin sulfate and of carboxy propeptides of type II procollagen for diagnosis of osteochondral fragmentation in horses. *American Journal of Veterinary Research* 60, 306–309.

Frisbie, D.D., Arthur, R., Blea, J., Baker, V., Duffy, E., Billinghurst, R.C. and McIlwraith, C.W. (2005) Prospective clinical study assessing serum biomarkers for musculoskeletal disease in 2- to 3-year-old racing Thoroughbreds. In *Proceedings of the 51st Annual Convention of the AAEP*, pp. 301–302.

Frisbie, D.D., Al-Sobayil, F., Billinghurst, R.C., Kawcak, C.E. and McIlwraith, C.W. (2008) Changes in synovial fluid and serum biomarkers with exercise and early osteoarthritis in horses. *Osteoarthritis and Cartilage* 16(10), 1196–1204. doi:10.1016/j.joca. 2008.03.008.

Frisbie, D.D., Lu, Y., Kawcak, C.E., DiCarlo, E.F., Binette, F. and McIlwraith, C.W. (2009) In vivo evaluation of autologous cartilage fragment-loaded scaffolds implanted into equine articular defects and compared with autologous chondrocyte implantation. *American Journal of Sports Medicine (Supplement)*, 37(S1), 71S–80S.

Kawcak, C.E., McIlwraith, C.W., Norrdin, R.W., Park, R.D. and Steyn, P.S. (2000) Clinical effects of exercise on subchondral bone of carpal and metacarpophalangeal joints in horses. *American Journal of Veterinary Research* 61, 1252–1258.

Kawcak, C.E., McIlwraith, C.W., Norrdin, R.W., Park, R.D. and James, S.P. (2001) The role of subchondral bone in joint disease: a review. *Equine Veterinary Journal* 33, 120–126.

Kawcak, C.E., Frisbie, D.D., Werpy, N.M., Park, R.D. and McIlwraith, C.W. (2008) Effects of exercise versus experimental osteoarthritis on imaging outcomes. *Osteoarthritis and Cartilage* 16(12), 1519–1525. doi:10.1016/j.joca.2008.04.015.

Lagoni, L., Butler, C. and Hetts, S. (1994) *The Human–Animal Bond and Grief.* W.B. Saunders, Philadelphia, PA.

McIlwraith, C.W. (2005a) Frank Milne Lecture: From arthroscopy to gene therapy – 30 years of looking in joints. In *Proceedings of the 51st Annual Convention of the AAEP*, pp. 65–113.

McIlwraith, C.W. (2005b) Use of synovial and serum biomarkers in equine bone and joint disease. *Equine Veterinary Journal* 37, 473–482.

Norrdin, R.W., Kawcak, C.E., Capwell, R.A. and McIlwraith, C.W. (1998) Subchondral bone failure in an equine model of overload arthrosis. *Bone* 22, 133–139.

Peterson, M.L. and McIlwraith, C.W. (2008) The effect of major track maintenance on the mechanical properties of a dirt racetrack. *Equine Veterinary Journal* 40, 602–605.

Peterson, M.L., McIlwraith, C.W. and Reiser, R.F. (2008) System development for in-situ characterization of horse racing track surfaces. *Biosystems Engineering* 101, 260–269.

Rogers, C.W., Firth, E.C., McIlwraith, C.W., Barneveld, A., Goodship, A.E., Kawcak, C.E., Smith, R.K.W. and van Weeren, P.R. (2008) Evaluation of a new strategy to modulate skeletal development in Thoroughbred performance horses by imposing track-based exercise during growth. *Equine Veterinary Journal* 40, 111–118.

Spindler, K. (2009) Sports medicine in the elite athlete. In *Proceedings of the 36th Annual Conference of the Veterinary Orthopaedic Society*, Steamboat Springs, CO.

Stover, S.M., Johnson, B.J., Daft, B.M. *et al.* (1992) An association between complete and incomplete stress fractures of the humerus in racehorses. *Equine Veterinary Journal* 24, 260–263.

Nutritional Management of the Horse

Joe D. Pagan

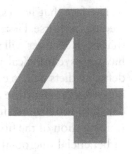

Horses have evolved over millions of years as grazers, with specialized digestive tracts adapted to digest and utilize diets containing high levels of plant fiber. They are capable of processing large quantities of forage to meet their nutrient demands. To maximize growth or productivity, many domesticated horses are fed rations that also contain grains and supplements. Striking the correct balance between forage and supplemental feed intake is the key to a successful horse feeding program.

4.1 Digestive Function of the Horse

Horses are classified anatomically as non-ruminant herbivores or hindgut fermenters. The large intestine of the horse holds about 21–24 (US) gallons (80–90 liter) of liquid and houses billions of bacteria and protozoa that produce enzymes that ferment plant fiber. Fermentation is the chemical reconfiguring of matter through microbial activity. These microbes are absolutely essential to the well-being of horses, since horses cannot produce these enzymes on their own. The by-products of this microbial fermentation provide horses with a source of energy and micronutrients.

The equine digestive tract is designed in this fashion to allow horses to ingest large quantities of forage in a continuous fashion. The small capacity of the upper part of the tract is not well suited for large single meals, a fact that is often misunderstood by horsemen. Horses typically eat small amounts for 14–20 hours each day. Large single meals of grain overwhelm the digestive capacity of the stomach and small intestine, resulting in rapid fermentation of the grain carbohydrates by the microflora in the hindgut. Such rapid-fire fermentation may result in a wide range of problems, including colic and laminitis.

Equine Welfare, First Edition. Edited by C. Wayne McIlwraith and Bernard E. Rollin.
© 2011 by UFAW. Published 2011 by Blackwell Publishing Ltd.

The fact that horses are hindgut fermenters has several implications for the person feeding the horse. First, since horses are designed to live on forages, any feeding program that neglects fiber will result in undesirable physical and mental consequences. Horses have a psychological need for the full feeling that fiber provides. Horses fed fiber-deficient diets will, in extreme cases, become chronic wood chewers capable of destroying wooden structures such as stalls and fences. It is also important to maintain a constant food source for the beneficial bacteria in the hindgut. Not only does hindgut fermentation of the fiber provide a great deal of energy for the horse, but the presence of beneficial microbials prevents the proliferation of potentially pathogenic bacteria.

Horses, like man, need a certain amount of bulk to sustain normal digestive function. As such, they have a capacious gastrointestinal system designed to process a large volume of feed at all times. Deprived of that bulk, the many loops of the gastrointestinal tract are more likely to kink or twist, resulting in colic or other abdominal disease.

4.2 Nutrients

Every horse requires the same nutrients. Life stage, however, determines which nutrients are most relevant and in what proportion they are necessary. Nutrients can be classified into six basic categories: water, protein, carbohydrates, fats, vitamins, and minerals.

4.2.1 Water

Water is the most essential nutrient, as it comprises approximately 65% of total body mass. In cool environments, horses at rest will typically drink 0.3–0.8 gallons of water per 100 pounds of body weight (25–70 ml/kg day), or 5.5–8.8 gallons (19–33 liter) of water for a 1100 pound (500 kg) horse. The amount of water needed will increase as the environmental temperature rises above 75°F (24°C). Common factors that may affect water intake include type and amount of feed and forage consumed (growing grass contains more moisture than hay), ambient temperature and humidity, physiological state, and physical activity of the horse. Sweat-inducing hard work or lactation may increase water requirements as much as 50–120% (NRC, 2007).

Horses need a constant source of fresh, clean water, and no restrictions should be placed on access to a reliable water source. The only exception to this may be immediately following intense exercise. In this instance, horses may be allowed sips of water during the cooling-out period, but unlimited or free-choice ingestion, particularly if the water is extremely cold, should not be allowed until horses are completely cooled out.

4.2.2 Protein

After water, the major constituent of the horse's body is protein. Some 80% of the horse's fat-free, moisture-free body composition is protein. Protein is the predominant component of all tissues in the body, as well as enzymes, hormones, and antibodies. Protein is a critical part of the horse's diet throughout its life (Pagan, 1998d).

Proteins are composed of 22 different amino acids. Although all of them are needed for synthesis of body protein, some can be produced in body tissues and do not need to be supplied in the feed. These are referred to as non-essential amino acids, while those that must be provided in the diet are called essential amino acids. There are 10 essential amino acids. The essential amino acid most likely to be deficient in the diets of growing horses is lysine. A great deal of research has been done on the requirement for lysine by growing horses. Studies have shown that horses fed diets deficient in lysine will grow more slowly than horses fed a diet high in lysine, even if the crude protein percentages of the diets are identical (Ott *et al.*, 1979, 1981; Ott and Kivipelto, 2002). Researchers have suggested that the second limiting amino acid for growing horses may be threonine (Graham *et al.*, 1994).

There are several sources of supplemental protein that are commonly used in horse feeds. These include milk proteins, alfalfa meal, and a number of by-product meals made from the production of oils, such as soybean meal, linseed meal, cottonseed meal, safflower meal, and sunflower meal. What is often overlooked, however, is the amount of protein and lysine that is supplied by the grain portion of a horse ration. Typically, cereal grains contribute about 40–50% of the total protein of a feed for growing horses. The amount of lysine supplied from these cereal grains, however, is only about 30–40% of the requirement, since cereal grains are fairly low in lysine. Therefore, the supplemental source of protein used in horse feeds should be of high quality. Alfalfa, milk proteins, and soybean meal are all good sources of quality protein for growing horses. Protein supplements that are deficient in lysine include linseed meal, cottonseed meal, and peanut meal (Pagan, 1998d).

Too little protein in the diet is cause for concern and may lead to sluggish growth, poor appetite, a dull hair coat, and a general unthrifty appearance. Overfeeding protein is also undesirable, especially when horses are housed indoors. A portion of the nitrogen in protein is excreted in the urine. This nitrogen, in the form of ammonia, can accumulate in poorly maintained or inadequately ventilated stalls. Ammonia fumes irritate the horse's respiratory passages, contributing to breathing problems, particularly in performance horses (Pagan, 1998d).

4.2.3 Carbohydrates

Carbohydrates are the primary source of energy in horse diets, so their importance as a nutrient cannot be underplayed. There are several different types of carbohydrates in horse feed, and how well horses digest and utilize each one varies considerably. In nutritional terms, carbohydrates can be divided into two broad categories, non-structural carbohydrates and structural carbohydrates (Pagan, 1998a).

Non-structural carbohydrates (NSCs) are those that either occur as simple sugars in the horse's feed or can be broken down by enzymes produced by the horse. Included in this category are glucose, fructose, lactose, sucrose, and starch. They range from being almost non-existent in a grass hay diet to comprising a high percentage of the total diet in a high-grain, low-fiber ration (Pagan, 1998a).

Structural carbohydrates are those that are resistant to the enzymes that populate the gastrointestinal tract. These carbohydrates occur in the cell wall portion of the plant and must be fermented by bacteria living in the hindgut before they can be utilized by horses. As a group, these carbohydrates are called plant fiber and they consist primarily of cellulose and hemicellulose (Pagan, 1998a).

4.2.4 Fats

Fats are triglycerides, which are composed of a glycerol molecule and three fatty acid molecules. They are very energy-dense, containing 2.25 times more energy than carbohydrates. Although fats are not a traditional component of horse diets, horses have the ability to digest fats efficiently. Therefore, high-fat feedstuffs such as vegetable oil and stabilized rice bran have a place in the diets of horses that have elevated energy needs. From a management perspective, fat is particularly useful when horses require large grain meals to sustain body condition. Under many circumstances, the amount of grain can be reduced if fat supplementation is started (Dunnett, 2005).

Other benefits of fats include improved energetic efficiency, diminished excitability, and metabolic adaptations that increase fat oxidation during exercise – as horses become accustomed to fats in the diet, their bodies will use them more efficiently to fuel exercise (Dunnett, 2005).

Researchers have focused their attention on two distinct families of fatty acids: the omega-3 family and the omega-6 family. The omega-3 family stems from alpha-linolenic acid (ALA), while the omega-6 family originates from linoleic acid (LA). ALA and LA are considered 'essential fatty acids' because they are instrumental in the lifecycle, yet they cannot be manufactured in the body and must be obtained from dietary sources. Significant members of the omega-3 family are eicosapentaenoic acid (EPA) and docosahexaenoic acid (DHA) (Dunnett, 2005).

Omega-6 and omega-3 fatty acids must be balanced in the body for both to be effective. Each class of fatty acid is necessary for the production and distribution of a diverse group of hormones called eicosanoids. Eicosanoids include thromboxanes, prostaglandins, and leukotrienes, which have diverse physiological effects, including inflammatory response, maintenance of cell membrane stability, development and function of central nervous system tissue, oxygen transfer, and immune functions (Dunnett, 2005).

The benefits of omega-3 fatty acids to the horse include improved sperm motility characteristics in frozen–thawed and cooled semen (Brinsko *et al.*, 2003). The improvement was attributed to an increase in the ratio of DHA to DPA (docosapentaenoic acid, an omega-6 fatty acid). Nutritionists have also demonstrated that omega-3 fatty acids benefit pregnant mares and their foals. The mares passed along the fatty acids to their foals in their milk. Researchers are also studying the effects of omega-3 fatty acids on estrous cycles and pregnancy rates of mares, with a possible connection to reproductive efficiency.

Table 4.1 Fatty acid composition of selected oils commonly used in horse diets.

	Selected fatty acids (% of total fatty acids)			
	Linoleic acid (LA)[a]	Alpha-linolenic acid (ALA)[b]	DHA and EPA[b]	Omega-3 to omega-6 ratio
Canola oil	22.1	11.1	—	Moderate
Corn oil	58.0	0.7	—	Low
Linseed oil	12.7	53.3	—	High
Safflower oil	74.1	0.4	—	Low
Soybean oil	51.0	6.8	—	Moderate
Sunflower oil	39.8	0.2	—	Low
Fish (menhaden) oil	2.0	1.5	26.4	High

[a] Omega-6 fatty acids.
[b] Omega-3 fatty acids.

Advantages of supplementing equine athletes with omega-3 fatty acids are coming to light. A reduction in joint inflammation in older arthritic horses was reported in horses supplemented with omega-3 fatty acids. Horses fed the supplement had lower synovial fluid white blood cell counts than those in the control group, indicating a lower level of inflammation (Manhart *et al.*, 2007).

Supplementation with omega-3 fatty acids has been hypothesized to reduce exercise-induced pulmonary hemorrhage (EIPH) in horses. Researchers have reported modulation of a decrease in erythrocyte membrane fluidity during exercise in horses fed a diet enriched with DHA and EPA (Portier *et al.*, 2006). Preliminary results from a study in 10 Thoroughbred horses at Kansas State University showed a reduction of EIPH after 83 and 145 days on a diet enriched with both DHA and EPA, but not with DHA alone (Erickson *et al.*, 2007).

The composition of fatty acids differs considerably in oils added to horse diets (Table 4.1). LA is greatest in safflower, corn, soybean, and sunflower oils, respectively, and is lowest in fish oil (menhaden), while linseed oil is rich in ALA. Fish oil has achieved popularity as an equine feed component, due in part to its concentration of the omega-3 fatty acids DHA and EPA.

4.2.5 Vitamins

Vitamins are complex organic compounds, present in minute amounts in natural foodstuffs, that are essential to normal metabolism. Lack of vitamins in the diet results in deficiency disease. Vitamins are a mixed group of compounds that are not similar to each other but are grouped by function, and are differentiated from trace elements by their organic nature. There are two general categories of vitamins, fat-soluble and water-soluble.

4.2.5.1 Fat-soluble vitamins

The fat-soluble vitamins are A, D, E, and K. These vitamins occur in nature in association with lipids and are absorbed with dietary fats. Conditions favorable to fat absorption would also be favorable to absorption of fat-soluble vitamins. Because of their lipid nature, fat-soluble vitamins can be stored in appreciable amounts in the body and are excreted in the feces via the bile. However, the relative ease of accumulating fat-soluble vitamins makes them more likely to cause problems in excessive amounts, particularly A and D (Crandell, 2001).

Vitamin A

Carotenes are the natural source of vitamin A for horses, since they are found in abundance in green forages. Unfortunately, much of the carotene content is destroyed by oxidation in the process of field curing. Horses are not able to absorb sufficient quantities of beta-carotene from hay to meet their requirement, except possibly from well-made early-bloom alfalfa hay (Duren and Crandell, 2001).

Vitamin D

Vitamin D is actually a hormone, and adequate sunlight results in the production of sufficient vitamin D in the skin. Hence, vitamin D is not required in the diet if sufficient amounts of sunlight are received. Adequate vitamin D must be present for calcium and phosphorus to be absorbed; a vitamin D deficiency markedly reduces absorption of both minerals (Crandell, 2001).

Vitamins E and K

Vitamin E functions as an antioxidant, protecting cell membranes from peroxidative damage. Vitamin K is necessary for blood coagulation (Crandell, 2001).

4.2.5.2 Water-soluble vitamins

Water-soluble vitamins include the B-complex vitamins and vitamin C (ascorbic acid). Because these vitamins are not soluble in fat, they are not stored to any great extent in the body. Thus, daily production or supplementation is required. These vitamins can be either synthesized in the body (vitamin C) or produced by microflora in the large intestine (B vitamins), but supplementation is probably still warranted since many performance horses consume high-grain rations that compromise fermentation in the hindgut (Crandell, 2001).

4.2.6 Minerals

Dietary minerals can be classified as either macrominerals or microminerals depending on the quantity required by the horse. Macromineral requirements are usually expressed as a percentage of the ration or in grams per day (g/day), while micromineral requirements are expressed as parts per million (mg/kg) or milligrams per day (mg/day) (Pagan, 2001).

4.2.6.1 Macrominerals

Macrominerals include calcium, phosphorus, magnesium, sulfur, sodium, chloride, and potassium. Calcium, phosphorus, and magnesium are major constituents of the skeleton. Nearly all of the body's calcium and 85% of the body's phosphorus are in bone. About 60% of the body's magnesium is in the skeleton, while 30% is contained in muscle (NRC, 2007).

Horses must not only receive adequate quantities of calcium and phosphorus in their rations, but also consume them in an appropriate ratio. High levels of phosphorus inhibit the absorption of calcium and may lead to a deficiency (Schryver et al., 1971), even if the amount of calcium is normally adequate. The calcium : phosphorus ratio in the rations of young horses should never be below 1 : 1 and ideally should be 1.5 : 1. Too much calcium may affect phosphorus absorption, particularly if the level of phosphorus is marginal, and may cause skeletal abnormalities. Calcium : phosphorus ratios greater than 2.5 : 1 should be avoided if possible. Forage diets with high calcium levels should be supplemented with phosphorus (Pagan and Nash, 2006).

Electrolytes are macrominerals that dissociate in solution into electrically charged particles called ions. In the horse, electrolytes play an important role in maintaining osmotic pressure, fluid balance, and nerve and muscle activity. During exercise, sodium (Na^+), potassium (K^+), and chloride (Cl^-) are lost in the sweat and urine. Loss of these electrolytes causes fatigue and muscle weakness, and decreases the thirst response to dehydration. Electrolytes should be supplemented in the horse's diet at levels that are adequate to replace losses in sweat (Pagan, 1998c).

4.2.6.2 Microminerals

As their name implies, microminerals are required by horses in trace amounts. The most relevant microminerals for horses are iron, manganese, selenium, iodine, copper, and zinc.

Iron

The majority of the iron in the body is contained in the red blood cells in the form of hemoglobin. Iron plays an important role in oxygen transport and cellular respiration (Schryver, 1990). Iron is the trace mineral most often associated with exercise, even though its true relevance is questionable since there are few instances when practical diets would result in iron deficiency anemia. Small amounts of iron are lost in sweat, and performance horses synthesize more hemoglobin and myoglobin than mature sedentary horses, resulting in a higher iron requirement (Pagan, 2001).

Manganese

The best-known function of manganese is its role in the formation of bone and connective tissue. Manganese is required for carbohydrate and fat metabolism, either as a coenzyme or as an activator of enzymes (NRC, 2007).

Selenium

Selenium is best known as an essential component of the selenium-dependent enzyme glutathione peroxidase, and functions as part of the cellular antioxidant defense system. Selenium, often in combination with vitamin E, serves as a defense mechanism against the ill effects of oxidation. Some forages tend to be low in selenium due to insufficient quantities of the nutrient in native soils. Inadequate levels of selenium and vitamin E in the diet may lead to muscle problems, lower conception rates in broodmares, and impaired immune function (NRC, 2007). Well-fortified feeds often contain sufficient selenium to compensate for shortfalls in the forage.

Iodine

Iodine is essential in the production of the thyroid hormones thyroxine and triiodothyronine. A deficiency or toxicity of iodine may result in goiter (Pagan, 2001).

Copper

Copper is essential for several copper-dependent enzymes involved in the synthesis and maintenance of elastic tissue and dispersal of iron stores throughout the body. Inadequate copper has been implicated as a cause of developmental orthopedic disease (DOD) (Bridges and Harris, 1988; Hurtig et al., 1993).

New Zealand researchers studied the effect of copper supplementation on the incidence of DOD in Thoroughbred foals. Pregnant Thoroughbred mares were divided into copper-supplemented and control groups. Live foals born to each group of mares were also divided into copper-supplemented and control groups. Copper supplementation of mares was associated with a significant reduction in the physitis scores of the foals at 150 days of age. Foals from mares that received no supplementation had a mean physitis score of 6, whereas foals from supplemented mares had a mean score of 3.7. A lower score means less physitis. Copper supplementation of the foals had no significant effect on physitis scores. A significantly lower incidence of articular cartilage lesions occurred in foals from supplemented mares. However, copper supplementation of the foals had no significant effect on articular and physeal cartilage lesions (Pearce et al., 1998a, b).

Zinc

Zinc is involved as a cofactor in a multitude of enzyme systems, particularly those involved in protein and carbohydrate metabolism. It is a vital nutrient for the health of eyes, skin, hair, and hooves. In conjunction with insufficient copper, deficiency of zinc might be a factor in certain cases of DOD. Reduced appetite and subsequent slow growth may result in young horses with a zinc deficiency (NRC, 2007).

4.3 Energy

While energy cannot technically be classified as a nutrient, it is one of the most important measures of a horse feed's value. Energy density determines how much feed must be supplied to meet an animal's energy requirement. Level of intake in turn dictates the concentration of all other nutrients in the feed. Therefore, horse feeds cannot be properly formulated without knowledge of their energy contents.

Digestible energy is provided by four dietary components, all of which were discussed previously: non-structural carbohydrates, fiber (structural carbohydrates), fats, and protein. Non-structural and structural carbohydrates are the primary sources of energy in horse diets. Fats are typically used to increase the energy density of a diet or to substitute for a portion of non-structural carbohydrates (from cereal grains, for example). Protein can be used as a source of energy, but it is most efficiently used for tissue accretion and repair.

4.4 Sources of Essential Nutrients

Aside from water, the basic components of horse diets include forages (as hay, pasture, or a combination of both), grains and concentrates (fortified or unfortified), and supplements.

4.4.1 Forages

Hay and pasture are the primary forage sources for horses and provide many of the nutrients required by the horse. Forages should remain the foundation of all feeding programs, regardless of where horses are raised or how they are used. Additional straight grains, fortified concentrates, or vitamin–mineral supplements should be used only to supply essential nutrients not contained in the forage. This method is the most logical and economical way to approach feeding horses because it eliminates the needless duplication or dangerous excess of fortification.

4.4.1.1 Forage composition

Horses consume forage either as fresh pasture or as cured, dry hay. The amount of each forage eaten will depend on season and availability. The nutrient composition of both types of forage will vary depending on species, stage of maturity, and season. Table 4.2 illustrates the effect that stage of maturity has on selected nutrients in various types of hay. Neutral detergent fiber (NDF) and acid detergent fiber (ADF) values are linked to forage consumption and digestibility, respectively. Generally speaking, as NDF increases, consumption decreases; and as ADF increases, digestibility decreases. These data can be used as a guide for selecting hay, but in practice it is worthwhile to have the actual hay that is being fed analyzed for the nutrient profile.

Table 4.2 Effect of maturity on the nutrient value of selected forages on a dry matter basis.

Forage/stage of maturity	Digestible energy		Crude protein (%)	Neutral detergent fiber (%)	Acid detergent fiber (%)
	(Mcal/kg)	(MJ/kg)			
Grass hay, cool season					
immature	2.36	9.88	18.0	49.6	31.4
mid-maturity	2.18	9.13	13.3	57.7	36.9
mature	2.04	8.54	10.8	69.1	41.6
Legume forage hay					
immature	2.62	10.97	20.5	36.3	28.6
mid-maturity	2.43	10.17	20.8	42.9	33.4
mature	2.21	9.25	17.8	50.9	39.5
Mixed grass and legume hay					
immature	2.46	10.30	19.7	45.4	30.8
mid-maturity	2.30	9.63	18.4	50.8	35.8
mature	2.11	8.83	18.2	56.0	40.1

Source: NRC (2007).

Hay can be classified into two general categories, legumes and grasses. The most popular legume hay fed to horses is alfalfa, but other legumes such as clover are available. When properly cured, alfalfa is the best of the legumes from a nutrient standpoint. Its high energy, protein, and calcium content make it especially useful in balancing rations for late-gestating and early-lactating broodmares and young growing horses. Many clover varieties are used alone or in combination with grass hays for horses. Red clover is similar to alfalfa and can be substituted for it, though it is lower in protein and usually has a higher ratio of stems to leaves than alfalfa.

4.4.1.2 Forage intake

To calculate accurately how forage contributes to the overall feeding program of horses, forage intake as well as composition must be known. Hay intake can be determined simply by recording the total weight of hay offered minus any hay wasted or refused. This record does not take into account the differences in composition between hay that is eaten and not eaten, but is accurate enough to do an adequate evaluation in the field. Pasture intake is more difficult to estimate. Pasture intake will vary depending on the season, species, and quality of pasture grazed, and the total amount of time horses are allowed to graze.

Distinction should be made between absolute minimum, recommended minimum, typical, and maximal forage intake. Absolute minimum forage requirement is 1% of body weight (10 pounds forage for a 1000-pound horse), though the

Table 4.3 Typical nutrient analysis of different feeds suitable for varying classes of horses.

Name of feed[a]	Phase I	Phase II	Phase III	Phase IV	Phase V	Balancer pellet
Class of horse	Foals and weanlings	Yearlings and broodmares	Performance horses	Mature, idle horses	Senior horses	All classes
DE[b] (Mcal/kg)	3.0	3.0	3.2	2.8	3.2	2.7
Fat (%)	4.5	6.0	8.0	4.0	8.0	3.1
Protein (%)	16.0	14.0	13.0	12.0	14.0	25.0
Lysine (%)	0.8	0.7	0.6	0.6	0.8	1.5
Calcium (%)	1.2	0.9	0.7	0.6	0.9	3.0
Phosphorus (%)	0.8	0.7	0.6	0.5	0.7	2.0
Magnesium (%)	0.2	0.2	0.3	0.2	0.4	0.4
Selenium (mg/kg)	0.7	0.6	0.7	0.4	0.6	2.1
Copper (mg/kg)	65.0	60.0	45.0	30.0	50.0	175.0
Zinc (mg/kg)	195.0	180.0	160.0	120.0	190.0	500.0
Vitamin A (IU/kg)	13200.0	11000.0	8800.0	6600.0	11000.0	44000.0
Vitamin D (IU/kg)	1320.0	1100.0	880.0	660.0	1100.0	4400.0
Vitamin E (IU/kg)	120.0	120.0	250.0	90.0	200.0	800.0

[a] Phase feeds formulated by Kentucky Equine Research (www.ker.com).
[b] DE = digestible energy.

recommended minimum is 1.5% of body weight. Typical forage intake is 1.8–2.2% of body weight. For most horses, maximal forage intake is 3–3.5% of body weight, though lactating mares and other horses with extreme energy needs might consume 5% of body weight daily.

4.4.2 Grains and concentrates

Cereal grains such as oats, corn, and barley are traditional feeds for horses. These grains are good sources of energy, but are typically deficient in protein, vitamins, and minerals for most classes of horse. Fortified grains or grain mixes are enriched with protein, vitamins, and minerals, with the level of fortification dependent on the class of horse for which the feed is intended (Table 4.3). Typically, fortified mixes are formulated to be fed at a level of intake between 3 and 6kg/day. A common mistake

Table 4.4 Expected daily feed consumption by horses.

Horse	Percent of body weight		Percent of diet	
	Forage	Concentrate	Forage	Concentrate
Maintenance	1.0–2.0	0–1.0	50–100	0–50
Pregnant mare	1.0–2.0	0.3–1.0	50–85	15–50
Lactating mare (early)	1.0–2.5	0.5–2.0	33–85	15–66
Lactating mare (late)	1.0–2.0	0.5–1.5	40–80	20–60
Weanling	0.5–1.8	1.0–3.0	30–65	35–70
Yearling	1.0–2.5	0.5–2.0	33–80	20–66
Performance horse	1.0–2.0	0.5–2.0	33–80	20–66

Source: Adapted from Pagan (1998b).

Table 4.5 Three classes of supplements, with examples and commentary.

Description of supplement	Example of a supplement	Commentary
Provides core nutrients such as vitamins and minerals	Balancer pellet for a grain-based diet[a]	When fed according to recommendations, this is an excellent way to properly fortify a diet that does not provide sufficient vitamins and minerals. When fed improperly, there is risk for insufficient or excessive supplementation
Provides nutritional support factors	Protected hindgut buffer[b]	Used to buffer excessive acid production in the hindgut that is often the result of large grain meals
Provides support for specific problem	Biotin[c]	Though biotin is synthesized in the intestine, certain horses with poor-quality hooves respond positively to biotin supplementation, growing healthy hooves

[a] All-Phase™, Kentucky Equine Research (www.ker.com).
[b] EquiShure™, Kentucky Equine Research (www.ker.com).
[c] Bio-Bloom™, Kentucky Equine Research (www.ker.com).

made with these types of products is to feed less than the minimum recommended level, a practice that results in vitamin and mineral deficiencies. There are more concentrated balancer-type products available which are designed to be fed at lower intakes when horses do not need the additional calories provided by a grain mix.

Complete feeds are generally composed of grains as well as hay or another forage source. These feeds are meant to be used as the complete diet for horses without additional grains, hay, or pasture. However, horses without access to at least a token amount of long-stem forage will sometimes develop habits such as wood chewing or coprophagy. Complete feeds are used when forage is unavailable or quality is poor.

Expected daily feed consumption by different classes of horses is shown in Table 4.4. Values are given for forage and concentrate as a percentage of body weight and as a percentage of diet.

4.4.3 Supplements

The use of supplements has grown tremendously over the last several years. Many supplements are relevant, even critical, to proper nutrition. Table 4.5 describes three distinct classes of supplements: substances that provide core nutrients; substances that provide nutritional support factors, though not necessarily nutrients; and substances, either nutrients or non-nutrients, that treat specific problems.

4.5 Feeding Different Classes of Horses

4.5.1 Feeding young horses

4.5.1.1 Sucklings

If the broodmare has been fed properly during late pregnancy, it is unnecessary to supplement the suckling with minerals until it reaches 90 days of age. At this time, moderate amounts of a well-fortified foal feed can be introduced and gradually increased until the suckling is consuming around one pound (0.5 kg) daily per month of age. It is critical that the suckling be accustomed to eating grain before it is weaned. If it is not, there is a very good chance that there will be a dramatic decrease in growth rate at weaning. When the weanling finally starts eating again, a compensatory growth spurt occurs that may result in developmental orthopedic disease.

4.5.1.2 Weanlings

The most critical stage of growth for preventing developmental orthopedic disease is from weaning to 12 months of age, when the skeleton is most vulnerable to disease, and nutrient intake and balance is most important. Weanlings should be grown at a moderate rate with adequate mineral supplementation. In temperate regions, the contribution of pasture is often underestimated, leading to excessive growth and developmental orthopedic disease.

The performance or growth rate of foals decreases in the period immediately following weaning. If foals have been on a solid nutritional program, the post-weaning slump (growth slump) will be minimal, as the foals will be accustomed to eating feed on their own. One of the critical aspects of feeding the weanling is to minimize the post-weaning slump. Many times the appearance of growth problems in young horses is linked to a severe growth depression followed by a period of rapid growth. If foals are being routinely weighed, handlers can record growth rate during this critical time and can head off some potential problems. The goal of feeding both the weanling and the yearling is to keep growth at an even pace, thus avoiding any significant growth slowdowns or spurts.

4.5.1.3 Yearlings
Once a horse reaches 12 months of age, it is much less likely to be affected by DOD than a younger horse. Many of the lesions that become clinically relevant after this age are typically formed at a younger age. Still, proper nutrient balance remains important for the yearling. It is best to delay the increased energy intakes that are required for show conditioning or sales prepping as long as possible because the skeleton is less vulnerable to developmental orthopedic disease as the yearling ages.

Feeding for sound growth
Orthopedic problems are often a major concern with yearlings that have been pushed for rapid growth. In the Thoroughbred industry, large, well-grown yearlings are desirable when offered for sale at public auction, since selling price is influenced by body size. Yearlings that sold higher than the median of the session in which they were sold were heavier and taller than yearlings that sold below the session median (Pagan et al., 2007). In addition, Thoroughbreds that were heavy and tall as yearlings had the most earnings, graded stakes wins, and grade-1 stakes wins (Brown-Douglas et al., 2007). Because of the premium price paid for mass, young Thoroughbreds are often grown rapidly to achieve maximal size. Excessive energy intake can lead to rapid growth and increased body fat, which may predispose young horses to developmental orthopedic disease.

A Kentucky study showed that growth rate and body size might increase the incidence of certain types of developmental orthopedic diseases in Thoroughbred foals (Pagan et al., 1996). Yearlings that showed osteochondritis dissecans (OCD) of the hock and stifle were large at birth, grew rapidly from three to eight months of age, and were heavier than the average population as weanlings.

The source of energy for young horses also may be important, because hyperglycemia or hyperinsulinemia have been implicated in the pathogenesis of OCD (Glade et al., 1984; Ralston, 1995). Foals that experience an exaggerated and sustained increase in circulating glucose or insulin in response to a carbohydrate (grain) meal may be predisposed to develop OCD (Pagan et al., 2001). In a large field trial, 218 Thoroughbred weanlings (average age 300 ± 40 days, average body weight 300 ± 43 kg) were studied (Pagan et al., 2001). A glycemic response test was conducted by feeding a meal that consisted of the weanling's normal concentrate at a level of intake equal to 1.4 g non-structural carbohydrate per kilogram of body mass. A single blood sample was taken 120 minutes after feeding to determine glucose and insulin levels. A high glucose and insulin response to a concentrate meal was associated with an increased incidence of OCD. More research is needed to determine whether the incidence of OCD can be reduced through feeding foals concentrates that produce low glycemic responses.

Feeding practices that contribute to developmental orthopedic disease

Several feeding scenarios may contribute to DOD. Once identified, most can be corrected easily through adjustments in feed type and intake. Several of the most common mistakes made in feeding young growing horses are explained. One of the most common problems of feeding young horses is excessive intake that results in accelerated growth rate or fattening. Both conditions may contribute to DOD. Unfortunately, there are no simple rules about how much grain is too much, because total intake of forage and grain determines energy consumption. Large intakes of grain are appropriate if the forage is sparse or poor quality, as often is the case in tropical environments. For example, grain intakes as high as 2–2.5% of body weight may be necessary to sustain reasonable growth in weanlings that have access to no forage other than tropical pasture. Conversely, grain intakes higher than 1% of body weight may be considered excessive when weanlings are raised on lush temperate pasture or have access to high-quality alfalfa hay.

The surest way to document excessive intake is by weighing and using condition scoring in the growing horse. Based on a body condition scoring system commonly used today (see Table 4.6), horses are scored from 1 to 9 (1 denoting extreme thinness and 9 indicating obesity). In a Kentucky study, fillies tended to have higher condition scores than colts, and the difference was greatest at four months of age (fillies 6.48; colts 6.0). These condition scores are considered moderate to fleshy according to the body condition scoring system. By 12 months of age the condition scores of the colts and fillies had dropped to 5.3 and 5.4, respectively. Both sexes increased condition score slightly from 14 to 18 months.

Managing the growth in horses becomes a balance between producing a desirable individual for a particular purpose without creating skeletal problems that will reduce a horse's subsequent athletic ability. Growing a foal too slowly results in the risk of it being too small at a particular age or never obtaining optimal mature body size. Therefore, it is widely recommended to maintain a steady growth rate by regularly weighing and measuring horses during the growth period (Pagan, 2005).

If growth rate cannot be measured, excessive intake can often be assessed by ration evaluation. For example, a six-month-old Thoroughbred weanling (250 kg body mass; 500 kg mature body mass) was being fed 4 kg/day of a 16% protein sweet feed and 2 kg of alfalfa hay, with access to high-quality fall Kentucky pasture. To support a reasonable rate of growth (0.80 kg/day), this weanling required about 17 Mcal (71 MJ) of digestible energy per day. The hay and grain intake of this foal alone would supply about 17.5 Mcal (73 MJ) of digestible energy, which is slightly above the weanling's requirement. If a reasonable level of pasture intake were included (1% body mass or 2.5 kg dry matter), this weanling would be consuming 135% of its digestible energy requirement, a level likely to cause problems.

To reduce intake, the alfalfa hay should be eliminated, if the pasture is indeed adequate. If hay were needed when the weanling was stalled, grass hay would be more appropriate. Grain intake should be reduced to a level of about 3 kg/day. At this level of grain intake, the weanling would need to consume about 3.3 kg of pasture dry matter to support a growth rate of 0.80 kg/day, and the ration would be nicely balanced.

Occasionally the concentrate offered to a growing horse is incorrectly fortified to complement the forage that is being fed. The problem occurs particularly when the forage is mostly alfalfa or clover. Most concentrates for young horses are formulated with levels of minerals and protein needed to balance grass forage.

For example, a 12-month-old yearling (315 kg body mass; 500 kg mature body mass; 0.50 kg/day average daily growth) is raised without access to pasture, and the only forage available is alfalfa hay, which is fed at a level of intake equal to 1.5% of the yearling's body mass (4.72 kg/day). At this level of forage intake, the yearling would only require about 2.5 kg of grain per day. If a typical 14% protein sweet feed that was formulated to balance grass forage were used, the ration would be inappropriate, for a number of reasons. Calcium would be 183% of the yearling's requirement, with a calcium:phosphorus ratio of 2.9:1. This would not be a problem, except that phosphorus and zinc are marginal in the ration. Because calcium may interfere with the absorption of these minerals, the yearling may be at risk of DOD from a zinc or phosphorus deficiency. The solution is to feed a concentrate that is more appropriately balanced for legume hay. For example, a 12% protein feed with 0.4% calcium, 0.9% phosphorus, and 180 ppm zinc would be more suitable.

The most common reasons for inadequate fortification are using unfortified or under-fortified grain mixes, using correctly fortified feeds at levels of intake that are below the manufacturer's recommendation, or using fortified feeds diluted with straight cereal grains. These errors in feeding can be corrected by incorporating a highly fortified grain balancer supplement.

For example, a six-month-old weanling (200 kg body mass; 400 kg mature body mass; 0.60 kg/day average daily growth) is fed 3 kg/day of a 10% protein sweet feed that is intended for adult horses. To compound matters, the weanling is also fed grass hay, with an estimated intake of 2.3 kg/day. This ration is deficient in protein, calcium, phosphorus, zinc, and copper. The foal would be prone to a rough hair coat and physitis. There are two ways to correct this problem. A properly formulated 14–16% protein grain mix with adequate mineral fortification could be used, or 1 kg of a grain balancer pellet could be substituted for 1 kg of the 10% sweet feed. This type of supplement is typically fortified with 25–30% protein, 2.5–3.0% calcium, 1.75–2.0% phosphorus, 125–175 ppm copper, and 375–475 ppm zinc. This is an extremely useful type of supplement to correct under-fortified rations.

4.5.1.4 Two-year-olds
The nutritional needs of two-year-old horses that are in training have not been thoroughly investigated. Requirements for these horses are derived largely from combining information about the nutritional needs for growth and performance.

Typically, most high-quality concentrates contain adequate protein, calcium, and phosphorus for two-year-olds since they are fed at a fairly high level of intake to supply extra energy required for exercise. If a two-year-old is a particularly easy keeper (maintains optimal body condition on little feed), then vitamin and mineral supplementation might be warranted.

4.5.2 Feeding broodmares

The nutritional requirements of a broodmare can be divided into three stages based on stage of production. The first stage begins at conception and lasts through approximately the first seven months of gestation. Barren mares and pregnant mares without sucklings by their sides fit into this category. The second stage encompasses the last trimester of pregnancy, which is from around seven months of pregnancy through foaling. The final stage is lactation, a period that lasts four to six months after foaling. The most common mistakes made in feeding broodmares are overfeeding during early pregnancy and underfeeding during lactation.

4.5.2.1 Early pregnancy

The equine fetus does not grow at a constant rate throughout the entire 11 months of pregnancy. The fetus is small during the first five months of pregnancy. Even at seven months of pregnancy, the fetus is only about 20% of its weight at birth. Because this equals less than 2% of the mare's weight, the fetus's nutrient requirements are minuscule compared with the mare's own maintenance requirements. Therefore, the mare can be fed essentially the same as if she were not pregnant. Mare owners often increase feed intake after the mare is pronounced in foal, reasoning that she is now 'eating for two.' Increased feeding is unnecessary and may lead to obesity and foaling difficulties, especially if the mare has access to high-quality pasture during early pregnancy.

4.5.2.2 Late pregnancy

The fetus begins to develop rapidly after seven months of pregnancy, and its nutrient requirements become significantly greater than the mare's maintenance requirements; therefore, adjustments should be made to the mare's diet. Digestible energy requirements increase only about 15% over early pregnancy. Protein and mineral requirements increase to a greater extent. This is because the fetal tissue being synthesized during this time is quite high in protein, calcium, and phosphorus. Trace mineral supplementation is also critical during this period because the fetus stores iron, zinc, copper, and manganese in its liver for use after it is born. The fetus has developed this nutritional strategy of storing trace minerals during pregnancy because mare's milk is quite low in these elements.

Mares in late pregnancy are often overfed energy in an attempt to supply adequate protein and minerals to the developing foal. If the pregnant mare becomes fat during late gestation, she should be switched to a feed that is more concentrated in protein and minerals so that less can be fed per day. This will restrict her energy intake while ensuring that she receives adequate quantities of other key nutrients.

4.5.2.3 Lactation

A mare's nutrient requirements increase significantly after foaling. During the first three months of lactation, mares produce milk at a rate equal to about 3% of their body weight per day. This milk is rich in energy, protein, calcium, phosphorus, and vitamins. Therefore, the mare should be fed enough grain to meet her greatly increased nutrient requirements. Mares in early lactation usually require from 10 to 14 pounds (4.5–6.5 kg) of grain per day depending on the type and quality of forage they are consuming. This grain mix should be fortified with additional nutrients to meet the lactating mare's needs. Trace mineral fortification is not extremely important for lactating mares because milk contains low levels of these nutrients and research has shown that adding more to the lactating mare's diet does not increase the trace mineral content of the milk. Calcium and phosphorus are the minerals that should be of primary concern during lactation. Grain intake should be increased gradually during the last few weeks of pregnancy so that the mare is consuming nearly the amount that she will require for milk production at the time she foals. A rapid increase in grain should be avoided at foaling because this may lead to colic or founder. Milk production begins to decline after about three months of lactation, and grain intake can be reduced to keep the mare in a desirable body condition.

4.5.2.4 Post-weaning management

The time immediately after weaning is an important one in the condition management of the mare. Because of the heavy demands placed on the mare during lactation, it may be necessary to allow the mare to rebuild energy stores. To encourage the mare to dry up (i.e., cease milk production), feed intake should be decreased for a week prior to and two weeks after weaning. If the mare is in satisfactory condition, she may be turned out on good pasture and managed as other barren or early pregnant mares. If the mare is thin, however, this is an excellent time to encourage some weight gain so that she enters the next foaling–lactation cycle with adequate energy stores.

4.5.3 Feeding performance horses

When feeding the performance horse, the primary nutritional component of concern is energy. For horses involved in moderate or intense activity, forage alone will not meet the energy requirement. Energy provided to the performance horse should be a blend of energy sources and should include non-structural carbohydrates (starch), fermentable fiber, and added fat.

Performance horses should be fed to meet the needs of the type of exercise they perform. For exercise of high intensity and short duration (Thoroughbred and Quarter Horse racing), starches and fats are the desired energy sources. Conversely, horses involved in exercise of low intensity and long duration (endurance riding) benefit most from energy sources rich in fat and fiber. Horses engaged in exercise that is of moderate intensity and moderate duration (show jumping, three-day eventing, and reining) perform optimally when given a combination of starches, fats, and fibers.

The best approach to meeting the horse's requirements is to use a well-fortified base feed rather than to top-dress cereal grains or grain mixes with vitamin–mineral supplements. For most feeding programs for the performance horse, protein is not a critical concern. If feed is adequate to meet energy requirements, then protein requirements are generally met as well. Trouble areas with respect to evaluating feeding programs for the performance horse are inadequate energy intake, inadequate intake of micronutrients, and suboptimum intake of hay or pasture.

4.5.4 Feeding geriatric horses

Though many geriatric horses, those over 20 years old, are able to maintain their body condition and health on normal maintenance rations, weight loss is not uncommon in old horses. Dental problems, parasitism, pituitary dysfunction, and chronic pain are a few problems that may hinder intake or digestion of feedstuffs.

If horses have no medical conditions other than dental abnormalities (but not a substantial number of missing teeth) or pituitary dysfunction, a concentrate specifically formulated for old horses is probably the wisest choice. Typically referred to as 'senior' feeds, these concentrates are generally supplemented with more water-soluble vitamins, calcium, and phosphorus than other feeds. They typically contain 12–16% protein and a high-quality source of fiber. Alternative energy sources such as beet pulp and oil are frequently used in these feeds.

If horses are unable to chew long-stem hay, they might be given moistened hay cubes as a source of forage. If a geriatric horse is afflicted with renal or hepatic dysfunction, a diet with a lower protein concentration and higher carbohydrate concentration should be offered. For horses with hepatic disease, beet pulp is a suitable source of fiber, though it should not be used for horses with renal disease because it is too rich in calcium. Vegetable oil can be fed to increase the caloric density of a ration for horses with renal disease, but it is not appropriate for those with hepatic dysfunction due to the risk of hyperlipidemia.

4.6 General Rules of Nutritional Management

Allow horses unlimited access to fresh, clean water at all times. A possible exception to this is following intense exertion, when water intake should be monitored closely, with horses drinking small measures periodically until body temperature returns to normal.

The diet of horses should be composed primarily of forage, either pasture or hay. Many horses stay in optimal body condition when kept on pasture full-time. When grazing is limited by space or season, horses can be given grass or legume hay, depending on life stage, to fulfill their fiber needs.

All feedstuffs given to horses should be of high quality and free from dusts, molds, and foreign debris. This is true of grains and grain mixes as well as hays. When evaluating hays, choose bales with more leaves than stems. The leaves of plants contain the most nutrients and are easier to digest than stems.

Table 4.6 Condition scoring system for horses.

Score	Description
1 Poor	Animal extremely emaciated; spinous processes, rubs, tailhead, tuber coxae, and ischii projecting prominently; bone structure of withers, shoulders, and neck easily noticeable; no fatty tissue can be felt
2 Very thin	Animal emaciated; slight fat covering over base of spinous processes; transverse processes of lumbar vertebrae feel rounded; spinous processes, ribs, tailhead, tuber coxae, and ischii prominent; withers, shoulders, and neck structure faintly discernible
3 Thin	Fat buildup about halfway on spinous processes; transverse processes cannot be felt; slight fat cover over ribs; spinous processes and ribs easily discernible; tailhead prominent, but individual vertebrae cannot be identified visually; tuber coxae appear rounded but easily discernible; tuber ischii not distinguishable; withers, shoulders, and neck accentuated
4 Moderately thin	Slight ridge along back; faint outline of the ribs discernible; tailhead prominence depends on conformation, fat can be felt around it; tuber coxae not discernible; withers, shoulders, and neck not obviously thin
5 Moderate	Back is flat (no crease or ridge); ribs not visually distinguishable but easily felt; fat around tailhead beginning to feel spongy; withers appear rounded over spinous processes; shoulders and neck blend smoothly into body
6 Moderately fleshy	May have slight crease down back; fat over ribs spongy; fat around tailhead soft; fat beginning to be deposited along the side of withers, behind shoulders, and along the sides of neck
7 Fleshy	May have crease down back; individual ribs can be felt but noticeable filling between ribs with fat; fat around tailhead soft; fat deposited along withers, behind shoulders, and along neck
8 Fat	Crease down back; difficult to feel ribs; fat around tailhead very soft; area along withers filled with fat; area behind shoulder filled with fat; noticeable thickening of the neck; fat deposited along the inner thighs
9 Extremely fat	Obvious crease down back; patchy fat appearing over ribs; bulging fat around tailhead, along withers, behind shoulders, and along neck; fat along inner thighs may rub together; flank filled with fat

Source: NRC (2007). Reproduced with permission from the National Academy Press.

Monitor body condition at regular intervals. Condition scoring is the best way to evaluate caloric adequacy of a diet. Generally, horses that do not consume sufficient calories to meet physiologic demands become thin and those that consume more calories than necessary become overweight. An accepted condition scoring system for horses is shown in Table 4.6.

While an all-forage diet might be suitable for certain horses, many will need grain meals to provide energy and nutrients for growth, work, or reproduction. Keep grain meals small by not feeding more than five pounds (2.5 kg) in one feeding (for a 1000-pound horse). Gastrointestinal disturbances may occur if more grain is fed at one time.

Feed horses on a regular schedule. If horses do not have continual access to forage, it should be offered at least two or three times daily. Depending on the total amount fed, grain can be given once a day (if five pounds or less) or split into two or three feedings.

Make dietary changes slowly, ideally over a period of seven to ten days. Start by mixing a small portion of the new feed into the old ration, gradually increasing the new feed and decreasing the old until the changeover is complete. This practice allows the microbes in the hindgut to adapt to the new feed, minimizing the chance of colic or other digestive upsets.

Disclosure

This article contains some recommendations of products sold by Kentucky Equine Research. Dr. Pagan is the President of that company.

References

Bridges, C.H. and Harris, E.D. (1988) Experimentally induced cartilaginous fractures (osteochondritis dissecans) in foals fed low-copper diets. *Journal of the American Veterinary Medical Association* 193, 215–221.

Brinsko S.P., Varner, D.D., Love, C.C., Blanchard, T.L., Day, D.C. and Wilson, M.E. (2003) Effect of feeding a DHA-enriched nutriceutical on motion characteristics of cooled and frozen–thawed stallion semen. In *Proceedings of the 49th American Association of Equine Practitioners Annual Convention*, New Orleans, LA, pp. 350–352.

Brown-Douglas, C.G., Pagan, J.D., Koch, A. and Caddel, S. (2007) The relationship between size at yearling sale, sale price and future racing performance in Kentucky Thoroughbreds. In *Proceedings of the 20th Equine Science Society Symposium*, Hunt Valley, MD, pp. 153–154.

Crandell, K. (2001) Vitamin requirements in the horse. In *Advances in Equine Nutrition II*, Pagan, J.D. and Geor, R.J. (eds), pp. 305–315. Nottingham University Press, Nottingham, UK.

Dunnett, C. (2005) Dietary lipid form and function. In *Advances in Equine Nutrition III*, Pagan, J.D. (ed.), pp. 37–54. Nottingham University Press, Nottingham, UK.

Duren, S.E. and Crandell, K. (2001) The role of vitamins in growth of horses. In *Advances in Equine Nutrition II*, Pagan, J.D. and Geor, R.J. (eds), pp. 169–177. Nottingham University Press, Nottingham, UK.

Erickson, H.H., Epp, T.S. and Poole, D.C. (2007) Review of alternative therapies for EIPH. In *Proceedings of the 53rd American Association of Equine Practitioners Annual Convention*, Orlando, FL, pp. 68–71.

Glade, M.J., Gupta, S. and Reimers, T.J. (1984) Hormonal responses to high and low planes of nutrition in weanling Thoroughbreds. *Journal of Animal Science* 59, 658.

Graham, P.M., Ott, E.A., Brendemuhl, J.H. and TenBroeck, S.H. (1994) The effect of supplemental lysine and threonine on growth and development of yearling horses. *Journal of Animal Science* 72, 380–386.

Hurtig, M., Green, S.L. Dobson, H. Mikuni-Takagaki, Y. and Choi, J. (1993) Correlative study of defective cartilage and bone growth in foals fed a low-copper diet. *Equine Veterinary Journal* 16, 66–73.

Manhart, D.R., Scott, B.D., Miller, E.M. Honnas, C.M. Hood, D.M. Cloverdale, J.A. and Gibbs, P.G. (2007) In *Proceedings of the 20th Equine Science Society Symposium*, Hunt Valley, MD, pp. 11–12.

NRC (2007) *Nutrient Requirements of Horses*, 6th rev. edn. National Research Council. National Academy Press, Washington, DC.

Ott, E.A., Asquith, R.L., Feaster, J.P. and Martin, F.G. (1979) Influence of protein level and quality on growth and development of yearling foals. *Journal of Animal Science* 49, 620–626.

Ott, E.A., Asquith, R.L. and Feaster, J.P. (1981) Lysine supplementation of diets for yearling horses. *Journal of Animal Science* 53, 1496–1503.

Ott, E.A. and Kivipelto, J. (2002) Growth and development of yearling horses fed either alfalfa or coastal bermudagrass hay and a concentrate formulated for bermudagrass hay. *Journal of Equine Veterinary Science* 22, 311–319.

Pagan, J.D. (1998a) Carbohydrates in equine nutrition. In *Advances in Equine Nutrition*, Pagan, J.D. (ed.), pp. 29–41. Nottingham University Press, Nottingham, UK.

Pagan, J.D. (1998b) Computing horse nutrition: how to properly conduct an equine nutrition evaluation. In *Advances in Equine Nutrition*, Pagan, J.D. (ed.), pp. 111–123. Nottingham University Press, Nottingham, UK.

Pagan, J.D. (1998c) Electrolytes and the performance horse. In *Advances in Equine Nutrition*, Pagan, J.D. (ed.), pp. 201–204. Nottingham University Press, Nottingham, UK.

Pagan, J.D. (1998d) Protein requirements and digestibility: a review. In *Advances in Equine Nutrition*, Pagan, J.D. (ed.), pp. 43–50. Nottingham University Press, Nottingham, UK.

Pagan, J.D. (2001) Micromineral requirements in horses. In *Advances in Equine Nutrition II*, Pagan, J.D. and Geor, R.J. (eds), pp. 317–327. Nottingham University Press, Nottingham, UK.

Pagan, J.D. (2005) Managing growth for different commercial end points. In *Advances in Equine Nutrition III*, Pagan, J.D. (ed.), pp. 319–326. Nottingham University Press, Nottingham, UK.

Pagan, J.D. and Nash, D. (2006) Managing growth to produce a sound athletic horse. In *Proceedings of the 15th Annual Kentucky Equine Research Conference*, Lexington, KY, pp. 71–81.

Pagan, J.D., Jackson, S.G. and Caddel, S. (1996) A summary of growth rates of Thoroughbreds in Kentucky. *Pferdeheilkunde* 12, 285.

Pagan, J.D., Geor, R.J., Caddel, S.E., Pryor, P.B. and Hoekstra, K.E. (2001) The relationship between glycemic response and the incidence of OCD in Thoroughbred weanlings: a field study. In *Proceedings of the 47th American Association of Equine Practitioners Annual Convention*, San Diego, CA, pp. 322–325.

Pagan, J.D., Koch, A. Caddel, S. and Nash, D. (2007) Size of Thoroughbred yearlings presented for auction at Keeneland sales affects selling price. In *Proceedings of the 19th Equine Science Society Symposium*, Tucson, AZ, pp. 234–235.

Pearce, S.G., Firth, E.C., Grace, N.D. and Fennessy, P.F. (1998a) Effect of copper supplementation on the evidence of developmental orthopaedic disease in pasture-fed New Zealand Thoroughbreds. *Equine Veterinary Journal* 30, 211–218.

Pearce, S.G., Grace, N.D., Firth, E.C., Wichtel, J.J., Holle, S.A., and Fennessy, P.F. (1998b) Effect of copper supplementation on the copper status of pasture-fed young Thoroughbreds. *Equine Veterinary Journal* 30, 204–210.

Portier, K., DeMoffarts, B., Fellman, N.J., Kirschvink, N., Motta, C., Letellierw, C., Ruelland, A., Van Erck, E., Lekeux, P. and Couder, J. (2006) The effects of dietary omega-3 and antioxidant supplementation on erythrocyte membrane fatty acid composition and fluidity in exercising horses. *Equine Veterinary Journal (Supplement)* 36, 279–284.

Ralston, S.L. (1995) Postprandial hyperglycemia/hyperinsulinemia in young horses with osteochondritis dissecans lesions. *Journal of Animal Science* 73, 184 (abstract).

Schryver, H.F. (1990) Mineral and vitamin intoxication in horses. *Veterinary Clinics of North America: Equine Practice* 6, 295–318.

Schryver, H.F., Hintz, H.F. and Craig, P.H. (1971) Phosphorus metabolism in ponies fed high phosphorus diet. *Journal of Nutrition* 101, 259–264.

Equine Psychological Needs and Quality of Life

Marthe Kiley-Worthington

5

5.1 Introduction

Veterinary science has, until very recently, concentrated on the treatment of physical diseases in horses and donkeys and (for various historical reasons concerning whether or not they have minds and can feel) largely ignored psychological ill-health. This has been the case despite the fact that, as long as equines have been involved with humans, they have clearly shown that they have emotions and feelings, and make decisions, and consequently do not always behave as the human handler would like. I am discussing both emotions and feelings, very important in mammalian lives, and which affect all cognitive world views. Emotions are generally considered to have a cognitive component (memory, predictions, etc.), whereas feelings have been separated as sensations (e.g., feeling pain or hot or cold), but feelings are often tied in with emotions. We must take both interrelated experiences into account.

It was the 'horse whisperers' who helped with psychological and behavioral problems. The first 'horse whisperer' who published was Rarey (1858), and many of his ideas have been brought back into fashion today by the modern 'natural horsemen' – Roberts, Parelli, Lyon and many others (see e.g. Roberts, 1992; Parelli, 1999). Today, with the growing development of animal welfare science, equine psychological problems are becoming of some concern to the veterinary profession. After a lifetime of research in the theory and practice of equine behavioral problems, it is becoming increasingly obvious that, provided horses' needs are fulfilled throughout their lives, and human handlers are trained appropriately, behavioral problems need not exist in the next horse generation. Thus, rather than listing the problems and their causes, it is more important to outline *how to prevent them* by pointing out what the needs of equines are, and how and why we know this, giving the equines the benefit of any remaining doubt.

Equine Welfare, First Edition. Edited by C. Wayne McIlwraith and Bernard E. Rollin.
© 2011 by UFAW. Published 2011 by Blackwell Publishing Ltd.

Although there are undesirable, often unnecessary, and sometimes cruel practices in training and riding, for the majority of modern horses, ponies, and some donkeys (excluding working donkeys), training and use is a very small part of their lives, usually less than 10–20%, albeit that this may be unpleasant and even traumatic. For 80% of their lives (often more), these animals live in their home environments. But whether or not they suffer during this time, and the effect that this is likely to have on their learning, is given little attention by those interested in training and equine welfare – see the various British Horse Society training manuals, Roberts (1992), and Parelli (1999).

The emphasis here is on whether horses suffer for much of their lives as a result of inappropriate husbandry, as well as training, which do not recognize or allow for all their needs. Can we ensure that horses under our care show no distress? Or, better, can we ensure that, from their point of view, they have a life of quality? I argue that, even given the present state of knowledge concerning equine ontology, we can outline how this can be achieved. If horses have a life of some quality, then the likelihood is that they will have fewer physical as well as psychological problems, live longer, and be more successful in their work. It will therefore make economic sense. This has been shown by the experimental Druimghigha Stud[1] over the past 20 years.

More knowledge is always needed, and nowhere is this more evident than when considering another species ontology; those interested in bettering equines' lives, whether scientists or practitioners, must therefore begin to ask questions to advance from what we already know (whether or not this is the result of scientific investigation). If we are serious about finding out anything new concerning equine needs, then folk knowledge (critically assessed practitioners' knowledge using the simplest possible explanation) is just as important as 'scientific' results. Here, we outline how this can be achieved.

5.2 The Interrelationship of the Body and the Mind

In light of neuroscientific and other physiological evidence, a belief in the existence of a separate body and mind is today considered outdated by many scientists and others. This is no place to discuss this issue; rather, I wish to point out that, even if the mind might exist independently of the body, inevitably one is formed and affected by the other, at least while they make up the physical/mental being alive on the Earth, whether man or mouse. We now know that some physical illnesses are

---

[1]The Druimghigha Stud is an experimental group of Arab and part-bred Arab horses whose behavior and welfare have been studied and monitored since 1964. They live in groups inside or outside, the stallions breed by running with the mares, contraceptives are often used, the foals are not weaned, and they begin their education with humans slowly from two weeks old. Their education is based on ideas from infant psychology. They compete up to international level. To date, 56 horses have been bred, educated, and sold, and eight individuals have competed internationally in many disciplines. See Druimghigha blog at http://eco-etho-research.blogspot.com/.

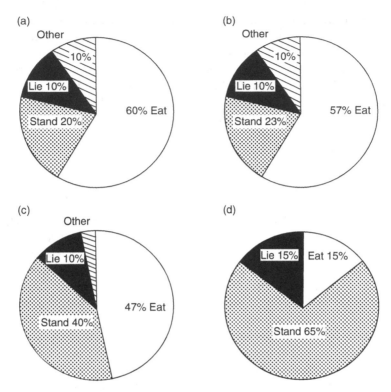

Figure 5.1 Time spent in the major activities for equines in different environments from 24 hour observations. (a) Feral horses in the Camargue, France. (b) Druimghigha experimental herd kept in mixed age and sex groups in yards. (c) Three Druimghigha horses in individual stables but able to see and touch each other and with *ad libitum* hay. (d) Stabled competitive horses kept in individual stables, able to see but not touch others, and fed rationed hay.

often the result of psychological ill-health, problems or pressures (e.g., ulcers), and that physical ill-health can give rise to psychological problems. Therefore, in order to advance our understanding of diseases and their treatment, a more careful consideration of all the various factors in a human or non-human mammal's life need to be considered. Thus, although it may be simpler to divide equines' needs into physical, social and psychological, since each is interrelated and mutually dependent, it can only be a summarized shorthand.

An example of the interrelatedness of these needs is shown by the large-scale changes in time budgets (Figure 5.1), as a result of equines being confined in isolation in single stables with rationed roughage. Although 'well nourished,' all the eating they could do was over in 4–5 hours, a third of the normal time (16–18 hours) equines spend eating when they have the opportunity, as shown by Kiley-Worthington (1987) and others since. This, coupled with monotonous, isolated, and restricted environments, results in 'boredom' or lack of environmental stimulation. To compensate, the individuals may develop ways of self-stimulation by performing behavioral abnormalities, such as pacing back and forth, eating or chewing wood, or behavioral pathologies such as stereotypes, or become aggressive or overreactive (Hutt and Hutt, 1965; Broom and Johnson, 1993; Hughes and Duncan, 1988; Kiley-Worthington and Wood-Gush, 1987).

5.2.1 Are horses needs fulfilled in modern husbandry systems?
There are many beliefs and preconceptions concerning equine psychological needs. The task is to separate the chaff from the oats, and to develop some measure to identify when we have got it wrong, because the animals are suffering for long periods of time – i.e., they are distressed. Distress is defined here as evidence for prolonged stress reflected in both physical and behavioral changes. The term is adapted from the work of Selye (1950), who pointed out that physical changes as a result of stressors are in the first place adaptive (now known as the 'general adaptive syndrome'). However, when these stressors continue for prolonged periods, their effects are detrimental to health – they are no longer adaptive, in fact they cause suffering. There is now a considerable amount of information concerning how to measure distress in many animals, including equines (Broom and Johnson, 1993; Hughes and Duncan, 1988; Kiley-Worthington, 1990, 1998b). Giving the benefit of any remaining doubt to the equines, we can summarize these indicators.

5.2.2 Indicators of distress (prolonged stress)

(1) Persistent evidence of ill-health, including wounds, poor nutrition, overgrown feet, etc.
(2) Evidence of frequent occupational diseases and/or wounds (e.g., frequent lameness as a result of jumping, rubs and wounds from harness, asotauria, laminitis, strained tendons, etc.).
(3) The need for the use of drugs (e.g., phenylbutazone, tranquillizers, other analgesics, antibiotics, corticoids, and hormones) and/or surgery (e.g., sewing up the vulva, and various fertility treatments, tracheotomy, and castration without serious consideration of the benefit to the individual) to maintain the animals in good health.
(4) Behavioral changes:
　(a) Performance of abnormal behaviors (those not normally in the species repertoire), and which appear to be of little direct benefit to the individual (e.g., pacing, box licking, rug eating, wood eating and chewing, persistent licking objects, tongue protrusion, etc.).
　(b) Stereotypes – behaviors repeatedly performed, fixed in all details, and apparently purposeless (e.g., crib biting, weaving, wind sucking, head tossing, and head nodding). The fitting of bars over the stable door to prevent weaving, for example, is admittance that the animals kept in these stables will perform stereotypes!

Table 5.1 The frequency of distress (identified as in the text), in 10 minute/horse observational periods in some top-of-the-market teaching and competing UK stable yards.

	Racing stables		Teaching stables	
	Number	**Percent**	**Number**	**Percent**
Establishments	5		12	
Horses	76		150	
Treated with drugs or surgically changed				
On phenylbutazone	5	6.5	43	28
Denervated	20	26.5	6	4
Total	25	33	49	32
Evidence for behavioral distress				
Wood chewing	79	92.0	50	33.0
Crib biting or wind sucking	6	7.8	9	6.0
Weaving or stable walking	12	15.7	10	6.6
Repeated head throwing or tossing in stable	10	13.1	20	13.3
Stable kicking	8	10.7	15	10.0
High levels of aggression	30	39.4	35	23.3
Different stable neuroses	26	34.0	47	31.3
Total	162	212.7	186	123.5

Source: from Kiley-Worthington (1990).

(c)   Substantial increases in aggression between individuals compared to feral or groups in large pastures. The normal occurrence of aggression is 0.068 per horse per hour; four times this (0.3 per horse per hour) can be considered an indicator of distress; and greater than 1.0 per horse per hour is very high.

(d)   Large differences in time budgets from the pastured or feral animals (see Figure 5.1, where there is a significant increase in time spent standing, and a decrease in lying behavior in stabled equines). Significant increases in behaviors related to frustration and conflict situations. This often includes increases in behavior in origin related to locomotion (pawing, leaping, rearing, or pacing), or skin irritation (Bindra, 1959; Andrews, 1963; Manning and Dawkins, 1998), head tossing, shaking, rubbing, scratching or licking self or an object (Kiley-Worthington, 1998b).

(e)   Ontological behavioral changes. Inability of foals to behave in ways characteristic of their age groups (e.g., foal not recognizing their mother or suckling after three days, the result of inappropriate experiences, or two-year-olds' inability to relate socially to others). Mature stallions being unable to court mares and know when to approach to avoid injury.

(f) Behavioral restrictions that are significantly greater than for feral or large pastured equines (see Table 5.3).

These simple measures of distress can be quickly performed by any trained observer, and give an indication of whether or not the way in which the equine is kept is acceptable. The results from a survey of a number of top racing, teaching, and competing yards using these measures indicated that, in these stables (which were often used as showcases of how to keep equines well), on average, every animal showed some indication of distress, and many more than one (Table 5.1).

It is safe to conclude, therefore, giving the horses the benefit of any doubt, that the behavioral needs of these animals were not being fulfilled, albeit they were being fed, watered, and brushed, and their wounds and maladies were treated. Let us then outline what the needs of equines are, as far as we know them today.

5.3 Physical Needs of the Horse

The physical needs of equines can be summarized as freedom from frequent diseases (e.g., colic and lameness) and occupational diseases (e.g., frequent use of drugs, protective clothing, or equipment to keep the animal performing). In addition, the following should be considered:

(1) Appropriate nutrition for the work done.
(2) *Ad libitum* fiber to allow them to eat for at least 16 hours per day.
(3) Clean, acceptable drinking water.
(4) Appropriate treatment for parasites, wounds, illnesses and feet.
(5) Sufficient exercise (at least 4 hours per day out of box, while able to move in all gaits).
(6) Ability to groom all parts of the body at all times.
(7) Sufficient acceptable bedding so the animals can choose to lie down in comfort when they want.
(8) Freedom from restriction for prolonged periods to areas polluted with odors, noises or other chemicals, particularly their own manure and urine.
(9) Sufficient shelter from wind, rain, snow, sun, heat, flies and other parasites that they can choose to enter.

5.4 Social Needs of the Horse

Equines are social, gregarious beings. In modern management, lack of free social contact between horses that are kept in single stables is another factor that contributes to insufficient environmental stimulation, i.e., boredom.

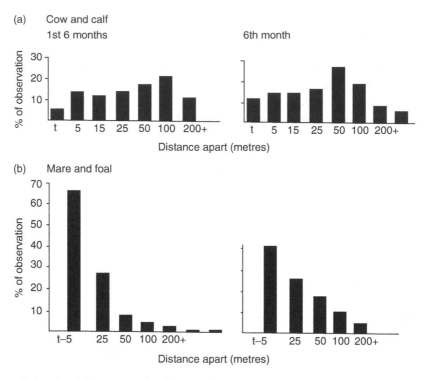

Figure 5.2 The differences in the distances apart of cows and their calves, and mares and their foals. Mares and foals are closer together for more of the time, even when the foals are six months old. Ten individual pairs of each species and total of observations over 4000 hours. Redrawn from Kiley-Worthington (1987).

There is another widespread behavioral pathology. The ability to integrate socially is, as we know from humans, the result of the individual's lifetime experiences. Although the individual may have innate tendencies to learn species-specific social behavior, whether s/he does or does not depends on having sufficient and appropriate social experiences. The lack of such an opportunity results in socially inept horses that are unable to be safely integrated into groups. The origin of this problem can often be traced back to the traumatic experience of weaning, followed by the youngsters being kept in similar aged groups, isolated from older animals who know the social rules. Indeed, sometimes (e.g., many competing yards) equines are kept isolated for the rest of their lives from any free unsupervised social intercourse with other equines.

Although many studs keep youngsters in similar aged groups, which is appropriate for humans and cattle (Reinhart, 1980), it is inappropriate for equines, because equines are a follower species, and the youngsters spend little time in peer groups, preferring association with their mothers or other older equines (Figure 5.2).

Table 5.2 Number and percentage of total behavior related to 'sticking' (group cohesion) and 'splitting' (group dispersive) behavior in a group of 13 horses of mixed age and sex recorded for over 2000 hours.

	Number	Percent
Cohesive behavior: 'sticking'		
Deflammatory (withdraw, ignore)	3625	29.79
Cohesive (approaching, show interest and affiliate behavior)	5379*	44.11
Total	9004*	73.9
Dispersive behavior: 'splitting'		
Inflammatory behavior (aggression, irritation, ears back, tail swish, kick, bite)	2213	18
Dispersive (avoidance)	900*	8
Total	3189*	26

Source: after Kiley-Worthington (1998a).
* Significant differences at $p > 0.001$, t-test.

One of the evolutionary reasons for these innate tendencies appears to be to facilitate social learning from older survivors. For centuries, social learning has been exploited by horse trainers, who use an older horse to show the youngster how to behave or work, and give them confidence in unfamiliar situations or places. In effect, equines have an innate tendency to have strong and long-lasting inter-generation contact and bonds, rather than spending much time with their peers (intra-generation bonds). Consequently, raising young horses in similar aged groups with no older individuals is likely to result in inappropriate behavior, which is the result of their particular social needs not being properly fulfilled. But from the welfare point of view, worse than this, is that many studs isolate the youngsters (particularly males kept for breeding) at weaning (at several months old). Under such conditions, they are unable to learn how to behave socially at all, and particularly stallions are often never allowed free contact with others for the rest of their lives. Such individuals (and there are many of them today) have very little or no opportunity of learning equine social rules and social contract. Many ordinary riding horses, mares and geldings, as a result of a lack of social education, behave inappropriately in social contacts, often attacking out of defensive threat (i.e., fear), and they are then branded as unable to live in a group. Indeed, because of ignorance of the importance of learning for successful social intercourse in equines, as well as humans, many believe that horses are always going to be aggressive with others, therefore at risk when in groups. In fact, affiliate behavior occurs 1.72 times more commonly than that involved with aggression or avoidance (Table 5.2).

But it is in the breeding of horses that probably today is where much of the common cruelty (that is, distress and suffering, a word used after careful consideration) occurs, and usually on some of the 'best run' studs. The techniques are even recommended in many veterinary texts (e.g., Morel and Davis, 1993)! The rationale for this statement is that the majority of top-of-the-market stud mares are consistently 'raped,' that is, mating is enforced by physical restraints. Mares are tied up with straps around their legs, often held with a twitch so they cannot escape the stallion. They also have to suffer daily internal examinations of their vulvas by veterinarians and are treated with a range of drugs. Even then, only 68% become pregnant (Rossdale, 1983)! These very widely spread breeding practices need to be severely investigated, if equine welfare is a priority, and if it is believed that equines are sentient. There is certainly evidence that equines do care about forced mating, that it matters to them – otherwise, after all, these restraints would not be necessary. The argument usually used against any change in these practices is that, if the stallion runs with mares, there would be injuries. Perhaps it is time to reflect that if such accidents and deaths were frequent during mating, how is it that equines have managed to survive and reproduce (indeed, feral equine populations often grow too rapidly)?

Of course, stallions and mares who have had no opportunity to learn how to behave socially will have a high risk of injuring each other, but this can be changed in one generation. Legislation against the forced mating (raping) of mares is surely one of the top priorities to reduce cruelty to equines today. When socially educated equines are allowed to court and cover each other freely, even with first-time covering, conception rates are much higher (Bristol, 1982). To date, in the experimental herd (Druimghigha stud, 132 coverings to date, 90% conception on first covering), there have been no severe injuries related to reproductive behavior (Kiley-Worthington, 2005).

Although, by their nature, equines are extremely adaptable and can learn to cope with a range of social environments, it is nevertheless possible to outline their fundamental social needs from studies of feral and domestic free-living populations.

(1) To have free social contact with other equines (not just one other) for at least part of each day.
(2) To have free social contact for at least part of the day with equines of different ages and sex groups.
(3) To have experience during their growing up of being able to learn social discourse and the equine social contract.
(4) To allow mares to wean their own foals, but ensure that the foals and youngsters have contact with other older equines.
(5) To ensure that future breeding stallions have acquired the necessary social knowledge to be able to safely court and copulate with mares as they and the mares choose.
(6) Ideally, to allow groups of one male with several mares and youngsters. In this case, unless all mares are expected to breed each year, some form of contraceptive must be used (e.g., for females, some suppression of ovulation; for males, vasectomy, or other male contraception not involving gross changes in physiology and personality, such as castration).

5.5 Emotions and Private Lives of the Horse

Anyone with horses is well aware that they have emotions or feelings. It is argued that all the behavior within the species' normal repertoire has a function, that is, it has evolved to aid survival in the long run. Emotions are a key player in survival and cognitive development (e.g., Evans and Cruse, 2004; and many others). Indeed, learning can only be acquired by the involvement of motivation (Dickinson, 1994), that is, some sort of feeling, e.g., pleasure or pain/fear. In addition, without fear, the equine would not show the physiological responses enabling the necessary behavioral responses, running away, for example (Selye, 1950). But other emotions, such as pleasure, aggression, attraction, hate, and frustration, also aid the survival, learning, and reproduction of all individuals. All mammals (and birds at least) 'mind' about things; they care (Dawkins, 1993).

But the problem is that emotions or feelings are private affairs. It is not possible to feel the feelings of another, even of our own species, and this has given rise to many debates concerning whether or not it possible to understand the subjectivity or ontology of a member of another species (Nagel, 1974). But, if this is the case, then it is also impossible to know what another human is feeling, yet in all our social intercourse we do have some idea of this. We do this by understanding shared experiences, and assessing what another is feeling from their behavior and expressions (Merleau-Ponty, 1962). Equines do just this – indeed, they are particularly good at reading what another is feeling from very slight changes in muscle tension, movements or expressions, as we learnt from Clever Hans (Candland, 1993). They can do this not only with their own species, but with others – humans, for example. Thus, if a human is feeling fearful, the horse may well pick up on this and react accordingly, a frightened human often resulting in a frightened horse. This is something that 'natural horse trainers' have understood and consequently they teach humans a visual language to help with their relationship with horses. We also know now (Wemelsfelder, 2008) that even naive humans who know nothing about another species interpret their feelings as a result of their behavior and agree on this.

One of the particularly attractive features of horses is that they are emotional beings, they display their emotions, and react to humans, often demonstrating that they understand our emotions. In some cases, since we are verbal beings, and use visual signals less than words, we may have more difficulty understanding their visual signals than they understand ours. Nevertheless, we can communicate our emotions to each other, which indicates that the private life of emotions and experiences is not always so private, because they are shared and can be recognized in others. Both humans and horses can make mistakes, but if we try, we can begin to understand what another is feeling much of the time (Kiley-Worthington, 2005).

To increase the quality of life of horses, we should first change their environments to better fulfill their needs if they show prolonged stress or distress (a sort of feeling). But should we ensure that they never display fear, or any of the other so-called negative emotions? The problem with emotions is that the threshold for their activation often changes, so that if the individual never experiences anything seriously uncomfortable, the threshold for 'discomfort' changes, and soon (as with the princess who feels a pea through a thick mattress) s/he feels uncomfortable (or a negative emotion) because the threshold for its activation has dropped. Thus, it is impossible to experience positive emotions such as joy or pleasure all the time. To experience positive emotions, there needs to be some sort of contrast with negative ones, or at least less joy or pleasure. Perhaps all we can say at this stage is that equines should have the possibility of experiencing a great variety of things during their lives, so that they can also experience a great variety of emotions, although not extreme or prolonged negative ones. This is the approach often adopted when bringing up children in order for them to be able to cope with life, be emotionally balanced, be able to adapt to many situations, and not to over-react to slight changes.

Experiences and feelings such as accompany motherhood and being mothered, or courtship and sex, are considered important for humans. Why, on the one hand, do we admit that horses feel (that is, are sentient) yet, on the other, disallow them from having the experiences that we value, such as courtship and sex? It may be that, since equines are not technological manipulators of the world, they feel emotions or their absence more strongly than humans. The jury is still out, but if we consider that horses feel, then we are in no position to argue rationally that certain pleasurable experiences such as courtship, sex, mothering, and being mothered are not as important to them as they are to us, whether they know this themselves or not. This means that we must carefully review whether or not we castrate males, wean foals, and disallow sex, among other things, if we are seriously interested in their welfare. Guidelines to help achieve a quality of life for horses and fulfill their emotional needs can then be drawn up.

(1) To be able to have varied experiences so that a range of emotions are felt, and the threshold of their activation does not become unduly low. For example, equines raised in very restricted environments lack experiences and become frightened and over-reactive as a result of very slight changes.
(2) An emotionally balanced equine should be able to adapt rapidly to a great variety of situations without experiencing high negative emotions, as well as having an opportunity to display a range of different emotions.

5.6 Cognitive Needs of the Horse

Since horses care about things, learn, perform voluntary acts, and acquire knowledge, they must also have 'mind needs' or cognitive needs. In order to find out the cognitive capability of equines, we can, of course, carry out experiments, but there are considerable problems with these, not the least being that negative results tell us very little, and experiments are expensive and need to be repeated to be sure the results hold.

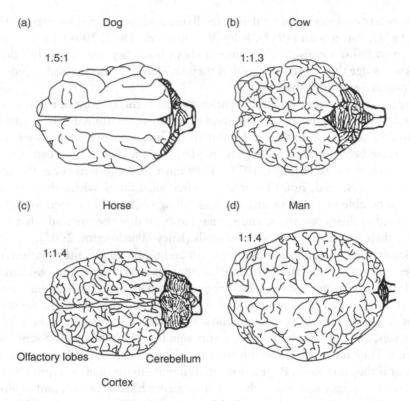

(a)   Dog   (b)   Cow

1.5:1   1:1.3

(c)   Horse   (d)   Man

1:1.4   1:1.4

Olfactory lobes   Cerebellum

Cortex

Figure 5.3 A comparison of the dorsal view of the brains of equines, dogs and humans. The numbers refer to the scale: the dog brain is enlarged 50%, the others reduced 50%. The cerebral cortex shows striking differences in convolutions between the dog and the other two. Redrawn from Kiley-Worthington (1987).

Another way of assessing the cognitive capabilities of horses is to study their brains and the lives they live and have evolved to live. If we do this, then it is clear that, in order to survive and breed, equines have evolved first of all a relatively large brain – although the relationship between size and cognitive abilities is anything but clear (see Jerison, 1973). Most importantly, the cerebral hemispheres, which control much of the voluntary behavior and decision-taking, are well developed and highly convoluted (Figure 5.3) when compared, for example, with dogs.

Little neurophysiological research has been done on the brains of equines, but there is no reason to believe that equines' brains function in an essentially different way from those of other mammals such as primates, cats or humans, who have been so studied. Until proved otherwise, we must assume that the equine brain functions fundamentally in a similar way to those of other mammals.

From behavioral studies of feral and free-living domestic horses by Berger (1977), Tyler (1972), Rubenstein (1981), Kiley-Worthington (1987, 2005) and many others, we now know a considerable amount about how they live, what they do, and what knowledge they have to acquire if they are going to survive and breed – that is, the cognitive abilities they have.

One area that has received little attention to date is the amount of environmental knowledge that an equine has to acquire. Like many other animals, they must learn what to eat, and where to find it, be able to tell one species from another, and to predict their behaviors (e.g., different predators), and when they can approach lions and when not to (Klingel, 1975). They must find and remember the way to shelter from heat, cold, sun, flies or wind. They must know where they can safely walk; and be able to avoid hazards such as falling objects. They need to find their way around in their own areas, know what has been there before and what is new, and find their way home even without trails (Kiley-Worthington 2005).

We know something about how they learn and retain all this information, using all types of learning: trial and error, instrumental, silent/cognitive, and observational/social learning. The point is that they are provided with both the hardware and the software to acquire large amounts of information, and they have the innate tendencies to use it. Exactly what they know is, however, the result of their lifetime experiences, and they make mistakes, a sure sign that the behavior is not pre-wired or innate. They must retain the information to make decisions about what, how, where, or if they do things. Populations in different environments acquire different information: equines raised in urban environments have very different ecological knowledge from feral mustangs; and mustangs have different ecological knowledge from the feral Namibian Thoroughbreds who have recently colonized the Namibian deserts. We moved our stud from a farm on mild Dartmoor, England, with rolling terrain and acid soil, to alkaline limestone mountains in La Drome, France, with cliffs, screes, precipices, deep valleys, forests, and montane grassland. On arrival, the horses ate only the few familiar species of vegetation that occurred in both areas and did not venture far. Two years on, they had acquired new ecological knowledge, and travel around the 172 hectares like mountain goats, and eat an enormous variety of different plants they had never encountered before.

Many domestic horses today have little chance of acquiring such ecological knowledge, but this does not mean that we should open all the stable doors and let them run off into the sunset. But, we must recognize that they have a mental need to acquire a great deal of knowledge, and ensure they have the facilities to do this. The belief of convenience that horses are slow learners and unable to learn to solve relatively complex problems results in a large number even of performing horses not having their cognitive needs fulfilled, and consequently showing distress. Performing in a specialized discipline, doing the same thing daily, is well known to 'sour' equines. It is in our interests, as well as theirs, to give them a great variety of things to learn and do.

As we have already mentioned, horses have also to acquire social knowledge and know the social rules. Again, they have an innate tendency to do so. Detailed work measuring many more behaviors than is usually done on the social organization of the experimental herd indicates that, in the experimental herd of equines living in a semi-wild environment, they all had different roles in the society (Gartlan, 1968) and complex personalities which we can begin to measure (Kiley-Worthington, 1998a, 2005) rather than the simplistic and metaphysical idea of 'dominance orders' (Bernstein, 1981; Moore, 1993; and many others). The predominant behavior was to help stick the group together, rather than the behaviors that tend to split the group, such as aggression and avoidance (Kiley-Worthington, 1998a; Table 5.2). This may be because, in a large grazing herbivore, there is little need to compete for resources for the majority of the time, since grazing is equally available, or not, for all. It has previously been pointed out that in some large herbivores dominance hierarchies are the result of restricted food or space resources, which are the result of the domestic environment (see above references), rather than a reflection of the species' innate social tendencies. But, whatever the details of the organization of their society, in order to live within it, each individual must have an idea of what the other is feeling to predict his or her next action and respond appropriately to stay in the group. In other words, they have to have a 'theory of mind,' that is, an awareness that others have intentions and desires (Kiley-Worthington, 2005).

Thus to provide horses with a life of quality, all these cognitive needs must be fulfilled, in some way or another.

(1) Opportunities to learn and acquire information about a whole variety of things within their world:
  (a) The local ecology, to become natural botanists, zoologists, geographers, geologists, and meteorologists: good natural ecologists.
  (b) To learn how to live in the society and how to behave toward each individual. This requires an acknowledgment of different age and sex classes, recognition of each individual in the group, and information about his/her personality and role within the society.
(2) If the animals are kept in suburban or urban-type environments:
  (a) They may have to be restricted, but specialized work such as competitive jumping, dressage, driving, racing, dancing, Western riding, showing in hand, etc., may not provide sufficient opportunities for the equine to acquire sufficient new knowledge to satisfy all his/her cognitive needs. In which case, it will be necessary to work with the equine in a variety of ways and disciplines.
  (b) To satisfy his/her social needs, which may also be restricted, work on developing and strengthening bonds between individual equines and humans can help to increase the emotional bonds and complexity required in social interactions, although relationships with humans may never completely satisfy the equines' social needs (see above).
(3) A greater variety of experiences should be provided for the equine so that s/he becomes familiar with a large range of places and situations (e.g., visiting new

and different places, towns, cities, roadways, paths, mountains, rivers, etc., on his/her own feet or being transported). Living and working with other equines and other species, including humans (e.g., long rides, drives, and camping out). Developing exercises and skills to work from the ground (such as 'join up', liberty work or lungeing, free jumping, etc.), as well as working at other competitive equine disciplines.

A measured comparison of whether some of the most common equine environments provide for these needs can be simply achieved, and can be the first step in assessing quantitatively as well as qualitatively the individual equine's welfare. First, the general welfare needs must be assessed:

(1)   absence of frequent illnesses;
(2)   long life;
(3)   lack of drug use to maintain the system; and
(4)   show no distress (as measured by the criteria given in Table 5.1).

Until we have substantiated evidence that the performance of some naturally occurring behaviors are unnecessary or even harmful for the individual, we must conclude that 'equines should be able to perform all the behaviors in their natural repertoire that they have an innate tendency to perform, provided they do not cause suffering to another (since the other also has rights).' Only in this way will it be possible to cater for the physical, social, emotional, and cognitive needs of the species. Thus, the next step is to quantify the degree of behavioral restriction that is inevitable within different common equine husbandry systems. This will give an indication of the relative degree to which the different husbandry systems fulfill equines' needs, and provide for a life of quality (Table 5.3).

Of course, the relative importance of the various behaviors in relation to the benefits to the individual must be discussed. For example, if not castrated, the colt could be kept isolated, and enclosed, and thus have a high restriction score. In such a case, for that individual, castration might be a preferable alternative.

The point of this exercise is to start responsible discussion concerning these issues, which have been remarkably absent in the animal welfare literature. As a result of lifetime experiences, different individuals may have different requirements, but, nevertheless, reduced behavioral restriction is something to be aimed at for the next generation, even though, in some places, substitution may have to be used. The Druimghigha Experimental Stud illustrates that this is possible for top competing equines. The stud has now bred seven generations that have been kept and bred in the husbandry system with the lowest restriction since 1970. They have also demonstrated that long life, lack of occupational or other diseases, and little need for drugs to maintain the system are possible for top national and international competitive equines (Kiley-Worthington, 2005; see Druimghigha blog at http://eco-etho-research.blogspot.com/).

Table 5.3 Minimum (0), maximum (5), and the possible range (e.g., 1–3) of behavioral restrictions in different common equine husbandry systems.[a] (In this table, it is assumed that the husbandry of all the animals under human jurisdiction is adequate in terms of the food they are fed, shelter provided, diseases and wounds treated, etc.)

				Type of husbandry			
Activity	Feral[b]	Large pasture[c]	Yard[d]	Small pasture[e]	Loose box (O)[f]	Loose box (I)[g]	Stalled alone[h]
Predominantly physical needs							
Sufficient exercise, move as far as s/he wants	0	0	2	2	4	4	5
Perform all gaits	0	0	1	2	4	4	5
Feed always available	1–4	0	0	0–1	0	4–5	4–5
Water always available	1–3	0	0	0	0	0	0
Liberty to go where s/he wants	0	0–1	2–3	2–3	4	4	5
Can groom all body parts	0	0	0	0	0	0	2–3
Shelter always available	2–4	0–1	0	0	0	0	0–1
Treatment of diseases, etc.	5	0	0	0	0	0	0
Social needs							
Free contact with others	0	0	0	3–5	3–5	4–5	4–5
Mixed age groups	0	0	0–5	5	5	5	5
Constant group	0–1	0–1	0–3	5	5	5	5
Courtship and sex possible	0	0–2	0–4	5	5	5	5
Mothering and being mothered	0	0	0	2–5	2–5	2–5	5
Natural weaning	0	0	0	5	0–5	0–5	5
Emotional needs							
Experience whole range of emotions	0	0	0	3–5	3–5	3–5	3–5

(continued)

Table 5.3 (Cont'd).

Activity	Feral[b]	Large pasture[c]	Yard[d]	Small pasture[e]	Loose box (O)[f]	Loose box (I)[g]	Stalled alone[h]
				Type of husbandry			
Cognitive needs							
Opportunity to learn	0	1-3	2-3	3-5	3-5	3-5	3-5
Allowed to make choices	0	0	0	2-5	2-5	2-5	2-5
Acquire ecological knowledge	0	1-3	3-5	5	5	5	5
Acquire social knowledge	0	0-2	2-3	5	5	5	5
Opportunities to solve problems	0	0-2	0-3	3-5	3-5	3-5	5
Interesting/changing environment	0	0-2	0-3	1-4	3-4	4-5	5
Total	9-12	2-17	12-35	53-70	56-76	62-80	78-88

Source: adapted from Kiley-Worthington (1990, 2005).

[a] The variations in restrictions within one group show the minimum and maximum restriction that is the result of the husbandry system itself and the constitution of the groups. The Druimghigha experimental herd has been kept in these husbandry systems – summer (large pasture, c) and winter (yard, d) – for 25 years now, with a minimum restriction score for most individuals. Breeding is controlled, and they are kept in enclosed areas, but it can be seen that it is possible to keep equines where the behavioral restrictions are as low as in many feral conditions. In other words, the 'quality of life' can be as good as, if not better than, for feral animals in terms of behavioral restrictions. It is possible to reduce further the restrictions in some of the other environments depending on the time spent out of the home environment, and the learning, training, and work performed.

[b] Wild equine populations allowed to breed at will, etc., in either unenclosed areas, or fenced within very large areas.

[c] Groups of at least five individuals kept with at least one stallion, with females and young of all ages in areas of over 10ha with shelter and fed when required.

[d] Similar sized mixed groups kept in a yard for part of the year and fed.

[e] Animals kept isolated in small pastures of maximum 1ha (a common husbandry technique for all sexes and ages), but able to see others.

[f] Outdoor looseboxes where they have access to ad libitum fiber feed and are able to see and touch adjacent neighbors.

[g] Looseboxes inside a large building with grids all around without ad libitum fiber feed, and able to see but not touch neighbors.

[h] Animals kept tied in lines for at least 8 hours per day, able to see and touch neighbors, but without ad libitum fiber food.

References

Andrews, R.J. (1963) The origin and evolution of the calls and facial expressions of the primates. *Behaviour* 20, 1–20.

Berger, J. (1977) Organizational systems and dominance in feral horses in the Grand Canyon. *Behavioral Ecology and Sociobiology* 2, 91–119.

Bernstein, I.S. (1981) Dominance: the baby and the bathwater. *Behavioral and Brain Sciences* 4, 419–429.

Bindra, D. (1959) *Motivation, a Systematic Reinterpretation*. Ronald Press, New York.

Bristol, J. (1982) Breeding behaviour of a stallion at pasture with 20 mares in synchronized oestrus. *Journal of Reproduction and Fertility (Supplement)* 32, 71–77.

Broom, D.M. and Johnson, K.G. (1993) *Stress and Animal Welfare*. Chapman & Hall, London.

Candland, D.K. (1993) *Feral Children and Clever Animal*. Oxford University Press, Oxford.

Dawkins, M.S. (1993) *Through Our Eyes Only? The Search for Animal Consciousness*. W.H. Freeman, San Francisco, CA.

Dickinson, A. (1994) Instrumental conditioning. In *Animal Learning and Cognition*, MacIntosh, N.J. (ed.). Academic Press, San Diego, CA.

Evans, D. and Cruse, P. (2004) *Emotion, Evolution and Rationality*. Oxford University Press, Oxford.

Gartlan, J.S. (1968) Structure and function in primate society. *Folia Primatalogica* 8, 89–120.

Hughes, B.O. and Duncan, I.J.N. (1988) The notion of ethological 'need'. Models of motivation and animal welfare. *Animal Behaviour* 36, 1696–1707.

Hutt, C. and Hutt, S.J. (1965) The effect of environmental complexity on stereotyped behaviour of children. *Animal Behaviour* 13, 1–4.

Jerison, M. (1973) *Evolution of Brain Size and Intelligence*. Academic Press, London.

Kiley-Worthington, M. (1987) *The Behaviour of Horses in Relation to Management and Training*. J.A. Allen, London.

Kiley-Worthington, M. (1990) *Animals in Circuses and Zoos. Chiron's World?* Little Eco Farms Publishing, Basildon, UK.

Kiley-Worthington, M. (1998a) *Cooperation or competition. A detailed study of communication and social organization in a small herd of horses (Equus caballus)*. Eco Research Centre Publ. 024.

Kiley-Worthington, M. (1998b) *Equine Welfare*. J.A. Allen, London.

Kiley-Worthington, M. (2005) *Horse Watch. What Is It to Be a Horse?* J.A. Allen, London.

Kiley-Worthington, M. and Wood-Gush, M.D. (1987) Stereotypes in horses. In *Current Therapy in Equine Medicine*, Robinson, N.E. (ed.). W.B. Saunders, London.

Klingel, H. (1975) Die soziale organization der Equiden. *Verhandlungen der Deutschen Zoologischen Gesellschaft* 71–80.

Manning, A. and Dawkins, M.S. (1998) *An Introduction to Animal Behaviour*. Cambridge University Press, Cambridge.

Merlau-Ponty, M. (1962) *The Phenomenology of Perception*. Routledge & Kegan Paul, London.

Moore, A.J. (1993) Towards an evolutionary view of social dominance. *Animal Behaviour* 46, 594–596.

Morel, M. and Davis, G.G. (1993) *Equine Reproduction Physiology, Breeding and Stud Management*. Farming Press, Ipswich, UK.

Nagel, T. (1974) What is it like to be a bat? *Philosophical Review* 83, 435–450.

Parelli, P. (1999) Natural horsemanship. In *L'Équitation, le Cheval et l'Éthologie*. L'École National d'Équitation, Saumur. Editions Belin, Paris.

Rarey, J.S. (1858) *The Modern Art of Taming Wild Horses*. Routledge, London.

Reinhart, V. (1980) Social behaviour of *Bos indicus*. In *Reviews in Rural Science IV. Behaviour in Relation to Reproduction, Management and Welfare of Farm Animals*, Wodzicka-Tomaszewska, N., Edey, T.N. and Lynch, J.J. (eds), pp. 153–156. University of New England, Armidale, NSW.

Roberts, M. (1992) *The Man Who Listens to Horses*. Hutchinson, London.

Rossdale, P.D. (1983) *The Horse from Conception to Maturity*. J.A. Allen, London.

Rubenstein, D.I. (1981) Behavioral ecology of island feral horses. *Equine Veterinary Journal* 13, 27–34.

Selye, H. (1950) *The Physiology and Pathology of Exposure to Stress*. Acta, Montreal.

Tyler, S. (1972) Behaviour and social organization of New Forest ponies. In *Animal Behaviour Monographs*, Cullen, J.M. and Beer, C.G. (eds), vol. 5, part 2, pp. 85–196. Bailliere Tindall, London.

Wemelsfelder, F. (2008) Curiosity, sentience, integrity: why recognizing the 'whole animal' matters. Wood-Gush Lecture. In *Proceedings of the International Society for Applied Ethology*, Dublin.

Spirit and Wellness in the Horse

Andrew F. Fraser[1]

6.1 Introduction

With standard husbandry, the quality of life for domestic animals usually varies from subsistence to satisfactory. Wellness, on the other hand, requires a higher level of animal care, which additionally involves preventive medicine and fundamental behavioral facility for each individual animal. Wellness is a state of holistic health. In the *Shorter Oxford English Dictionary* of 1933, the word 'wellness' was defined as 'the state of being well, or in good health.' Some of the modern management of horses has now reached that level, and shows how horse welfare can be improved to give our animals better conditions and better standards of living. The end-results of such policies are reduced suffering, improved well-being, and better physical health in the animals we own. A comprehensive state of health is therefore intended to be the ultimate outcome of humane animal care. Comprehensive health is the broad meaning of the term *wellness*. With its reference to animals, it means good

---

[1]Sections of this chapter are extracted from the author's monograph *Humane Horse Care* (Fraser, 2003) published by Canadian Farm Animal Care Trust, Barrie, Ontario.

Editors' Note
Andrew Fraser is one of the pioneers of farm animal ethology in Europe and North America, both in his scholarship and in his formation of the Society of Veterinary Ethology, and subsequently when he served as founding editor-in-chief of the *Journal of Applied Ethology*. In this contribution, Dr. Fraser draws upon his sixty years of experience with horses as clinician and ethologist to provide a striking and lyrical portrait of equine well-being, one that synthesizes material drawn from equine science with an equally valuable subjective account of spirit and wellness that will elicit instantaneous recollection from anyone who has enjoyed an empathic relationship with horses.

Equine Welfare, First Edition. Edited by C. Wayne McIlwraith and Bernard E. Rollin.
© 2011 by UFAW. Published 2011 by Blackwell Publishing Ltd.

body condition, the expression of normal behavior, signals of special health, with containment in satisfactory accommodation. In brief, the animal's body and behavior can reveal the signs of wellness, where this has been established.

In common use among human-health exponents, *wellness*, as a term, refers to good health physically and psychologically, i.e., sound in both body and mind. It denotes a comprehensive state of health. This is the meaning that is used in this text in relation to our companion horses. It is taken that the minds of these animals are reflected in their behavior. The complete picture of the animal's behavior is like an assembled jigsaw puzzle of the individual's sundry activities, its particular manner of living, and welfare (Webster, 1994).

All the modern developments in the three fields of preventive veterinary medicine, applied animal behavior, and animal welfare allow *wellness* to become a feasible target in animals. The condition can be identified in an animal when given a suitable inspection. One major proviso in animal wellness is that the subject must be treated as an individual. Since horses are usually managed individually and have their conditions and characteristic behavior well known to those who care for them continuously, they can easily become subjects of wellness. With wellness, the animal is in harmony with its circumstances, and this is the main objective in humane animal care. In their domestication, our horses have two simple goals: they live for self-maintenance and service. They are essentially good-natured (de Waal, 1996).

The term *wellness* with its concept has also been picked up recently in veterinary medicine, as a fresh objective. But perhaps it is not so new – perhaps this state of total well-being in animals was always the ultimate objective in veterinary work. The term *well-being* is often misused as a synonym for *welfare*. For this further reason, the use of the term *animal wellness* has become necessary for its distinct meaning.

The Angell Memorial's *Book of Wellness and Preventative Care for Dogs*, edited by Darlene Arden (2003), is a technical book that has an editorial team of great veterinary authority, plus seven renowned contributing editors. A detailed program for canine wellness has thus been expertly launched by the Angell Memorial Animal Hospital in Boston, Massachusetts, a world leader in modern veterinary medicine. The ice is now broken in a discipline that has long been focused on corporeal matters; the incorporeal field in animal health has now been opened. Wellness creates quality of life, and there is a wellness motive in the animal for this purpose. In health, the horse shows a determination to live and to live well. Animal wellness is a union of factors. Its components are physical health, dynamic capability, sensory satisfaction, ingestive sustenance, body comfort, and appropriate accommodation. Proper animal care establishes all of these things (Broom and Fraser, 2007).

Good-quality care for a horse can not only assure its welfare, but also establish sound health and permit full expression of natural behavior, including play (Bekoff and Byers, 1998). The combination of these two properties forms a constitution of wellness in a horse. With a state of wellness established in a horse, it may not remain permanently, like a brand, for example. Its persistence will rely heavily on

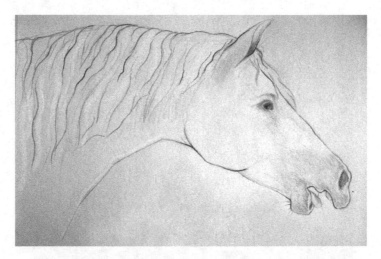

Figure 6.1   Expression of a 'hot-blooded' type. (Drawing by Christina Rees.)

continuity of humane management and good bodily care of the subject. Preservation of wellness in a given horse depends on a policy of preventive husbandry being practiced by those who are the animal's caregivers. The primary factors for this purpose are obviously proper nutrition, health care, parasite control, accommodation, and use. These topics are addressed in other chapters, but additional aspects of equine preventive husbandry are of importance and are addressed here in principle, namely environment management, grooming, and vaccination.

6.2 Equine Spirit

When European horse fanciers first took stock of Arabian and Levant horses, they perceived them as being very spirited or high-spirited in their natures. It was evident that, in contrast to British types of draught horses, the typical Arabian was a fast runner, quick in responsiveness, and keen to act. These features were seen to be the result of an inherent high spirit that generated such active characteristics in this variety of horse.

The spirit of a horse is commonly regarded as that vital animating essence of the animal, or that non-physical and non-material property that has a motivational role in the animal's typical expressiveness. This property of spirit is reflected in the horse's kinetic behavior and is apparent at various, individual levels of reactivity. The most spirited horses of Arabian type were termed 'hot-blooded' (Figure 6.1). Those horses that had phlegmatic temperaments were therefore classified as 'cold-blooded' (Figure 6.2) in order to distinguish them in their differing behavioral traits. These blood classes were given so imaginatively by early horse fanciers. Breeds of horses

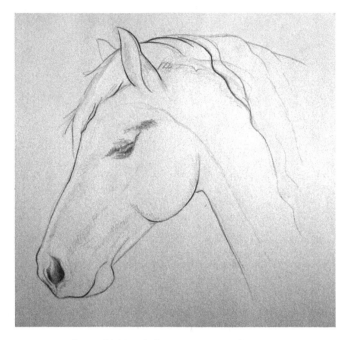

Figure 6.2   Expression of a 'cold-blooded' type. (Drawing by Christina Rees.)

that have emerged from a mixture of these two contrasting, equine, behavioral types have become termed 'warm-blooded' (now warmblood). These terms continue to be understood by horse workers even in this time of modern ethology (McDonnell, 2002). All equine blood, in its true sense, is the same, of course.

6.2.1 Foundation

In temperament, the 'cold-blooded' horse was characteristically phlegmatic, even dour. The temperament was not flighty, perhaps lacking in overt emotions all around. It did not show fear very readily. The 'hot-blooded' horse looked and acted differently. It had a more upright stance, extended neck, long slender limbs and a tail of high carriage. These were the shapes of Mediterranean and Arabian varieties of horse, which, with extravagant spirits, imparted a 'hot-blooded' image to them, by comparison with their cold-spirited northern, distant cousins. Our modern knowledge of horse character makes it obvious that the basic temperaments of the pony and the heavy horse are different. In terms of 'spirit' then, ponies lie somewhere between 'warm' and 'cold.'

In this text the term *temperament* is used to label the animal's characteristic spirit, as shown in its overall behavior. The term *disposition* is used in reference to a given attitude emerging from the animal's general temperament. Disposition is attitude. The use of this equine terminology is consistent with their modern common usage.

6.2.2 History

The true cold-blooded horses had some potential for enormous bulk, although, paradoxically, an essential compactness coexisted. This bulky potential came into its own in the benign grazing environment of the Low Countries. This one branch of the equine family gave gigantic specimens after it had migrated to the western edge of the continent of Europe. No doubt, mutation was at work. The world's largest type of horse was bred thereafter by Belgian farmers. The horse was now the result of selection by man. The great horse of the Low Countries was duly produced by selectively breeding a trait for great potential size, which had resided in this type of cold-blooded horse. Its steady selection by farmers eliminated some other variables. The result was the world's largest horses, very uniform in their characteristics, including a very limited color range and coat type.

The smaller horse from the Nordic latitudes went on its way as a pony. Types were evidently naturally produced. They retained all the genes for every known horse color. They also possessed various types of hair covering, including seasonal coats. Their hooves were small. As they took up residence here and there, they adapted by degree. By these, the body took on forms suited to the location. They lived by foraging, and poor grazing in winter meant reduced intake of food. Bodies adjusted to this as time passed. Local types became the established variety, region by region. They must have had resilience to flourish so well. As a special race, the ponies duly became established across Asia and Europe, on a corridor 50–60° north, along which they slowly spread. By finally arriving on the islands of Iceland, Britain, and Ireland in their primitive forms, the ponies had spread widely.

The warm-blooded corridor for the horse was 30–40° north, across Asia and Europe. These two corridors of evolution, on either side of the 40–50° north niche, were the common, early ancestors of all types of horse, and the Przewalski. They roamed their European and Asian territories. In the meantime, the prehistoric horse on the American continent had become extinct, for reasons unknown.

Four forms of general temperament in the domestic horse can now be recognized, namely, the quick and spirited hot-blooded, the cold-blooded heavy draft, the warm-blooded breeds resulting from earlier crossbreeding with the Arabian and large horses, and the cool-blooded adaptable pony (see Figures 6.1 and 6.2). Perhaps 100 different pony breeds now exist. The ponies on their evolutionary corridor across northern Europe, in the post Ice Age, evidently had much uniformity. They had similar physique and, presumably, similar temperament to maintain their well-being. The classification of temperament by 'blood' can be broadened to accommodate pony 'blood.' Metaphorically, ponies could be classed as cool-blooded.

6.2.3 Adaptation to niche

Within broad latitude, dispersal took place to the east and the west, allowing fresh scope to the adapted herds. Evidently, full adaptation to this cold niche was not the answer for all the strains, and some went south, driven by forces of well-being, finding more benign temperatures in the lands of the Mediterranean, Arabia, Persia, and the subcontinent of India. So there came to exist, about two million years ago, immediate ancestors of *Equus caballus* and of the wild horse, the Przewalski.

Animals with long extremities do not find favor with the elements where biting cold prevails. The Ice Age eliminated every animal that had great stature. Compact forms of 'cold-blooded' horse-kind, however, survived below the Arctic Circle along the 60° parallel of Europe, where many equine herds were located after roughly eight million years of continental evolution.

6.3 Wellness

6.3.1 Physical features

The appraisal of animal wellness is based on both the dynamics and the physical appearance of the animal by assessment of the particular individual. The physical features of relevance include the coat, the eyes, the flesh, and the bones. With grooming (Table 6.1), the coat, from head to tail, should lie naturally with its normal direction of flow. It should not appear to be of a dry, harsh condition, or be dishevelled, or tangled, or soiled. The eyes should have some sparkle, some glistening appearance. They should not be sunken or fast moving. The physical features of the whole body are of primary importance.

A degree of fleshiness should be detectable over the back. The thighs also should be firm, and they should be as muscular as is appropriate for the type of horse and its age. Protruding ribs should not be noticeable and the bones along the back should not be prominent (Table 6.2). Very obvious fat does not indicate a good physical condition. Extra fat will be noticeable over the trunk, between the thighs, over the root of the tail, and along the side of the neck. Fatness is very easily acquired in ponies. It may predispose them to laminitis and should be controlled.

Well-developed musculature is the result of proper exercise and is evident in the clear outlining of numerous muscles, particularly from the shoulder to the knee in the fore leg, and from the hip to the stifle in the hind. A sharp division between two well-developed muscles in the hindquarters creates a visibly indented narrow groove

Table 6.1 Grooming.

Type of grooming	Procedure
Basic	Quartering: wiping face and dock
Routine	Head to feet brushing: body massaging; wiping face, dock; rough combing of mane, tail, and limbs; cleaning sloes and hoof walls
Special	As above, plus fine combing of all long hair; full body brushing; special attention to face, belly, thighs, and lower limbs; hoof rasping as necessary
Extra	Trimming mane and tail; clipping body and limbs; washing legs; painting hoof walls with protectant

Table 6.2 Spectrum of equine body conditions.

General appearance	Factors indicative of body condition
Poor/emaciated	Bony projections of vertebrae, ribs, tailhead, and points of hips and buttocks are prominent. No fat present anywhere on body. Sunken orbits
Very thin	Spinal vertebrae, ribs, tailhead, and points of hips and buttocks are prominent. Withers, shoulders, and neck bones faintly evident
Thin	Slight fat cover over ribs. Spinal vertebrae and ribs easily discernible. Tailhead prominent, but individual vertebrae not visible. Hip appears rounded, but easily seen. Points of buttock, withers and shoulder bones evident
Lean	Slight ridge along the back and outline of ribs visible. Points of hips not evident. Withers, shoulders, and neck not obviously thin
Good physique	Back level. Ribs cannot be visually distinguished, but can be easily felt. Fat around tailhead feels spongy. Withers rounded, shoulders, and neck blend smoothly into body
Well-built	Slight dip along back. Fat over ribs feels spongy. Fat around tailhead feels soft. Slight fat along the sides of the withers, behind the shoulders, and along the sides of the neck
Overweight	Shallow crease down back. Individual ribs can be felt, but fat between them. Fat around tailhead is soft. Fat deposited around withers, behind the shoulders, and along the sides of the neck
Fat	Indented crease down back. Difficult to feel ribs. Fat around tailhead very soft. Area along withers filled with fat, and area behind shoulders filled in flush. Noticeable thickening of neck, fat deposits on inner buttocks
Extremely fat to obese	Noticeably indented crease down back. Patchy fat over ribs. Bulging fat around tailhead, along withers, behind shoulders, and along neck. Inner buttock fat deposits touching each other

Source: adapted from Henneke et al. (1983).

down the postero-lateral aspect of the haunch. This is also the location of the so-called 'poverty line' seen in impoverished horses. The division between the biceps femoris and semitendinosis muscles becomes wider and very obvious due to atrophy or shrinkage of these adjacent thigh muscles to create the so-called poverty line.

Young horses less than two years old do not, as a rule, show great muscularity. However, with physical development, the breasts should become fleshy and the general area from the hips to the tailroot should become leveled off with muscle.

Table 6.3 Physical signs of wellness.

Item	Satisfactory findings
General physique	Well muscled, good abdomen, rounded trunk and rump
General mobility	Moves freely in all gaits, backs, and turns
Reaction	Reacts with alert and cooperative responses
Stance	Firm; relaxed flexion occasionally in alternate hind legs
Skin condition	Sleek coat, parasite-free, no scurf, plucks easily
Eyes	Clear and bright, evidence of good sight
Mouth membranes	Salmon pink in color, moist
Teeth	Age estimation, absence of sharp-edged molars
Body surface	Absence of lesions, lumps, injuries or dirt
Natural orifices	Clean, free of discharge
Respiration	Approx. 12 unbroken respirations per minute
Joints	Full flexion of limb joints and body regions, bends neck easily
Hooves	Intact and smooth walls, not ringed, dry frogs

Young horses, in a condition of good development, should have a degree of plumpness in front of the withers. At this site, the elastic tissue of the ligamentum nuchae, stretching from the poll to the withers, should be well enough developed to be grasped easily by the hand and found to be large and firm, not thick and cord-like. Such latter findings are an early sign of malnutrition affecting this fibro-fatty tissue.

All horses are not exactly alike. In addition to physical variations, there are great differences in abilities, temperament, tolerance, patience, and other properties of a non-physical nature. All the individual characteristics of a horse can become revealed with intimate knowledge of the animal. When any horse is appraised, most obvious is its body form, in such characteristics as height, conformation, body size, breed type, stages of body development, weight, and general appearance. The latter relates to body condition (Table 6.3). Good physical form is a primary factor in the assessment of the horse's health and welfare. Physique is the first dimension of the horse. The second is its behavior, particularly its output of action. Its chief domesticated purpose is compliant performance in all its uses. The output of power takes particular forms in racing, ridden performance, driving, and hauling. The horse is a uniquely strong and mobile domestic animal. Its generous muscling ensures its powerful mobility.

6.3.2 Handling

Stabled horses require daily care and attention. Grazing horses also require daily inspection. Such daily management refers literally to each day of the year. The daily routines in management include: feeding, cleaning out of stalls, changing water, bedding, grooming, walking outdoors or otherwise exercising, cleaning rugs, utensils, etc., and ventilation of premises. The horse is large, strong, and liable to react defensively or aggressively when disturbed suddenly or handled carelessly. All personnel should take due precaution against bites and kicks when dealing with horses, since horses are often very reactive (Fraser, 1974).

6.3.3 Special factors in outdoor management

Optimal outdoor environmental conditions should take the following factors into account:

(1) Outdoor buildings for horses must provide shelter and shade for each animal, and must also ensure safety for the staff handling them.
(2) Fences should be made so that horses can clearly see them. This is particularly important with an electric fence.
(3) It is necessary to keep horses in groups of the same or similar age.
(4) More feeders should be provided than the number of animals, and these should not be placed in corners where fleeing horses can become trapped.
(5) Strange horses should be allowed to make their first contact across a safe fence before putting them together.
(6) Horses that are apparently friendly in stalls may not be so at pasture. The opposite is also possible.

6.3.4 Preventive management

Much humane protection against illness can be given to horses by good management. Although there are numerous forms of sickness in horses, many of these can be prevented. Four good rules of management that can contribute a great deal towards the prevention of illness in any horse facility are given in the following subsections.

6.3.4.1 Guard against overstocking

When horses are crowded together, either indoors or outdoors, dormant illness can flare up and transmissible infections can become widespread and extensive. Also, injury is more likely in crowded situations.

6.3.4.2 Maintain a high level of hygiene

This point cannot be overstressed. Cleanliness is needed at every level of care. Feed boxes and troughs must be kept free of old food. Buckets and drinking vessels must be hygienic. Grooming items have to be kept clean and periodically disinfected. Drains must be kept open and flushed regularly. Windows have to be clean and permit good ventilation. Dust must be controlled as much as possible. Premises must be kept rodent-free. A hygienic environment should be the general objective in all aspects of stable management.

6.3.4.3 Turn out each horse in a stable on a daily basis

This should include wintertime, although severe weather such as a snowstorm, heavy rain or a driving cold wind would obviously be exceptions. An outdoor facility should have a windbreak such as a section of boarding or natural shelter. Fresh air and free movement are health aids.

6.3.4.4 Establish a close connection with a veterinary service

This is a most important requirement of management. It is a usual practice to call a veterinarian to treat a sick or injured horse or to administer vaccinations, but a better system of veterinary attendance can be arranged. The connection between management and veterinarian can be set out in a clear, contractual arrangement. This could deal with routine horse care matters on a scheduled program of visitation. The visits can be for a prescribed time during which routine matters could be addressed. Matters such as pregnancy testing, nutrition review, teeth checking and floating, health checks, special examination, blood and fecal sampling, worming, vaccination, and advice can be dealt with on a routine basis. A pre-set fee agreement for such a visit, plus materials, could be understood by both parties, and this would assist in budgeting. Emergency visits would likely be reduced, but any of these would be outside the 'contract' of course.

A wellness program can emerge from such a system, and this could incorporate any new information of great value on an extensive range of health-care topics. A health and welfare program could provide assurance and guidance on matters of preventive medicine for the horse caregiver (Fraser, 2003).

6.3.5 Disease control

An important part of infectious disease control is a vaccination program. Vaccinated animals have a very good prospect of resisting the common infections of horses. Vaccinations against the viruses of equine influenza and rhinopneumonitis, plus the bacteria of tetanus and strangles, are considered to be of basic importance. Only a veterinarian working the area would know of any need for additional vaccination. Regional illnesses must also be borne in mind when shipping any horse in, or taking it out of its home base. To attend a show, competition or any event where horses will be gathered, consideration must be given, at least a month before, to protection against infection. Incoming animals can be quarantined for a month.

Normality of general and vital signs of health together with norms of physiological factors are all consistent with a general state of wellness. These features must be sought and determined in the course of an examination for soundness of function (see the 20 items in Table 6.4 to be included in a suggested comprehensive examination).

6.3.6 Conditioning

During winter, it is common for idle horses to be fed only a maintenance diet. Any idle horse that is due to be given some form of activity should be put on gradually increasing rations. Before the scheduled work or recreational activity, the grain

Table 6.4 Equine examination protocol to determine clinical wellness.

Examination item	Satisfactory findings
Skin condition	Sleek coat, parasite-free, no scurf, plucks easily
Eyes	Clear and bright, evidence of good sight
Mucous membranes	Salmon pink in color, moist, quick filling time
Teeth	Age estimation, absence of sharp-edged molars
Body surface	Absence of lesions, lumps, injuries or dirt
Natural orifices	Clean, free of discharge
Respiration	Approx. 12 unbroken respirations/minute, clear lung sounds
Temperature	38°C ± 0.5°C (100.5°F ± 0.5°F)
Pulse/heart rate	40 ± 5 beats/minute, normal heart sounds
Joints	Full flexion of limb joints and body regions, bends neck easily
Hooves	Intact and smooth walls, not ringed from laminitis
Sole of foot	Full-sized frog, dry, no offensive odor, free of corns in heels
Blood samples	Norms of blood chemistry and cell picture
Fecal sample	Non-significant helminth egg count; normal consistency
General physique	Well muscled, good abdomen, rounded trunk and rump
General mobility	Moves freely in all gaits, backs, and turns easily
Reaction	Reacts to examination with alert and cooperative responses
Tail	Not flaccid or stiff, may move side to side in the walk
Ears	Freely mobile, no excess movement or stiffly laid back
Stance	Relaxed with comfort shifts, especially in alternate hind legs

ration should be slowly built up to full work level. It is an important component of conditioning to have the horse harnessed on several occasions and exercised before real use. This can build up until the horse is performing a half-day of light work, then a half-day of full work. For all of this conditioning to be complete, about two or three weeks would be required. An unfit horse, although healthy, should never be made to do a full day of work of any kind. Apart from fitness, the horse's skin must be allowed to become toughened by harness contact. Even carrying a saddle needs hardening of the skin of the back and girth area.

6.3.7 Individuality
While the primary behavioral nature of free-living horses can be seen in the wild, the secondary nature of each horse, or individuality, is obscured there. With handling and close surveillance in custody, a horse's temperament can be recognized. In addition, the individual can often be seen to have its own ways, its 'personality.' Each individual may have its own variety of behavioral characteristics in habits, traits, and disposition. It may possess such individuality to a greater or

lesser extent as a secondary nature. Some of this behavioral individuality is learned, some is inherited.

Horses show many of the moods, wants, and emotional states that are known so well in human life. Some of their senses are much keener than the human equivalent. Although horses do not possess intelligence as it is known at the human level, they seem to have some basic 'feelings' that resemble human feelings to some extent. Their 'feelings' go beyond the well-acknowledged ones of pain, hunger, fear, and rage. Some individual horses do show greater intelligence than others; some show more emotions than others. Among themselves, they show fluctuations of moods in their social behavior.

The activities of horses show that they have both sense and feelings. Their show of sense indicates their intelligence. This is of a type and level much lower than the human form due to a much smaller cerebral cortex in the horse's brain. However, feelings are largely processed in the elaborate limbic system in the brain of both humans and horses. The horse has a very functional limbic system that enriches its life and its nature.

A major component of the horse is its individuality. Behavior, together with individuality, make up this feature. Horse husbandry involves special forms of control. By this controlled custody, the animal's natural behavior is suppressed or managed to a great extent. This is much less so, of course, where space and freedom are provided at pasture.

Once a horse's nature is fully recognized by someone, it cannot ever again become unseen by that person. When the richness of a horse's self, with its sensitive properties and its firm characteristics, become fully recognized by its caregiver, the horse then becomes and remains appreciated as a being of quality. This appreciation is the best basis for a good animal care policy.

6.3.8 Wellness and emotional balance

A horse's state of well-being features a component of emotional balance. The latter is expressed in the 'body language' of the relaxed and resting animal. This exists in both its covert and overt behavior. The expressions of satisfactory acceptance of its circumstances include minute actions. For example, the muzzle relaxes, the upper eyelids descend slightly, excessive ear movement or fixation is reduced, and the tail hangs still. More noticeable expressions of satisfaction may include nodding of the head, relaxation of one or another hind limb, and deep vocalizations. These body-based expressions, together with normality of behavior, are the principal source of evidence for emotional well-being in a horse. Comprehensive well-being has been likened to a state of 'global wellness' in the individual.

When viewed from outside the area of its own space, while given some freedom of movement in an accustomed environment and left undisturbed, a horse with well-being and fully awake should show alertness in its body language without any reactive excess. It should exhibit interest in any event in its vicinity and be observant of intrusion into its particular 'individual space.' In suitable circumstances of free mobility, an elevated carriage of the head and steady flexibility in back-and-forward ear movement will also demonstrate wellness.

The stance in a state of well-being will be altered freely and easily. In its sound and natural stance, the horse will variously distribute its weight on all four legs. It may bear its weight across both fore legs plus only one hind leg, while the other has its toe touching the ground. This single hind limb support alternates between legs several times in the course of a period of resting stance. It is normal for one fore foot to advance occasionally, while both hind limbs are evenly weight-bearing.

6.3.9 Equine dynamics

The dynamics of equine actions have to be fully appreciated in the care of this particular muscular and mobile subject. The horse has a kinetic constitution and this must be taken into account in all circumstances. In addition, there is great individuality in equine reaction. Breed, temperament, and the environment in which it was raised all affect the horse's behavior under management. Horses that have been raised on free range or away from people will have a large flight distance; they may panic and become agitated when a handler approaches within such a distance. Horses that have been raised in close confinement are usually more approachable and easier to handle and train. Anticipating a horse's reaction is undoubtedly the best means of exercising some control over its behavior. This is particularly true when training. Each method employed in the 'breaking' of a horse in a single session involves its frustrating control, with varying degrees and durations of enforcement, to the point of ceased reaction in the subject and its acceptance of the imposed circumstances.

The essence of the horse is sensitive power. Humane care has to focus rationally on this elemental factor. Although this equine quality is holistic in its nature, it can be examined analytically. Its various parts are to be found in the horse's physique, its actions, and its senses. Although these may be governed by the animal's individual circumstances – to some extent – they require appreciation as vital components of horse function. They have a direct influence on performance. General care requires knowledge of them.

It is the exceptional locomotor capacity of the horse that has been exploited in domestication. Even with the selection pressures imposed on breeds of horse, most of their original, innate, dynamic traits have been maintained and enhanced rather than diminished. Their kinetic character persists in their conventional uses for traction and running power. These natural properties can permit a state of wellness to coexist with work and age (Table 6.5), given proper care of the animal.

6.3.10 Birth and growth

When the foal is born, it remains recumbent, close by its mother, for 10–20 minutes, still connected to her, with the umbilical cord unbroken. This allows much of its blood to be retrieved from the placenta inside the mare. With this transfusion accomplished, the foal's blood volume is maximized. This creates a sound physiological base for vitality in the demands of the elemental work that follows.

Table 6.5 General wellness concerns in horse age groups.

Age group	Span (years)	Wellness concerns[a]
Infancy	birth–0.5	Suckling, navel, joints, infections, parasites, nutrition, custody
Juvenility	0.6–1.5	Weaning, nutrition, immunity, parasites, injury, custody
Youth	1.6–3	Nutrition, immunity, injury, parasites, infection, breeding, custody
Maturity	4–9	Parasites, infections, nutrition, breeding, injury, respiration, environment
Aged	10–17	Parasites, bowels, hooves, breeding, nutrition, legs, respiration, environment
Old age	18–25	Nutrition, parasites, hooves, joints, respiration, teeth, various organs, bowels, legs, environment
Extreme age	26+	Nutrition, parasites, hooves, joints, teeth, digestion, locomotion, bowels, other organs, mastication, respiration, environment

[a]Welfare monitoring with preventive measures and animal care address these concerns.

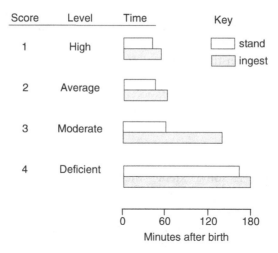

Figure 6.3 Four levels of neonatal vitality in foals: modal times taken for newborn foals to stand securely and suck successfully are shown as indices of vitality.

The newborn foal's life is in the balance unless it has the vitality or spirit to rise and stand within an hour, walk and locate the mare's mammary gland soon after, and ingest a feed of colostral milk before it is 3–4 hours old (see Figure 6.3) The normal foal shows determination in achieving each programmed step to reple-tion. Significant, inherent vitality (or spiritedness) in the neonate clearly maintains the progressive drive to survive its postnatal challenges. Without such vitality, the foal will fail to feed and will be dead by the following day if it does not receive

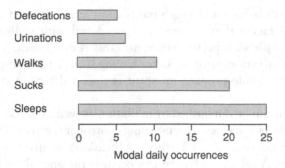

Figure 6.4 Neonatal functions in foals: incidences of basic functions are shown as indices of vitality in foals aged one to three days.

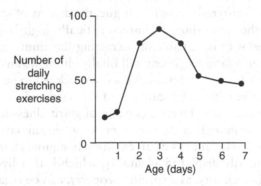

Figure 6.5 Exercise by stretching in foals up to seven days old.

human help. With the neonatal vitality consumed in the first critical work of graduating from a fetus to an ambulatory milk consumer, the foal spends most of the next few days ingesting and sleeping (see Figure 6.4).

While it may not be possible or easy to recognize or quantify spirit or vitality as a singular factor in neonatal behavior, the reality of its existence is illustrated in the example given above. That it is a component of wellness is also made clear. In the early days of life, the quantity and quality of pandiculations, or compound stretching exercises, provide an indication of neonatal wellness (see Figure 6.5).

6.4 Conclusion

6.4.1 Spirit and wellness

Although the equine spirit is a self-determined force, prevailing in the subject's conduct, the animal's display of spirit is linked to its general health – during illness, it is reduced or virtually eliminated. In optimal health, i.e., wellness, the animal's spirit is freely and fully displayed behaviorally. This non-aggressive spirit provides tone to the animal's behavior through motivation at an elevated level. It is therefore a behavioral factor that is positively correlated with wellness. The horse's principal output is physical performance, and this is dependent on a combination of wellness and motivation, with the latter having some basis in the subject's inherent spirit. This intangible property of spirit is thus a determinant in equine performance.

The equine spirit can be diminished by inhibition as well as illness. When a horse is being 'broken in' by enforcement of frustrating control, it is essentially its spirit that is 'broken' by the experience. Every method of 'breaking-in' involves enforcement of frustrating control. A rebound of spirit can occur if the animal finds itself liberated environmentally. This phenomenon is readily observed when a horse is first 'turned out' in an extensive pasture after a long period of restraint. In such circumstances, most horses will run and kick when freed, their spirit and wellness being expressed.

The horse's spirit is also reduced with fatigue, the display of spirit being dependent on energy. At the same time, a characteristically high level of spirit in the individual horse seems to be capable of energizing the animal at a time of incipient fatigue. However, a fatiguing event will finally eliminate any evidence of spirit within the horse's performance. Spiritedness is considered to be shown in the running horse's demeanor, with a high carriage of the head and elevated extension of the fore limbs. The lax and subjective concept of spiritedness in animal behavior is applied to the horse more than to any other domestic animal; in fact, it appears to be recognized by horse fanciers as an exclusively equine characteristic. Equine spiritedness is essentially displayed as vitality, which is that lively ability to support the subject's life. Vitality, as a specific property, can be regarded as the product of spirit in the horse. Vitality is therefore the evident output of spiritedness inherent in the animal in given circumstances. This intangible property of 'blood' or spirit is safely assumed to be an activating factor in the horse's characteristic expressiveness. As such, it serves as the dynamic foundation in much of the animal's usual kinetic behavior as vitality, including reactivity and locomotion. It also may be considered to have some role in the temperament of the individual horse, which, in fact, in a general non-specific way, is revealed in the overall expressiveness of the animal.

6.4.2 Suffering and stress

Suffering and wellness are opposite states, either tolerated or enjoyed by the horse's constitution. It is a valid clinico-behavioral rule that either state displaces the other. The imbalance between these two endogenous states demands the recognition of both states in behavioral manifestations. Suffering is also a component of more ambiguous conditions such as stress or distress. Distressful circumstances of husbandry can disturb the animal beyond its ability to adapt to them. Suffering can therefore result from psychological insults, independently of a physical cause. Certain acute behavioral signs such as intensive vocalizations, struggling, and trembling are clear evidence of a reactive variety of suffering. In addition, chronic forms such as passively depressed behavior show suffering. The latter varieties of suffering can therefore be classified as psychological. Forms of stereotyped behavior are widely assumed to indicate such suffering. Many of these forms have long been incorrectly known as stable vices and are now recognized as stereotyped syndromes that impair welfare (Mason and Rushen, 2006). All aspects of animal welfare now need attention in veterinary education to address both clinical and subclinical stressfulness in our animals (Fraser, 2008).

References

Arden, D. (ed.) (2003) *The Angell Memorial Hospital Book of Wellness and Preventative Care for Dogs*. McGraw-Hill, New York.

Bekoff, M. and Byers, J.A. (1998) *Animal Play*. Cambridge University Press, Cambridge.

Broom, D.M. and Fraser, A.F. (2007) *Domestic Animal Behaviour*, 4th edn. CABI Publishing, Wallingford, UK.

Fraser, A.F. (1974) *Farm Animal Behaviour*. Bailliere Tindall, London.

Fraser, A.F. (2003) *Humane Horse Care*. Canadian Farm Animal Care Trust, Barrie, Ontario.

Fraser, A.F. (2008) Veterinarians and animal welfare – a comment. *Canadian Veterinary Journal* 49(1), 8.

Henneke, D.R., Potter, G.D., Kreider, J.L. and Yeates, B.F. (1983) Relationship between condition score, physical measurements and body fat percentage in mares. *Equine Veterinary Journal* 15(4), 371–372.

Mason, G. and Rushen, J. (eds) (2006) *Stereotypic Animal Behaviour – Fundamentals and Applications to Welfare*, 2nd edn. CABI Publishing, Wallingford, UK.

McDonnell, S.M. (2002) Behaviour of horses. In *The Ethology of Domestic Animals*, Jensen, P. (ed). CABI Publishing, Wallingford, UK.

de Waal, F. (1996) *Good Natured*. Harvard University Press, Cambridge, MA.

Webster, J. (1994) *Animal Welfare: a Cool Eye Towards Eden*. Blackwell, Oxford.

Pain and its Management in Horses

Laurie Goodrich
and Khursheed Mama

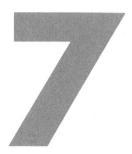

7.2 What is Pain?

Pain is a perception; unless there is a cerebral center, and an organized recognition of noxious stimulus, no response or adaptation in the patient will occur. In humans,

Equine Welfare, First Edition. Edited by C. Wayne McIlwraith and Bernard E. Rollin.
© 2011 by UFAW. Published 2011 by Blackwell Publishing Ltd.

it is important that the patient verbally express or communicate the presence of pain in some manner. A general lack of recognition of pain in animals, specifically horses, results from the absence of verbal communication that expresses pain perception. Dogs and cats often vocalize when in a painful state; however, the horse does not express pain in this manner, and this unfortunately may result in an unawareness of a painful state.

Pain is a complex multidimensional sensory experience normally generated by the activation of high-threshold pain receptors (nociceptors), which send electrical signals from the periphery to the spinal cord and brain via multiple pathways. This results in responses that warn and protect the host from impending tissue damage, which serves to maintain bodily integrity and survival (Muir, 2005). Nociceptive pain is frequently referred to as physiological pain because it minimizes tissue damage by activating reflex withdrawal mechanisms and modifies behavioral, autonomic, and neurohumoral responses that maintain body integrity, prevent tissue damage, and promote healing for survival. Maladaptive pain is pain associated with abnormal sensory processing due to damage to tissues (inflammatory pain) or the nervous system (neuropathic pain), or to abnormal function of the nervous system (functional pain). Maladaptive pain is pathological and described by an exaggerated and prolonged response to noxious (hyperalgesia) and non-noxious (allodynia) stimuli (Woolf, 2004). Maladaptive pain may result in stress that can lead to abnormal behavior, poor quality of life, and, if uncontrolled, distress and death (Muir, 2005). The last point is relevant to the equine practitioner due to the common practice of euthanasia in horses with uncontrollable or chronic pain.

7.3 Consequences of Pain

One of the most important reasons to control pain is to avoid the consequence of 'wind-up' phenomenon (Muir, 1998). Pain is usually the first and most dominant clinical sign in horses suffering from disease or injury. Pain and inflammatory responses induced by surgical procedures and anesthesia-related ischemia produce a series of behavioral, neurophysiological, endocrine, metabolic, and cellular responses (stress response), which initiate, maintain, and amplify the release of pain and inflammatory mediators (Figure 7.1) (Muir, 1998). Pain is normally produced by the mechanical, chemical, or thermal activation of small-diameter high-threshold sensory nerve fibers (Muir, 1998). When pain is uncontrolled, inflammation increases the sensitivity of peripheral nerve fibers, and stimulates the synthesis and release of nerve growth factor, substance P, and calcitonin gene-related peptide, all which contribute to the development of sensory hyperexcitability and hyperalgesia. Cumulative increases in positive feedback loops and neural sensitivity result in increases in excitability of spinal cord neurons and central nervous system 'wind-up' (Figure 7.2) (Muir, 1998). Uncontrolled pain produces a catabolic state, suppresses

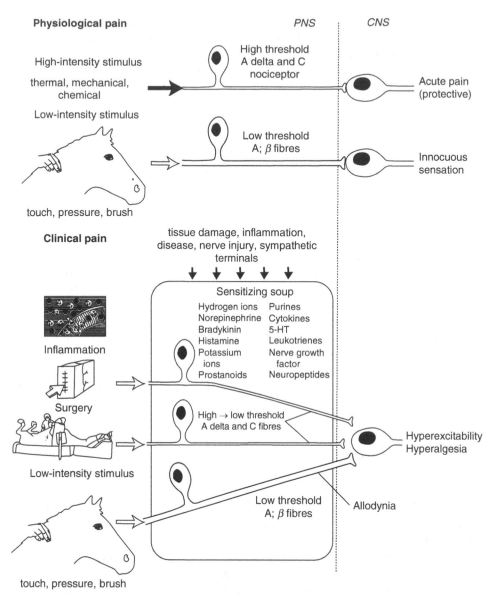

Figure 7.1 The differences between physiological pain and clinical pain. Tissue damage and inflammation can lead to hypersensitivity to mechanical, chemical, and thermal stimuli, resulting in increased sensation or 'hyperalgesia.' (From Muir (1998) *Equine Veterinary Education* **10**, 335–340, with permission.)

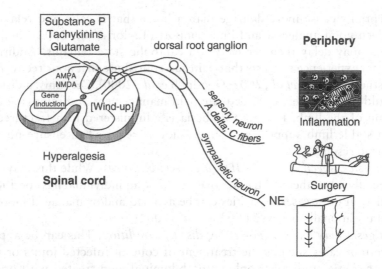

Figure 7.2 The result of chronic input of pain centrally causing up-regulation of gene induction and central nervous system 'wind-up.' (From Muir (1998) *Equine Veterinary Education* **10**, 335–340, with permission.)

the immune response, and promotes inflammation, which delays wound healing and predisposes the patient to infection and intensified medical care.

Although the clinician cannot control the degree of pain that the horse presents with, most commonly the procedure used to treat the condition will often cause similar or potentially worse pain, until the tissues and/or bones heal. Pre-emptive analgesia is a term used to denote the administration of analgesic drugs before extensive soft tissue or orthopedic surgery in an attempt to minimize the response to pain, particularly the development of central nervous system (CNS) hypersensitivity and resultant hyperalgesia and allodynia (Woolf and Chong, 1993).

Other consequences of ongoing, uncontrolled pain include weight loss, depression, immunosuppression, alterations of intestinal motility, and overuse of non-steroidal anti-inflammatory drugs (NSAIDs), leading to toxicity. Any of these consequences alone may also lead to the horse's demise, and are common sequellae to chronic pain.

7.4 Common Misconceptions Regarding Pain Management in Horses

Fortunately, the field of pain management is improving for the horse. Reluctance to use analgesics, however, still persists. Reasons often revolve around the following (from Taylor *et al.*, 2002):

(1) *Removing the pain in an injured body part will result in overuse of that limb and cause further damage.* This is a poor argument on humanitarian and practical grounds. An agitated horse in pain from a fractured limb could

potentially cause more damage than a horse that is calm and relaxed that is given good analgesia and limb support (Taylor *et al.*, 2002). Inappetent horses may delay their recovery if a catabolic state remains. Additionally, clinical experience suggests that pain can contribute to a poor recovery from anesthesia (Taylor *et al.*, 2002; Goodrich *et al.*, 2000). Certainly, a distinction should be made between adequate pain management and removing all sensation of the limb. If local anesthesia is administered to a fractured limb, then stable limb support and supervision is required to ensure no further damage results.

(2) *Analgesics, specifically NSAIDs, are toxic in horses.* While this may be true especially when the NSAIDs are overdosed or an individual has specific sensitivities, in most cases, toxicities can be avoided and/or managed more easily than traditionally believed (Taylor *et al.*, 2002).

(3) *Analgesia may mask a worsening disease condition.* This can be applicable in certain cases such as the treatment of colic or infected joints or tendon sheaths. In a study of people with abdominal pain treated with opioid or saline, the opioid-treated individuals had improved pain relief, and analgesia did not interfere with the diagnosis of their condition (Pace and Burke, 1996). In most cases, judicious use of analgesics will provide adequate pain management but also allow 'breakthrough' pain that the clinician will be able to appreciate.

(4) *The use of analgesia in horses is expensive and not economically viable.* This is rarely true, since some of the most commonly used analgesics (phenylbutazone and flunixin meglumine) are inexpensive. Furthermore, the costs associated with complications related to ongoing pain negate the monetary costs due to drug purchase.

The obvious benefits of controlling pain and improving the welfare of the horse should not need further mention. The negative implications associated with pain and the published reports on improved outcome from disease in people with adequate pain relief prove the benefits of good pain management (Taylor *et al.*, 2002; Singelyn *et al.*, 1998). In equine practice, it is well recognized that excellent pain control will positively influence a horse's outlook, particularly the willingness to eat. Pain relief will often reverse an injured horse's despondency, and improves recovery. An anabolic state is also needed for a functional immune system.

Besides the benefits of avoiding central sensitization and 'wind-up,' there now exists evidence where improved mobility was shown in people who received more profound analgesia perioperatively (Singelyn *et al.*, 1998; Capdevila *et al.*, 1999; Taylor *et al.*, 2002). Although no studies such as this exist in horses, it is likely that similar beneficial effects apply. Studies in people have also shown that the method of analgesia can affect the rate of return of bowel function, and this may be directly applicable to equine colic patients (Liu *et al.*, 1995; Thoren *et al.*, 1989).

7.5 Assessing Pain

Various methods exist that assist researchers and practitioners in assessing pain. None are extremely accurate; however, they do allow some objective measures to be documented so that progression or control of pain can be recorded. The literature is replete with various scoring methods (discussed in section 7.7) attempting to provide adequate assessment. But, because of the individual variation between animals and how they modify their behavior due to pain, no one method is used. The following are measurements that are used to interpret intensity of pain.

7.5.1 Heart rate

Heart rate is commonly used as an indicator of pain. However, various reasons exist that may also cause heart rate changes, such as excitement, certain drugs or drug combinations, and the temperament of the individual. In dogs, heart rate was not found to be a helpful indicator of degree of pain, and various equine studies have proved that heart rate can be variable after surgical procedures whether NSAIDs had been given or not (Raekallio *et al.*, 1997a). In horses with colic, an increase in heart rate was a good predictive value indication for surgical intervention; however, other factors such as shock and endotoxemia may have an influence on heart rate (Pascoe *et al.*, 1990). Furthermore, horses with colic pain treated with detomidine and xylazine may have a drug-induced drop in heart rate in contrast to horses receiving only flunixin or butorphanol. In a study of 43 horses, 40 revealed a significant correlation between orthopedic disease and heart rate (Courouce *et al.*, 1996). It is important, however, to be aware of drugs administered when assessing pain levels through heart rate, because some horses may be in pain and not have an elevated heart rate.

7.5.2 Beta-endorphin

Beta-endorphin is an endogenous neurotransmitter found in the neurons of the central and peripheral nervous system. Along with pain, beta-endorphin levels can be increased due to stress and shock; hence, increased levels do not always indicate pain. Studies have been done detecting elevated levels post-arthroscopy (Raekallio *et al.*, 1997a) and following more invasive surgeries (Raekallio *et al.*, 1997b).

7.5.3 Catecholamines and corticosteroids

Catecholamines and corticosteroids are markers of stress, and although horses in pain are often in stress, these can be elevated in periods of non-painful stress. Cortisol levels were shown to be increased in horses and ponies after anesthesia and surgery compared with a similar anesthetic protocol without surgery (Taylor, 1998). However, in another study, chronic pain actually caused a significant decrease in cortisol levels (Mills *et al.*, 1997). Overall, it appears that cortisol may be increased with acute pain, although there is a wide degree of variation, and chronic pain does not appear to be measured accurately with cortisol, and other parameters should be used.

7.5.4 Ground reaction force

The degree of lameness exhibited by a horse should be reflected by the ground reaction force. Various investigators have used ground reaction forces, force plate analysis, or an in-shoe pressure measurement system (Judy *et al.*, 2001; Merkens and Schamhardt, 1988; Willemen *et al.*, 1999). Although these systems appear to be accurate in assessing limb pain, few institutions have this technology available. For those that possess these technologies, they are a highly reliable measurement of limb pain in the patient able to tolerate this form of evaluation (Ishihara *et al.*, 2005).

7.5.5 Response to pressure

Using instruments to quantify what force is needed to cause a reaction to a painful stimulus is an attempt to obtain objective measurements of pain. Owens *et al.* (1995b) used compression thresholds from calibrated hoof testers in laminitic horses as an objective means of measuring foot pain. Following baseline measurements, alpha-2 adrenoreceptor agonist analgesia was used to measure the results of pain management. Recently, Haussler and Erb (2006) and Haussler *et al.* (2008) have published promising results from utilizing pressure algometry to assess musculoskeletal pain. This technique quantifies perceived pain using an instrument that measures response to pressure. In the future, this technique could prove valuable in assessment of many different forms of pain, such as back, skin, and incisional pain.

7.5.6 Gait analysis

High-speed treadmills allow observers to view movies to analyze components of motion and achieve objective data on speed, range, and displacement of different aspects of the body (Keegan, 2007; Keegan *et al.*, 2000, 2008). They offer excellent objective data, but the facilities, software analysis, and expertise needed to run such analyses make this method of pain assessment rare.

7.5.7 Thermographic imaging

Thermography reveals areas that have increased temperature due to an inflammatory response. This area has not had extensive study; however, useful localization of limb pain, cast sores, and back pain has been reported using this technique (Schweinitz *et al.*, 1999).

7.5.8 Electroencephalography

Although not useful in awake horses, electroencephalography (EEG) patterns have been useful for evaluating effectiveness of analgesics in horses (Johnson and Taylor, 1998; Johnson *et al.*, 1999; Otto *et al.*, 1996). One study examined the effect of detomidine and ketamine on EEG during surgical procedures, and concluded that these analgesics ameliorated any EEG arousal (Miller *et al.*, 1995).

7.5.9 Behavioral signs

Studies have begun to include behavioral signs of pain (explained in section 7.6) that are consistent with ongoing pain (Doria *et al.*, 2008; Rietmann *et al.*, 2004). More studies are needed regarding how these behavioral assessments are consistent with severity and duration of pain.

7.5.10 Response to analgesics

Most practitioners would probably agree that the most frequently used assessment of pain control is response to analgesics. Although variable from horse to horse, the behavior associated with analgesic administration highly influences the dose and frequency of administration of analgesics. An important consideration in this assessment, however, is that certain analgesics (such as alpha-2 agonists), in addition to providing excellent analgesia, also result in profound sedation, thus possibly eliminating behaviors that would exhibit the true severity of pain.

7.6 Behavioral Changes Associated with Pain in the Horse

Pain assessment in horses is usually interpreted through behavior. In addition to pain, various environmental factors such as a strange environment, separation of herd mates, and anxiety over a certain situation may change a horse's behavior. These confounding factors may make interpretation of pain difficult. Regardless of a horse's temperament, experience with horses and what their 'normal' state is remains essential to pain assessment. The horse is a flight animal; this often results in a 'flight' reaction to a painful stimulus that is one of escaping or 'running away' from pain.

Taylor *et al.* (2002) have described behavioral effects of pain in horses. Sudden, sharp pain will usually cause a reflex escape or attack reaction; thus, a horse may run or, alternatively, bite or kick at the source of stimulus. For instance, an insect bite may elicit a stomp, bite, or gallop in response to the associated pain. Head pain usually causes shaking of the head, snorting, and restlessness. Jaw or mouth pain may result in difficulty eating, drooling of saliva, and chewing on one side of the jaw.

Limb pain may cause lameness, unwillingness to bear weight, constant picking up and replacement of the limb, or stomping. Alternatively, the limb, or various aspects of the hoof, may have less load bearing. Severe limb pain may cause constant lifting of the leg, touching it down, and then lifting it again. Restlessness, agitation, and sweating can be marked, such as in a sustained fracture. Although fractures can be severely painful, in the 'flight' phase of fracture, horses may continue to gallop, jump or run for some time and not develop acute pain until minutes to hours later. This phenomenon has been compared to injuries of soldiers sustained on the battlefield.

Abdominal pain may cause general restlessness, kicking at the belly, rolling, and occasional tail swishing. Additionally, horses showing signs of colic will often look at their sides, play in the water trough with their muzzle without drinking, or repeatedly lie down, roll and get up again. Occasionally the horse may stay in lateral or partial dorsal recumbency for a few minutes in an abnormal or stretched out position. Throughout this restlessness, the horse may sweat sometimes to the point of dehydration. Lip curling may also occur during times of colic.

Back pain may cause behavioral changes that are uncharacteristic of the horse's temperament, such as tail swishing, grinding of the teeth, head shaking, and resentment of the saddle or grooming, sinking when mounted, failure to bend or yield to aids, stumbling, tripping, backing or bucking, and rearing. This may be superimposed on more subtle behaviors such as poor performance or appetite or even a sour attitude.

Severe and unrelenting acute pain will result in restlessness, tachypnea, tachycardia, agitation, and copious amounts of sweat and foam production. A gentle mannered horse can sometimes become difficult to communicate with. The horse's attitude changes and may take on a wild and distracted appearance, especially in its eye, and occasionally it may take little care to avoid knocking into a person or other animal.

Chronic pain can lead to a depressed horse that often stands with its head down, avoiding contact with other horses or humans. Tension in abdominal muscles may reveal a tucked up appearance. Mental alertness is decreased, and the horse's eye may appear dull, listless, and distant. Often these horses have a waning appetite and may spend long periods lying down. Chronic laminitis, navicular disease, peritonitis or rhabdomyolysis may cause such depression.

7.7 Pain Scoring and its Inconsistencies

Pain management in veterinary medicine is handicapped by the lack of validated methods of clinical assessment. Accurate assessment of pain is complicated because observations of pain are subjective, and developing a complete description of the various degrees of pain is difficult (Firth and Haldane, 1999). Also, it may be hard to differentiate the effects of general anesthesia from those of pain. A valid method of pain scoring should result in a complete, clear, and consistent means of describing the degree of pain in animals after acute injury or surgery, and should be able to discern differences in response to analgesic treatments. These scoring systems are used commonly in people and are the basis for most analgesic studies. Scoring systems used can be classified into three types: a visual analog scale (VAS), a simple descriptive scale (SDS), and the numerical rating scale (NRS).

The VAS usually consists of a 10 cm line that has statements such as 'no pain' at one end and 'severe pain' at the other end. The observer uses a pencil to place a mark somewhere along the line to interpret the degree of pain. The VAS is subject to a great deal of observer variation, but because it does not use defined categories, it is often considered to be more sensitive than an NRS or SDS. VAS scales are widely used in human hospitals for pain scoring.

The SDS uses a numerical scale with behavioral descriptions attached to each number, for example, four or five degrees of severity, such as no evidence of pain, mild, moderate, severe, and very severe. Such scales may not be linear, i.e., the difference in pain between a score of 3 and 4 may be quite different from the difference between a score of 5 and 6.

The third approach is to use an NRS on many different parameters (including objective data such as heart rate) and to add numbers together in some form of multidimensional scoring system (Taylor et al., 2002). This scoring system also suffers from the lack of linearity and needs to be tailored to the particular set of conditions (i.e., abdominal pain would be different from orthopedic pain).

There has been very little use of these pain scales in horses. Probably the most common lameness pain scale is that used by the American Association of Equine Practitioners (AAEP). In an attempt to 'standardize' lameness grades, the AAEP published a lameness scale on a 0 to 5 scale, with 0 being 'no lameness' and 5 being 'non-weight-bearing lameness' (Ross, 2003). Other clinical studies have used SDS, or NRS, to observe postoperative pain assessment, with variable results (Johnson et al., 1993; Raekallio et al., 1997a). Regardless of isolated studies, adequate pain scoring systems are in need of development for the horse. A recent study described a composite orthopedic pain scale in the horse that used behavioral and physiological criteria in determining equine orthopedic pain (Bussieres et al., 2008).

7.8 Management of Pain in the Horse using Specific Drugs

7.8.1 Non-steroidal anti-inflammatory drugs

Non-steroidal anti-inflammatory drugs (NSAIDS) are some of the most commonly used analgesics in equine practice. They reduce inflammation by inhibiting the production of prostaglandins and, as a result, are only effective in the face of an inflammatory process (Owens et al., 1996). The acidic nature of these compounds allows them to accumulate in inflamed tissues, which are also acidic. They are highly protein-bound, and therefore higher concentrations are found in the serum, although inflamed synovial joints have higher concentrations due to increased blood flow and vascular permeability induced during inflammation (Kallings, 1993). At the site of injury, they inhibit the cyclooxygenase pathway (COX), and prevent the formation of prostaglandins. The two enzymes that make up this pathway are COX-1 and COX-2. COX-1 is responsible for normal functions of the mucosa in the gastric stomach by increasing blood flow, decreasing acid production, and increasing mucus production. COX-2 is usually not present in most tissues but is inducible in injured tissues, which results in prostaglandin production and inflammation. NSAIDS that are currently used today block both COX-1 and COX-2 and can sometime result in toxicity.

Cyclooxygenase-2 inhibitors are emerging in the area of NSAID therapy. They specifically block the COX-2 pathway but do not inhibit the 'housekeeping' functions

Table 7.1 Doses of non-steroidal anti-inflammatory drugs.

Drug	Route	Dose
Flunixin meglumine	Oral or intravenous	1.1 mg/kg for up to 5 days
Ketoprofen	Intravenous	2.2 mg/kg for up to 5 days
Phenylbutazone	Oral or intravenous	4.4 mg/kg twice daily for 1 day, then 2.2 mg/kg twice daily for 2–4 days, then 2.2 mg/kg on alternate days
Naproxen	Oral	10 mg/kg once daily for 10–20 days
Firocoxib	Oral	10 mg/kg once daily for up to 30 days
Carprofen	Oral or intravenous	0.7 mg/kg IV once daily or 1.4 mg/kg orally once daily for 7 days

of prostaglandins such as mucus production and blood flow stimulated by COX-1 (Halverson, 1999). Theoretically, they should minimize the occurrence of NSAID-induced toxicities and will replace the NSAIDs associated with greater risks of toxicities.

Toxicity associated with NSAID administration is due to: oral, gastric, duodenal, and colonic ulceration and necrosis; renal papillary necrosis; altered clotting times; a decrease in plasma total protein; diarrhea; and perivascular irritation and necrosis (Geiser, 1990). Early signs of toxicity are depression, inappetency, anorexia, oral ulceration, and abdominal edema (Kallings, 1993). Clinicians should be aware of these toxicities and immediately stop NSAID administration if they are noted. A study by MacAllister *et al.* (1993) compared the adverse effects of phenylbutazone, flunixin, and ketoprofen, and found that phenylbutazone had the greatest toxic potential, followed by flunixin and ketoprofen.

NSAIDs provide effective analgesia for many orthopedic procedures that cause mild to moderate pain (Baller and Hendrickson, 2002). They are often given intravenously before or during anesthesia so that they will be effective in surgery and postoperatively. It should be noted that non-steroidal drugs are protein-bound and therefore may displace other protein-bound drugs and deepen anesthesia (Nolan, 2000).

The most common NSAIDs used perioperatively today are phenylbutazone, flunixin meglumine, ketoprofen, and to a lesser extent carprofen and firocoxib (Equioxx®). Specific dosages are found in Table 7.1.

7.8.1.1 Phenylbutazone (Equiphen®, Equipolozone®)
Pharmacokinetics
The efficacy, availability, and affordability of phenylbutazone (PBZ) continue to make it the most widely used NSAID in the horse. Classified as an enolic acid, it is highly protein-bound in plasma (>99%), metabolized in the liver, and excreted in

the urine. When PBZ is given intravenously (IV) at the recommended loading dose of 4.4 mg/kg, the plasma half-life is approximately 5.5 h in horses and ponies (Lees et al., 1985).

Oral administration is the most common method of dosing. Length of time to absorption can vary, depending on the amount of feed present in the stomach at the time of administration. Horses fasted for 1 h pre- and post-administration reach peak plasma levels at 6 h, in contrast to 13 h if free-choice hay is allowed (May and Lees, 1996). The time at which the highest plasma levels are desired is an important consideration to the veterinarian treating a horse in competition. A late peak could result in unacceptably high plasma levels during competition. Plasma levels decrease 6 h post-administration, but exudate half-life exceeds plasma, with the duration of action lasting up to 24 h (May and Lees, 1996).

Clinical applications

Phenylbutazone remains the most commonly administered NSAID in the horse. Its efficacy for musculoskeletal pain has stood the test of time, and, although it can have toxic effects on the gastrointestinal tract, when used at the appropriate dosage, most horses do not seem to exhibit toxic effects. Experimental work investigating the PBZ safety margin suggests that doses not exceeding 2.2 mg/kg or less twice a day are relatively safe (Collins and Tyler, 1984). The margin of safety is drastically reduced if this dose is exceeded. Obtaining an accurate weight using conventional methods such as a weight tape or body score system of scale is of utmost importance when calculating the amount to be administered. In the authors' experience, it is not uncommon to see toxicity in smaller horses or yearlings where a seemingly accurate dose of '1.5 g per horse, twice a day' actually exceeded the recommended daily dose. Furthermore, dosing can often be reduced to once a day, depending on the severity of pain. Clinicians should use caution, however, when administering phenylbutazone for horses at high risk of side-effects.

A study by Raekallio et al. (1997a) demonstrated improved pain scores measured postoperatively when horses were administered phenylbutazone at a dose of 4 mg/kg intravenously before surgery and 2 mg/kg every 12 h following surgery. This study proved that the intravenous route of administration of phenylbutazone, when used perioperatively for postoperative pain, was effective. The belief among many clinicians is that phenylbutazone is more effective than flunixin and ketoprofen at providing analgesia for musculoskeletal pain. This has been substantiated by studies where a synovitis model was utilized to test the efficacy of each of these NSAIDs, and phenylbutazone provided improved efficacy over the others (Owens et al., 1996; McMurphy, 1998). Although phenylbutazone has the highest risk of toxicity compared to flunixin and ketoprofen, practitioners generally agree that its efficacy for orthopedic pain appears greatest. Despite this, interestingly, a recent study by Erkert et al. (2005) revealed no differences in analgesic effects between phenylbutazone and flunixin meglumine in horses with navicular syndrome when evaluated with force plate analysis. A recent study by Hu *et al.* (2005) revealed that phenylbutazone administered at a higher dosage (8.8 mg/kg) is no more efficacious than a standard dose (4.4 mg/kg) once daily intravenously. This is important, since phenylbutazone toxicity is commonly a result of overdosage of the drug.

Toxicity

The most common side-effects seen with phenylbutazone in a study in 1993 were hypoproteinemia, renal crest necrosis, and ulcer formation in the gastrointestinal tract (MacAllister *et al.*, 1993). When comparing phenylbutazone, flunixin, and ketoprofen, the toxic potential was greatest for phenylbutazone, less for flunixin, and least for ketoprofen. PBZ should not be administered in quantities above the loading dose of 4.4 mg/kg twice daily for two days followed by 2.2 mg/kg twice daily. Doses exceeding this recommendation are toxic and may result in anorexia, neutropenia, hypoproteinemia, and eventually death (Snow *et al.*, 1980). Postmortem examination of horses, ponies, and foals that died from PBZ toxicosis revealed gastrointestinal ulceration, renal papillary necrosis, and vascular thrombosis. Oral ulceration may also occur as a result of local toxicosis of orally administered PBZ (MacKay *et al.*, 1983). Caution should be taken when administering phenylbutazone to patients that are at a higher risk in developing these side-effects, and it should be noted that toxic effects of multiple NSAIDs at the same time are additive, since many have a common ability to inhibit cyclooxygenase.

7.8.1.2 Flunixin meglumine (Banamine®)

Pharmacokinetics

Unlike PBZ, the half-life of flunixin is relatively short, ranging from 1.6 to 2.5 h (Chay *et al.*, 1982). Peak plasma levels are quickly reached within 30 min following oral administration if horses are withheld from feed. However, peak plasma levels can be extended up to 7.5 h in horses allowed free access to feed (Welsh *et al.*, 1992). Similar plasma concentrations between oral and IV administration suggest complete gastrointestinal absorption (May and Lees, 1996).

Clinical applications

Flunixin meglumine is the second most commonly used NSAID in horses. Flunixin is used clinically at a dose of 1.1 mg/kg, given once daily by IV or oral routes. Although the mechanism of action is similar by blocking the COX pathway, its efficacy has been determined to be greater for visceral than for musculoskeletal pain. Horses do not seem to be as sensitive to the kidney perfusion problems that dogs and cats are, and therefore it is commonly used perioperatively. Although it is used orally and intravenously, it should not be used intramuscularly due to its potential to result in clostridial myonecrosis (Peek *et al.*, 2003). The onset of analgesia usually occurs within 2 h of administration and can persist up to 30 h. It is theorized that the rapid accumulation of the drug at the inflammatory foci is responsible for the long duration of action compared to the short plasma half-life.

In addition to being a widely popular drug used in treating equine abdominal pain, flunixin meglumine is also useful in treating musculoskeletal problems such as osteoarthritis (OA), but the cost-effectiveness of PBZ means that it is often chosen over flunixin meglumine. In an early study, flunixin was administered daily to 262 horses with various musculoskeletal diseases for up to five days (Houdeshell and Hennessey, 1977). In a study comparing postoperative analgesia of PBZ, flunixin, and carprofen, flunixin had the longest duration of analgesic effect (12.8 h) compared to PBZ (8.4 h) and carprofen (11.7 h) (Johnson et al., 1993). Further, an in vitro study of flunixin, PBZ, and carprofen showed decreased inflammation measured by prostaglandin E_2 (PGE_2) in lipopolysaccharide-challenged synovial explants.

In a study comparing effects of analgesia between flunixin meglumine, detomidine, and xylazine, flunixin meglumine was not as effective as detomidine and xylazine for abdominal pain. However, one benefit of flunixin meglumine is that most horses that have a strangulating lesion will 'break through' the abdominal pain to indicate a need for surgical intervention (Jochle et al., 1989).

Toxicity
Flunixin is a relatively safe NSAID with toxicity reported only when approximately five times the daily recommended dose of 1.1 mg/kg is administered (Houdeshell and Hennessey, 1977). Only one horse out of five developed renal crest necrosis in a study by MacAllister et al. (1993) in which five horses were given 1.1 mg/kg three times daily (twice more than the recommend administration) for 16 days. The intramuscular (IM) use should not be practiced due to clostridial myonecrosis that may subsequently develop following injection via this route (Peek et al., 2003).

7.8.1.3 Ketoprofen (Ketofen®)
Pharmacokinetics
Although 2.2 mg/kg is the recommended dose of administration in the adult, studies recommend increasing the dose to 1.5 times the recommended amount in foals less than 24 hours of age due to a large volume of distribution (Wilcke et al., 1998). It appears that the inflamed joint in equine models of synovial disease serves as a site of sequestration for ketoprofen, which may result in an improved and extended efficacy in inflamed joints compared to normal joints; however, improved efficacy has not been demonstrated (Owens et al., 1995a). When phenylbutazone was compared to ketoprofen in an acute synovitis model, phenylbutazone was superior in reducing lameness, joint temperature, synovial fluid volume, and synovial PGE_2 (Owens et al., 1996). Furthermore, the plasma pharmacokinetics may be altered by inflammation in peripheral compartments such as the joint. Ketoprofen is restricted to IV and IM administration, since no oral formulations exist. In an experiment where ketoprofen was administered orally as a micronized powder or an oil-based

paste, ketoprofen was not bioavailable, regardless of the feeding schedule (Landoni and Lees, 1995).

Clinical applications
Ketoprofen was originally proposed as a dual inhibitor of cyclooxygenase and 5-lipoxygenase (Betley *et al.*, 1991). This property would potentially broaden keto-profen's anti-inflammatory effects, making it a more effective NSAID. However, multiple *in vitro* and *in vivo* studies measuring leukotriene B4 (LTB4) levels following ketoprofen treatment of inflammation have refuted its superiority (Dawson *et al.*, 1982; Landoni and Lees, 1995).

Ketoprofen is still used and, although it has less risk of toxicity compared to phenylbutazone, its efficacy for musculoskeletal pain is not as good compared to phenylbutazone (Owens *et al.*, 1996).

Toxicity
Ketoprofen appears to have low toxicity in the horse. Its margin of safety appears to be much wider than for other NSAIDs such as PBZ. In a study by MacAllister *et al.* (1993), ketoprofen, PBZ, and flunixin were administered three times daily rather than the once-daily recommended dose for 12 days. Necropsy confirmed that horses administered ketoprofen did not have lesions, unlike horses in the other two groups, which developed stomach and intestinal lesions along with renal crest necrosis. Ketoprofen's propensity to accumulate at sites of acute inflammation and clear rapidly from the body may partially explain the low degree of toxicity (Owens *et al.*, 1995b).

7.8.1.4 Naproxen (NM®, Equiproxen®)
Pharmacokinetics
In the horse, bioavailability of the drug is approximately 50% and has an elimination half-life of approximately 4–5 h. Peak plasma levels are 2–3 h following administration (Tobin, 1979).

Clinical applications
Naproxen is usually administered orally at a dose of 10 mg/kg but can also be administered IV. A granule formulation exists for horses (Equiproxen) and administration at 10 mg/kg twice or once daily is recommended (Kallings, 1993). Tablets also exist in 250, 375 and 500 mg dosages, in addition to an oral suspension of 125 mg/5 ml (Naproxyn, Syntex). Often, horses will be placed on 10 mg/kg every other day for several weeks with very low morbidity associated with this dose. Efficacy of naproxen in treating OA has not been compared to PBZ and flunixin; therefore, it is difficult to comment on its effectiveness compared to conventionally used drugs. The closeness between its anti-inflammatory and analgesic doses suggests that naproxen may have a greater anti-inflammatory effect than PBZ and aspirin due to its ability to decrease leukocyte migration more than other NSAIDs

(Higgs *et al.*, 1980). Naproxen was more effective than PBZ in providing analgesia in an induced model of myositis (Jones and Hamm, 1978). This may suggest that it is an appropriate NSAID for treating inflammatory swelling and associated lameness.

Toxicity

Naproxen has a wide margin of safety. Naproxen did not show any signs of toxicity when given at three times the recommended dose for 42 days (Tobin, 1979). Furthermore, naproxen given for three weeks, with the last seven days at twice the recommended dose, resulted in no change in protein.

7.8.1.5 Carprofen (Rimadyl®)

Pharmacokinetics

Carprofen's mechanism of action has not been fully elucidated (Armstrong and Lees, 2002). Studies show that moderate inhibition of COX occurs *in vitro* (Armstrong *et al.*, 1999), with *in vivo* studies showing only minimal inhibition (Lees *et al.*, 1994). Like ketoprofen, carprofen exists as two enantiomers but with a much longer half-life of 18–22 h (May and Lees, 1996). Pharmacokinetic studies revealed some COX-2 selective inhibition; however, various doses tested revealed different selective COX-2 inhibition (Beretta *et al.*, 2005).

Clinical applications

Carprofen is administered IV at a dose of 0.7 mg/kg or orally at 1.4 mg/kg (twice the recommended dose) in the horse. Currently, this drug is only licensed in the USA for use in dogs but it is commonly used 'off-label' in the horse. The existing pharmacokinetic data support once-daily dosing (May and Lees, 1996). Carprofen's efficacy has been shown in various *in vivo* trials using a heating element and balloon model to assess its effect on visceral pain (Schatzmann *et al.*, 1992). Carprofen's efficacy has also been compared with that of PBZ and flunixin in a clinical study that measured duration of analgesia for abdominal pain postoperatively (Johnson *et al.*, 1993). Carprofen provided adequate analgesia for 11.7 h, just behind flunixin at 12.7 h. PBZ provided only 8.4 h.

Carprofen may have a niche in treating OA. Unlike many NSAIDs, carprofen appears to have potentially beneficial effects on proteoglycan metabolism of equine chondrocytes (Armstrong and Mow, 1982). In an *in vitro* study, carprofen significantly decreased PGE_2 production by unstimulated chondrocytes, and antagonized the increase in PGE production induced by interleukin-1 (IL-1) (Armstrong and Lees, 1999). It also appears to increase proteoglycan synthesis and decrease glycosaminoglycan (GAG) release from cartilage. These findings have also been shown in canines, using both explants and chondrocytes in monolayer and measuring GAG synthesis, cell viability, and prostaglandin release following exposure to carprofen (Benton *et al.*, 1997). If these *in vitro* results can be repeated in the horse, carprofen may become the NSAID of choice in the future.

Toxicity
Carprofen is well tolerated at the recommended oral or IV dose of 0.7 mg/kg but is
not recommended for IM use because of muscle necrosis (Lees *et al.*, 1994). Three
out of six horses developed subcutaneous edema not related to hypoproteinemia on
day 7 when given carprofen at twice the recommended oral dose for 14 days (May
and Lees, 1996). Clinicians in our hospital often use carprofen in foals rather than
PBZ due to the ease of oral administration and its apparent lesser toxicity compared to PBZ.

7.8.1.6 Firocoxib (Equioxx®)
Pharmacokinetics
Firocoxib is a fast-acting COX inhibitor (coxib) highly specific for the type-2 inducible isoform and is the first highly selective inhibitor of COX-2 developed specifically for veterinary use in the horse. Its development and use are aimed at reducing
the side-effects associated with COX-1 and COX-2 inhibitors (Back *et al.*, 2009).

Clinical applications
Firocoxib appears to have value in its ability to adequately decrease lameness associated with chronic lameness in horses (Back *et al.*, 2009). In this study, 64 horses
were evaluated with chronic lameness using force plate analysis. Firocoxib appeared
to decrease lameness significantly within the first day of dosing. The effective dose
appeared to be 0.1 mg/kg orally once daily. No apparent side-effects were reported
in this study. In another large-scale field study, the analgesic effects on musculoskeletal pain were compared to PBZ, and comparable effects were noted (Doucet *et al.*,
2008). Currently the main disadvantage to firocoxib is its expense compared to
PBZ. If the cost ultimately is reduced, it is most likely that use of this NSAID will
be much more common.

Toxicity
In a toxicity study in the horse, firocoxib was not associated with gastrointestinal
tract ulceration when administered at recommended dosages, and increases in
prevalence of reversible oral mucosal lesions and classic NSAID-associated neph-
ropathy were detected only when dosages 3–5 times the recommended level were
administered for 30–90 days. Thus, firocoxib appears to be a safe alternative to the
long-term use of phenylbutazone (FDA, 2006).

7.8.2 Topical NSAIDs
While orally administered non-steroidal drugs remain one of the frontline treatments for lameness, recent studies suggest that the non-steroidal drug Surpass®
(diclofenac) has excellent absorbance into tissues through the skin (Lynn *et al.*,
2004; Caldwell *et al.*, 2004), and significantly reduces inflammation associated
with osteoarthritis (Frisbie *et al.*, 2009). In horses that had induced osteoarthritis,
the last study revealed significant improvement in glycosaminoglycan content and

reduction in subchondral bone sclerosis and cartilage erosion (Frisbie *et al.*, 2009). This non-steroidal drug is absorbed via a liposomal suspension that delivers the drug to deeper subcutaneous tissues. Little to no toxicity has been appreciated with this formulation, and it appears to be an excellent adjunct to oral NSAID administration.

7.8.3 Local anesthetics

Local anesthetic drugs have historically been administered to horses by many routes. They mediate analgesia by blocking neural conduction from the periphery and therefore reduce input to the central nervous system. Most commonly they are used subcutaneously to facilitate repair of a laceration, perineurally or intra-articularly during lameness examinations, and epidurally to facilitate perineal procedures. Their administration via these routes in the anesthetized horse as a means to provide perioperative analgesia is increasingly common. For example, anesthetics may be 'splashed' on or infiltrated in and around (e.g., intra-testicular prior to castration) the surgical site. While maximum doses of 1–2 mg/kg may be reached when administering the drug subcutaneously, they are rarely necessary for administration by other routes. Since residual proprioceptive deficits and/or motor blockade (which might influence anesthetic recovery) are possible with certain perineural blocks or epidural administration, many favor lidocaine, which has a short duration of action, and limit both the volume and dose (e.g., 5 ml of 2% lidocaine to an adult horse at sacrococcygeal location). When administered intra-articularly, a volume consistent with the size of the joint is recommended (e.g., 3–5 ml for smaller joints and 10 ml for larger joints). Chondrocyte toxicity when using this route is reported to be less with 1% and 2% lidocaine than with 0.5% bupivacaine (Karpie and Chu, 2007; Chu *et al.*, 2006).

Because of the success of these techniques in managing pain in horses, there is interest in utilizing them on a longer-term basis both in the postoperative period and in the management of chronic pain. A simple, non-invasive approach is application of the transdermal lidocaine patch similar to that available for diclofenac. Although application via this route does not provide sufficient uptake of local anesthetic for systemic effects, it may have local benefit over a site of injury. Epidural catheters have long been in use in horses but are not typically utilized with local anesthetics due to fear of motor blockade. With the development of local anesthetics with differential effects on sensory and motor actions (e.g., ropivacaine), this may become less of an issue in time. Recently, a novel technique of using a catheter for sustained perineural blockade of the limb has been described by Zarucco *et al.* (2007) and Driessen *et al.* (2008a). While currently experimental, this technique may provide an option for longer-term management of horses with diseases such as laminitis.

Systemic administration of local anesthetics has also been described. Owing to its cardiovascular safety in comparison to drugs like bupivacaine, lidocaine is most commonly administered when using this route. Its intravenous use was advocated upon its discovery as a prokinetic agent in horses, and it is now commonly administered to both awake and anesthetized horses at 30–70 μg/kg min (micrograms per kilogram per minute). While the mechanism remains unclear, many horses appear to benefit from systemic lidocaine administration, which is thought to be in part mediated through its analgesic actions. This belief has led to its widespread use as an intravenous analgesic, and at least one study in non-anesthetized horses supports its efficacy as a somatic analgesic (Robertson *et al.*, 2005). Dose reduction of the inhaled anesthetic has the added benefit of cost savings, especially with newer inhalants.

7.8.3.1 Lidocaine
Lidocaine is a short-acting anesthetic with a rapid onset of action. The effects last approximately 1.5–2 h, and onset is seen in less than 10 min. The most common use for lidocaine is peripheral nerve blocks and epidurals. It has been shown to significantly decrease the pain withdrawal reflex (Kamerling, 1993). Common CNS toxicity signs can include convulsions, coma, and respiratory arrest. The maximum safe dose is 4 mg/kg (0.4 ml/kg of a 1% solution, subcutaneously) (Baller and Hendrickson, 2002).

7.8.3.2 Mepivacaine
Mepivacaine is the most widely used local anesthetic in equine practice. Its duration is similar to lidocaine (slightly longer), but it has less vasodilatory effects and causes less local edema in tissues (Baller and Hendrickson, 2002). It is used frequently for nerve blocks, epidurals, and intra-articular anesthesia.

7.8.3.3 Bupivacaine
Bupivacaine is the most potent and longest-lasting local anesthetic. It tends to have a slower onset (longer than 10 minutes) but has a duration of action of 3–8 h. Bupivacaine is more commonly administered for postoperative musculoskeletal pain relief. It has been found to provide analgesia for extended periods of time, yet does not significantly interfere with motor function (Baller and Hendrickson, 2002). Bupivacaine has been found to be more cardiotoxic than other local anesthetics, however, and it can cause ventricular arrhythmias and myocardial depression (Nolan, 2000). The maximum safe dose has been found to be 1–2 mg/kg (0.4–0.8 ml/kg of a 0.25% solution, subcutaneously). This drug should not be administered intravenously.

7.8.4 Intra-articular analgesics
Intra-articular use of analgesics has been very successful at controlling joint-related pain. It offers direct control at the site of inflammation and does not interfere with proprioception. The agents covered in this section will be local anesthetics and opioids. Corticosteroids and hyaluronic acid formulations are also commonly used to decrease pain and inflammation, but are beyond the scope of this chapter,

and should not be classified as analgesics. For a thorough review of various steroid and hyaluronic acid formulations used intra-articularly, please see Goodrich and Nixon (2006). The mechanism of action of local anesthetics was covered in section 7.8.3, and they act similarly to peripheral nerve anesthesia by blocking neuronal signals. Opioids produce analgesia by binding the mu, kappa, or sigma receptors in the CNS. Mu receptor-selective opioids include morphine, fentanyl, and oxymorphone. Opioids reduce the sensation of pain and have been shown to produce analgesia when injected locally into a site of inflammation. Human trials have shown that low doses of morphine administered intra-articularly (0.5–6 mg) produced long-lasting periods (up to 48 h) of analgesia in patients following orthopedic surgery (Kazemi *et al.*, 2004).

7.8.4.1 Intra-articular mepivacaine, bupivacaine and lidocaine
Clinicians typically inject joints intra-articularly with mepivacaine to anesthetize them to aid in lameness diagnosis. The volume used is typically based on the volume of the joint to be injected. Effects usually last between 30 min and 1 h following injection. Recently, new data suggest that intra-articular lidocaine and bupivacaine may be toxic to cartilage (Chu *et al.*, 2008; Karpie and Chu, 2007). To date, no studies have been done to evaluate the most commonly used intra-articular anesthetic, mepivacaine, in the horse. Further evaluations need to be done in the horse joint to evaluate lidocaine, bupivacaine, and mepivacaine, and assess any potential toxic effects. To date, the authors recommend caution with using lidocaine and bupivacaine intra-articularly before dosing trials to establish any toxic effects that may exist.

7.8.4.2 Intra-articular morphine
Morphine has been used successfully in human clinical trials to provide intra-articular pain management. A recent study by Santos *et al.* (2009) compared intra-articular ropivacaine (similar properties of bupivacaine) to morphine and a ropivacaine–morphine combination. The horses had an experimentally induced synovitis and obtained the greatest level of analgesia with the morphine–ropivacaine combination. Morphine alone resulted in excellent analgesia for 24 h. The onset of action was delayed, however, and the authors concluded that an earlier onset of action could be achieved with a ropivacaine–morphine combination. This is the first study to evaluate intra-articular morphine in the horse. Analgesic effects suggest that mu receptors are present within the synovium. Advantages of using intra-articular morphine may be that it is inexpensive, easily administered, and specific for the surgical site.

7.8.5 Alpha-2 agonists
Many alpha-2 agonist drugs (xylazine, detomidine, romifidine, medetomidine, dexmedetomidine) are available to the equine practitioner. Alpha-2 agonists mediate their effects via receptors of the central descending inhibitory pain pathways. Receptors are also found in the periphery (e.g., joints). Their use is widespread, in

part because these drugs not only provide reliable sedation but also are among the most reliable analgesics available for horses. They are used by intravenous bolus and infusion to facilitate standing procedures and are the mainstay of anesthetic premedication, where they also provide a significant anesthetic sparing effect: xylazine (0.5–1 mg/kg IV) reduces the dose requirement for inhaled anesthetics by 25–35% at one hour post-administration (Steffey *et al.*, 2000). When given by infusion, these drugs provide sustained sedative and analgesic effects. For example, detomidine infusions reduce the dose requirement of halothane by up to 55% (Dunlop *et al.*, 1991). Medetomidine (3.5 µg/kg h) facilitates completion of painful procedures in standing horses (Bettschart-Wolfensberger *et al.*, 1999) and reduces the dose requirement for inhaled agent (Neges *et al.*, 2003).

Unfortunately, in addition to sedation, which may be considered a side-effect when only analgesia is required, alpha-2 agonists significantly decrease cardiac output when given by intravenous bolus. Additionally, urine output is increased and appetite and gastrointestinal motility reduced following these drugs. While these side-effects may be managed in most instances, they should be considered when using these drugs for long-term administration as analgesics. Intramuscular and epidural administration have been advocated as a means to reduce the systemic effects. Unfortunately, while side-effects are reduced following intramuscular administration of detomidine, beneficial effects were also of a lesser magnitude and lasted a shorter duration when compared to administration of the same dose intravenously (Mama *et al.*, 2009). When administered epidurally, lipophilic drugs such as detomidine tend to be systemically absorbed, whereas non-lipophilic drugs such as xylazine are not. Xylazine has been used intra-articularly and shows promise as an analgesic when administered by this route.

7.8.6 Opioids

Like alpha-2 agonists, opioids mediate their effects by receptors located both centrally and peripherally, and their analgesic efficacy is well documented in dogs and primates. While most would agree that opioids have a beneficial role in modifying behavior when used in conjunction with sedative (e.g., xylazine) or tranquilizing (e.g., acepromazine) drugs in the horse, the analgesic actions of the opioids appear to be inconsistent and have led to significant controversy among clinicians. When efficacy is shown, it is often at doses that are not clinically useful due to behavioral side-effects, ranging from excitation to recumbency. For example, butorphanol did provide analgesia for a short duration (1–2 h) at doses (0.1–0.2 mg/kg or 50–100 mg for a 500 kg horse) that most practitioners would not find either practical to administer or economically viable. However, there is also literature where results support the premise that opioids have analgesic benefits at clinically useful doses, and it is primarily these results that continue to fuel the ongoing use and study of opioids as analgesics in the horse. Results of one such study suggest that horses given morphine perioperatively needed less additional anesthetic medication and had better recoveries (presumed to be due to improved analgesia) than those receiving a standard analgesic protocol (Clark *et al.*, 2005, 2008). Another report states that butorphanol when given by infusion had lower cortisol levels and a shortened hospital stay in horses following colic surgery (Sellon *et al.*, 2004). Yet another (Thomasy *et al.*, 2004) suggests an analgesic effect of the fentanyl patch when used with NSAID.

When efficacy is not shown, much discussion is raised about whether the models used to test analgesia are appropriate. Until recently, most studies evaluating opioid analgesia used anesthetic dose reduction as an indicator of analgesia. Interestingly, when evaluated in this manner, none of the mu opioid drugs studied (alfentanil, morphine) showed a consistent effect on anesthetic dose requirement – in fact, in most cases the inhaled dose requirement was increased even at doses and plasma drug concentrations that have been shown to be analgesic in other species (Steffey *et al.*, 2003; Pascoe *et al.*, 1993; DiMaio Knych *et al.*, 2009). Butorphanol had a more variable effect on inhaled anesthetic dose requirement, raising it in some ponies and lowering it in others (Matthews and Lindsay, 1990). While it is possible that CNS stimulation as seen in non-anesthetized horses after opioid administration may mitigate the anesthetic sparing effect caused by analgesia, it is noteworthy that the addition of morphine to alpha-2 drugs did not change the anesthetic requirement beyond that noted for the alpha-2 agent alone (Bennett *et al.*, 2004). Similarly, a study in non-anesthetized horses using dental dolorimetry to test analgesia supports the lack of any additive or synergistic analgesic activity of alpha-2 and opioid combinations (Brunson and Majors, 1987). In a recent study evaluating intravenous fentanyl in non-anesthetized horses, the authors were not able to demonstrate any analgesic benefit using a thermal threshold or gastrointestinal distention model (Sanchez *et al.*, 2007).

Opioid-induced side-effects must also be weighed when considering their systemic use in the horse. Beside behavioral effects, perhaps the most significant side-effect of opioids in horses is gastrointestinal stasis, which, as reported by Boscan *et al.* (2006), can be of significant duration. Given these controversies, many individuals opt to use opioids via non-systemic routes such as epidurally or intra-articularly. Unlike with systemic opioids, epidural opioids (morphine, meperidine, methadone, etc.) have consistently been shown to have drug- and dose-dependent analgesic effects with minimal systemic side-effects. Intra-articular use has also been advocated, as evidence shows the presence of opioid receptors in equine joints.

7.8.7 Dissociatives

Equine veterinarians are familiar with the use of ketamine for induction of anesthesia in horses. It has also been used by many with inhaled anesthetics due to its anesthetic sparing effect. Recently, it has been suggested that, as in human and canine patients, it may be effective at reducing 'wind-up' or up-regulation of the nervous system during chronic pain states. This effect is seen in other species during infusions of extremely low doses (2–10 µg/kg min) and has been used clinically for this purpose in both the anesthetized and the non-sedated horse. The user should note that, while uncommon, an occasional non-sedated horse will manifest behavioral changes even at these low doses. Ketamine has also been recently advocated for use as part of standing chemical restraint protocols. Recent investigations (A.E. Wagner *et al.*, unpublished data) suggest that, while there may be a benefit in some horses, this is very transient, and ataxia (beyond that seen with alpha-2 agonist–butorphanol combinations) is a common side-effect.

7.8.8 Epidural analgesia

Epidural analgesia has grown in its popularity in the last ten years (Martin *et al.*, 2003; Sysel *et al.*, 1996, 1997; Goodrich *et al.*, 2002). The benefits of epidural analgesia are primarily focused on the hind limbs, since front limb pain does not seem to be reduced even with large volumes of drugs delivered through epidural catheters placed at cervical vertebrae C1–C2 (Martin *et al.*, 2003). Epidural analgesia is an excellent adjunctive way to provide analgesia and has several benefits when given preoperatively, such as reducing the need for intra-operative drug therapy, reducing the need for higher concentrations of gas anesthetics, and improved recoveries (Goodrich *et al.*, 2000). Many different drug combinations are reported for epidural analgesia, with xylazine, detomidine, and morphine being the most commonly used combinations. Advantages in using these drugs is that there is no loss of motor function to the hind limbs and excellent analgesia is provided (Sysel *et al.*, 1996). One of the most common combinations reported is morphine at 0.2 mg/kg and detomidine at 0.03 mg/kg, which is brought up to 20 ml with saline if administering through a needle or an epidural catheter (Sysel *et al.*, 1996; Goodrich *et al.*, 2002). One of the present authors (L.G.) has found that this dose of morphine may predispose to decreased gut motility and currently uses 0.1 mg/kg of morphine combined with detomidine at the above dosage, which provides excellent analgesia. When this combination was administered preoperatively to horses undergoing bilateral hind limb arthroscopies, significant analgesia was provided (Goodrich *et al.*, 2002). Furthermore, stress as measured by cortisol levels was significantly reduced intra-operatively (Goodrich *et al.*, 2000). The technique of administration is the standard approach to delivering epidural drugs through a needle placed in between coccygeal vertebrae 1 and 2 and advancing to the epidural space.

7.8.8.1 Analgesia through epidural catheters

If the clinician expects ongoing pain postoperatively, an epidural catheter can be placed preoperatively, and epidural drugs may be delivered by this route. One of the authors (L.G.) has placed more that 50 catheters preoperatively to deliver analgesic drugs, and has not had a problem with the catheters becoming dislodged during or post-recovery. Epidural catheter placement is an effective way to continue delivery of drugs postoperatively, and long-term placement for three weeks has not resulted in any long-term detrimental effects (Sysel *et al.*, 1997). Epidural catheter placement is easy and horses appear to tolerate them well (Figure 7.3). A detailed description of epidural catheter placement is available elsewhere (Goodrich and Nixon, 2003).

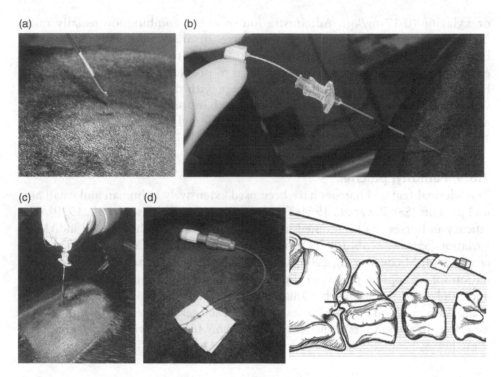

Figure 7.3 The insertion of an epidural catheter, which can be placed pre- or postoperatively to supply excellent analgesia for hind limb orthopedic or soft tissue pain.

There are many individual and combined analgesic drug choices available for perioperative epidural use. Common combinations are opioids such as morphine and alpha-2 agonists such as xylazine or detomidine (Muir, 1998). These combinations have proved to be excellent for providing good analgesia prior to general anesthesia, and a more in-depth coverage of the use of these drugs perioperatively is available (Bennett and Steffey, 2002).

7.8.8.2 Continuation of epidural analgesia

If an epidural catheter is placed for long-term pain management, administration of analgesics can be continued for several weeks through this route (Sysel *et al.*, 1997; Martin *et al.*, 2003). If not placed preoperatively, then postoperative placement should be considered for horses with ongoing moderate to severe pain of the hind limbs. The authors have placed many epidural catheters in horses with fractures, septic joints, and various conditions causing hind limb pain, with excellent results. The most common combination used in this situation is a combination of morphine (0.1 mg/kg) and either detomidine (0.03 mg/kg) or xylazine (0.17 mg/kg). Administration of either combination usually takes 20–30 minutes for the combination to have an analgesic effect and can last between 12 and 36 hours depending on the severity of pain. In the authors' experience, detomidine and morphine seem to provide greater analgesia and to last a longer length of time. The disadvantage with this combination is that the sedative effects of the detomidine are greater than for the xylazine and may last approximately 30–40 minutes, compared to the xylazine, which seems to last 10–15 minutes.

7.8.9 Fentanyl patches

Transdermal fentanyl patches have been used extensively in human and small animal patients (Sandler *et al.*, 1994; Franks *et al.*, 2000; Robinson *et al.*, 1999). The efficacy in horses has been tested in the last few years and has shown individual variation (Sanchez *et al.*, 2007; Orsini *et al.*, 2006; Mills and Cross, 2007; Thomasy *et al.*, 2004; Maxwell *et al.*, 2003; Kamerling *et al.*, 1985). The current recommendation for orthopedic pain is to clip the cephalic or saphenous region of the limb and apply two patches each 10 mg. The time for absorption can vary between 2 and 14 hours, and in some horses may not reach serum levels to have an analgesic effect. In the authors' experience, there seems to be individual variation, with some horses benefiting and some not.

7.8.10 Continuous peripheral nerve block

Methods to provide excellent analgesia to the front limbs continues to evade orthopedic surgeons, such that support limb laminitis continues to be a common sequella to ongoing front limb pain. A method to provide a continuous block with regional anesthesia has been investigated by implanting catheters subcutaneously at the medial and lateral palmar nerves (Driessen *et al.*, 2008b). The continuous infusion appears to be efficacious; however, distal limb swelling associated with the catheters appears to be problematic. Furthermore, if metal implantation is present, the risk of introducing infection subcutaneously may outweigh the benefit of placement of these catheters. Further study is needed in this particular instrumentation to provide analgesia; however, they may have a place in future management of orthopedic pain.

7.8.11 Continuous intravenous infusions

Continuous rate intravenous infusions of drugs such as ketamine, lidocaine, and butorphanol have been studied to supply analgesia in horses (Peterbauer *et al.*, 2008; Sellon *et al.*, 2004; Malone *et al.*, 2006). Most studies using these drugs have examined their effects on gastrointestinal pain and not orthopedic pain. The effects of these infusions appear to provide some benefit to the equine patient suffering from gastrointestinal pain. Studies need to be performed on horses with orthopedic pain before such infusions can be recommended.

7.8.12 Other analgesic drugs

7.8.12.1 Gabapentin

Gabapentin is an anticonvulsant drug used for treatment of partial seizures in human patients and has been suggested as a treatment for chronic and specifically neuropathic pain. Pharmacokinetic analysis in horses shows that the drug is absorbed when given orally (albeit to a lesser degree than in other species). Peak concentrations in plasma were reached at approximately 90 minutes after an oral dose of 5 mg/kg in four horses. The elimination half-life was 3.4 h (Dirikolu *et al.*, 2008). In addition to the pharmacokinetic data, there is one published report of the use of gabapentin in a clinical patient. The report discusses a beneficial effect and no side-effects following twice daily administration of 2.5 mg/kg to a near-term draft mare with a presumed neuropathy (Davis *et al.*, 2007).

7.8.12.2 Sarapin

Sarapin is a natural product distilled from the pitcher plant and has been used as a regional analgesic agent for control of pain of neuralgic origin. Its mechanism of action has not been elucidated. This product has been used for centuries in human medicine, but the literature largely consists of clinical experiences. A study by Harkins *et al.* (1997) compared the anesthetic effects of this agent to saline and bupivacaine on research horses in which the hoof withdrawal reflex was compared. In this study, sarapin was not found to be significantly different from saline. The authors concluded that, if sarapin had a significant effect on decreasing pain, it likely had a greater effect on reducing chronic pain rather than acute pain mechanisms tested in this study.

7.9 Summary

In the last decade, pain management has played a larger part in equine welfare. Epidural management of hind limb pain has played an important role in providing analgesic benefits to the equine patient. Furthermore, pre-emptive analgesia has been demonstrated to have beneficial effects on minimizing postoperative pain and some of the complications associated with ongoing pain. Equine clinicians are becoming aware of the benefits that well-planned analgesia initiated early in the pain process can improve, enhance, and extend the life of the horse. Further studies on more effective analgesia will hopefully be forthcoming and add more options to providing effective pain management to equine patients.

References

Armstrong, C.G. and Mow, V.C. (1982) Variations in the intrinsic mechanical properties of human articular cartilage with age, degeneration, and water content. *Journal of Bone and Joint Surgery* 64-A, 88–94.

Armstrong, S. and Lees, P. (1999) Effects of R and S enantiomers and a racemic mixture of carprofen on the production and release of proteoglycan and prostaglandin E$_2$ from equine chondrocytes and cartilage explants. *American Journal of Veterinary Research* 60, 98–104.

Armstrong, S. and Lees, P. (2002) Effects of carprofen (R and S enantiomers and racemate) on the production of IL-1, IL-6 and TNF-alpha by equine chondrocytes and synoviocytes. *Journal of Veterinary Pharmacology and Therapeutics* 25, 145–153.

Armstrong, S., Tricklebank, P., Lake, A., Frean, S. and Lees, P. (1999) Pharmacokinetics of carprofen enantiomers in equine plasma and synovial fluid. *Journal of Veterinary Pharmacology and Therapeutics* 22, 196–201.

Back, W., MacAllister, C.G., van Heel, M.C., Pollmeier, M. and Hanson, P.D. (2009) The use of force plate measurements to titrate the dosage of a new COX-2 inhibitor in lame horses. *Equine Veterinary Journal* 41, 309–312.

Baller, L.S. and Hendrickson, D.A. (2002) Management of equine orthopedic pain. *Veterinary Clinics of North America: Equine Practice* 18, 117–131.

Bennett, R.C. and Steffey, E.P. (2002) Use of opioids for pain and anesthetic management in horses. *Veterinary Clinics of North America: Equine Practice* 18, 47–60.

Bennett, R.C., Steffey, E.P., Kollias-Baker, C. and Sams, R. (2004) Influence of morphine sulfate on the halothane sparing effect of xylazine hydrochloride in horses. *American Journal of Veterinary Research* 65, 519–526.

Benton, H.P., Vasseur, P.B., Broderick-Villa, G.A. and Koolpe, M. (1997) Effect of carprofen on sulfated glycosaminoglycan metabolism, protein synthesis, and prostaglandin release by cultured osteoarthritic canine chondrocytes. *American Journal of Veterinary Research* 58, 286–292.

Beretta, C., Garavaglia, G. and Cavalli, M. (2005) COX-1 and COX-2 inhibition in horse blood by phenylbutazone, flunixin, carprofen and meloxicam: an in vitro analysis. *Pharmacological Research* 52, 302–306.

Betley, M., Sutherland, S.F., Gregoricka, M.J. and Pollett, R.A. (1991) The analgesic effect of ketoprofen for use in treating equine colic as compared to flunixin meglumine. *Equine Practice* 13, 11–16.

Bettschart-Wolfensberger, R., Clarke, K.W., Vainio, O., Aliabadi, F. and Demuth, D. (1999) Pharmacokinetics of medetomidine in ponies and elaboration of a medetomidine infusion regime which provides a constant level of sedation. *Research in Veterinary Science* 67, 41–46.

Boscan, P., Van Hoogmoed, L.M., Farver, T.B. and Snyder, J.R. (2006) Evaluation of the effects of the opioid agonist morphine on gastrointestinal tract function in horses. *American Journal of Veterinary Research* 67, 992–997.

Brunson, D.B. and Majors, L.J. (1987) Comparative analgesia of xylazine, xylazine/morphine, xylazine/butorphanol, and xylazine/nalbuphine in the horse, using dental dolorimetry. *American Journal of Veterinary Research* 48, 1087–1091.

Bussieres, G., Jacques, C., Lainay, O., Beauchamp, G., Leblond, A., Cadore, J.L. *et al.* (2008) Development of a composite orthopaedic pain scale in horses. *Research in Veterinary Science* 85, 294–306.

Caldwell, F.J., Mueller, P.O., Lynn, R.C. and Budsberg, S.C. (2004) Effect of topical application of diclofenac liposomal suspension on experimentally induced subcutaneous inflammation in horses. *American Journal of Veterinary Research* **65**, 271–276.

Capdevila, X., Barthelet, Y., Biboulet, P., Ryckwaert, Y., Rubenovitch, J. and d'Athis, F.
(1999) Effects of perioperative analgesic technique on the surgical outcome and duration
of rehabilitation after major knee surgery. *Anesthesiology* **91**, 8–15.

Chay, S., Woods, W.E. and Nugent, T. (1982) The pharmacology of nonsteroidal anti-
inflammatory drugs in the horse: flunixin meglumine (Banamine). *Equine Practice* **4**, 16–23.

Chu, C.R., Izzo, N.J., Papas, N.E. and Fu, F.H. (2006) In vitro exposure to 0.5% bupivacaine is cytotoxic to bovine articular chondrocytes. *Arthroscopy* **22**, 693–699.

Chu, C.R., Izzo, N.J., Coyle, C.H., Papas, N.E. and Logar, A. (2008) The in vitro effects of
bupivacaine on articular chondrocytes. *Journal of Bone and Joint Surgery (British Volume)*
90, 814–820.

Clark, L., Clutton, R.E., Blissitt, K.J. and Chase-Topping, M.E. (2005) Effects of perioperative morphine administration during halothane anaesthesia in horses. *Veterinary
Anaesthesia and Analgesia* **32**, 10–15.

Clark, L., Clutton, R.E., Blissitt, K.J. and Chase-Topping, M.E. (2008) The effects of
morphine on the recovery of horses from halothane anaesthesia. *Veterinary Anaesthesia
and Analgesia* **35**, 22–29.

Collins, L.G. and Tyler, D.E. (1984) Phenylbutazone toxicosis in the horse: a clinical study.
Journal of the American Veterinary Medical Association **184**, 699–703.

Courouce, A., Geffroy, O., Chatard, J.C. and Auvinet, B. (1996) Significance of high heart
rate recorded during standardized field exercise tests in the detection of orthopaedic
diseases in Standardbred trotters. *Pferdeheilkunde* **12**, 588–593.

Davis, J.L., Posner, L.P. and Elce, Y. (2007) Gabapentin for the treatment of neuropathic
pain in a pregnant horse. *Journal of the American Veterinary Medical Association* **231**,
755–758.

Dawson, W., Boot, J.R., Harvey, J. and Walker, J.R. (1982) The pharmacology of benoxa-
profen with particular to effects on lipoxygenase product formation. *European Journal of
Rheumatology and Inflammation* **5**, 61–68.

DiMaio Knych, H.K., Steffey, E.P., Mama, K.R. and Stanley, S.D. (2009) Effects of high
plasma fentanyl concentrations on minimum alveolar concentration of isoflurane in
horses. *American Journal of Veterinary Research*, **70**(10), 1193–1200.

Dirikolu, L., Dafalla, A., Ely, K.J., Connerly, A.L., Jones, C.N., ElkHoly, H., Lehner, A.F.,
Thompson, K. and Tobin, T. (2008) Pharmacokinetics of gabapentin in horses. *Journal of
Veterinary Pharmacology and Therapeutics* **31**, 175–177.

Doria, R.G., Valadao, C.A., Duque, J.C., Farias, A., Almeida, R.M. and Netto, A.C. (2008)
Comparative study of epidural xylazine or clonidine in horses. *Veterinary Anaesthesia and
Analgesia* **35**, 166–172.

Doucet, M.Y., Bertone, A.L., Hendrickson, D., Hughes, F., MacAllister, C., McClure, S.
et al. (2008) Comparison of efficacy and safety of paste formulations of firocoxib and
phenylbutazone in horses with naturally occurring osteoarthritis. *Journal of the American
Veterinary Medical Association* **232**, 91–97.

Driessen, B., Scandella, M. and Zarucco, L. (2008a) Development of a technique for continuous perineural blockade of palmar nerves in the distal equine forelimb. *Veterinary Anaesthesia and Analgesia*, **35**, 432–438.

Driessen, B., Scandella, M. and Zarucco, L. (2008b) Development of a technique for continuous perineural blockade of the palmar nerves in the distal equine thoracic limb. *Veterinary Anaesthesia and Analgesia* **35**, 432–448.

Dunlop, C.I., Daunt, D.A. and Chapman, P.L. (1991) Anesthetic potency of three steady-state plasma levels of detomidine in halothane-anesthetized horses. In *Proceedings of the Fourth International Congress of Veterinary Anesthesia*, 7.

Erkert, R.S., MacAllister, C.G., Payton, M.E. and Clarke, C.R. (2005) Use of force plate analysis to compare the analgesic effects of intravenous administration of phenylbutazone and flunixin meglumine in horses with navicular syndrome. *American Journal of Veterinary Research* **66**, 284–288.

FDA (2006) Freedom of information summary. Equioxx oral paste – 0.82% firocoxib (w/w). Food and Drug Administration, Rockville, MD.

Firth, A.M. and Haldane, S.L. (1999) Development of a scale to evaluate postoperative pain in dogs. *Journal of the American Veterinary Medical Association* **214**, 651–659.

Franks, J.N., Boothe, H.W., Taylor, L., Geller, S., Carroll, G.L., Cracas, V. *et al.* (2000) Evaluation of transdermal fentanyl patches for analgesia in cats undergoing onychectomy. *Journal of the American Veterinary Medical Association* **217**, 1013–1020.

Frisbie, D.D., McIlwraith, C.W., Kawcak, C.E., Werpy, N.M. and Pearce, G.L. (2009) Evaluation of topically administered diclofenac liposomal cream for treatment of horses with experimentally induced osteoarthritis. *American Journal of Veterinary Research* **70**, 210–215.

Geiser, D.R. (1990) Chemical restraint and analgesia in the horse. *Veterinary Clinics of North America: Equine Practice* **6**, 495–512.

Goodrich, L.R. and Nixon, A.J. (2003) How to alleviate acute and chronic hind limb pain in horses. In *Proceedings of the 49th Annual Convention of the AAEP*, pp. 262–267.

Goodrich, L.R. and Nixon, A.J. (2006) Medical treatment of osteoarthritis in the horse – a review. *Veterinary Journal* **171**, 51–69.

Goodrich, L.R., Butler, E., Donaldson, L., Warnick, L.R., Nixon, A.J., Fortier, L.A. *et al.* (2000) The efficacy of epidurally administered morphine and detomidine in decreasing stress levels under general anesthesia and the effect on anesthetic recoveries. *Veterinary Surgery* **29**, 463.

Goodrich, L.R., Nixon, A.J., Fubini, S.L., Ducharme, N.G., Fortier, L.A., Warnick, L.D. *et al.* (2002) Epidural morphine and detomidine decreases postoperative hindlimb lameness in horses after bilateral stifle arthroscopy. *Veterinary Surgery* **31**, 232–239.

Halverson, P.B. (1999) Nonsteroidal antiinflammatory drugs: benefits, risks, and COX-2 selectivity. *Orthopaedic Nursing* **18**, 21–26.

Harkins, J.D., Mundy, G.D., Stanley, S.D., Sams, R.A. and Tobin, T. (1997) Lack of local anaesthetic efficacy of Sarapin in the abaxial sesamoid block model. *Journal of Veterinary Pharmacology and Therapeutics* **20**, 229–232.

Haussler, K.K. and Erb, H.N. (2006) Pressure algometry for the detection of induced back pain in horses: a preliminary study. *Equine Veterinary Journal* **38**, 76–81.

Haussler, K.K., Behre, T.H. and Hill, A.E. (2008) Mechanical nociceptive thresholds within the pastern region of Tennessee Walking Horses. *Equine Veterinary Journal* 40, 455–459.

Higgs, G.A., Eakins, K.E., Mugridge, K.G., Moncada, S. and Vane, J.R. (1980) The effects of non-steroid anti-inflammatory drugs on leukocyte migration in carrageenin-induced inflammation. *European Journal of Pharmacology* 66, 81–86.

Houdeshell, J.W. and Hennessey, P.W. (1977) A new non-steroidal, anti-inflammatory analgesic for horses. *Journal of Equine Medicine and Surgery* 1, 57–63.

Hu, H.H., MacAllister, C.G., Payton, M.E. and Erkert, R.S. (2005) Evaluation of the analgesic effects of phenylbutazone administered at a high or low dosage in horses with chronic lameness. *Journal of the American Veterinary Medical Association* 226, 414–417.

Ishihara A., Bertone, A.L. and Rajala-Schultz, P.J. (2005) Association between subjective lameness grade and kinetic gait parameters in horses with experimentally induced forelimb lameness. *American Journal of Veterinary Research* 66, 1805–1815.

Jochle W., Moore, J.N., Brown, J., Baker, G.J., Lowe, J.E., Fubini, S., Reeves, M.J., Watkins, J.P. and White, N.A. (1989) Comparison of detomidine, butorphanol, flunixin meglumine and xylazine in clinical cases of equine colic. *Equine Veterinary Journal (Supplement)* June, 111–116.

Johnson, C.B. and Taylor, P.M. (1998) Comparison of the effects of halothane, isoflurane and methoxyflurane on the electroencephalogram of the horse. *British Journal of Anaesthesia* 81, 748–753.

Johnson, C.B., Taylor, P.M., Young, S.S. and Brearley, J.C. (1993) Postoperative analgesia using phenylbutazone, flunixin or carprofen in horses. *Veterinary Record* 133, 336–338.

Johnson, C.B., Bloomfield, M. and Taylor, P.M. (1999) Effects of ketamine on the equine electroencephalogram during anesthesia with halothane in oxygen. *Veterinary Surgery* 28, 380–385.

Jones, E.W. and Hamm, D. (1978) Comparative efficacy of phenylbutazone and naproxen in induced equine myositis. *Journal of Equine Medicine and Surgery* 2, 341–347.

Judy, C.E., Galuppo, L.D., Snyder, J.R. and Willits, N.H. (2001) Evaluation of an in-shoe pressure measurement system in horses. *American Journal of Veterinary Research* 62, 23–28.

Kallings, P. (1993) Nonsteroidal anti-inflammatory drugs. *Veterinary Clinics of North America: Equine Practice* 9, 523–541.

Kamerling, S.G. (1993) Narcotics and local anesthetics. *Veterinary Clinics of North America: Equine Practice* 9, 605–620.

Kamerling, S.G., Weckman, T.J., DeQuick, D.J. and Tobin, T. (1985) A method for studying cutaneous pain perception and analgesia in horses. *Journal of Pharmacological Methods* 13, 267–274.

Karpie, J.C. and Chu, C.R. (2007) Lidocaine exhibits dose- and time-dependent cytotoxic effects on bovine articular chondrocytes in vitro. *American Journal of Sports Medicine* 35, 1621–1627.

Kazemi, A.P., Rezazadeh, S. and Gharacheh, H.R. (2004) Pain relief after arthroscopic knee surgery – intraarticular sufentanil vs morphine. *Middle East Journal of Anesthesiology* 17, 1099–1112.

Keegan, K.G. (2007) Evidence-based lameness detection and quantification. *Veterinary Clinics of North America: Equine Practice* 23, 403–423.

Keegan, K.G., Wilson, D.A., Smith, B.K. and Wilson, D.J. (2000) Changes in kinematic variables observed during pressure-induced forelimb lameness in adult horses trotting on a treadmill. *American Journal of Veterinary Research* 61, 612–619.

Keegan, K.G., Messer, N.T., Reed, S.K., Wilson, D.A. and Kramer, J. (2008) Effectiveness of administration of phenylbutazone alone or concurrent administration of phenylbutazone and flunixin meglumine to alleviate lameness in horses. *American Journal of Veterinary Research* 69, 167–173.

Landoni, M.F. and Lees, P. (1995) Influence of formulation on the pharmacokinetics and bioavailability of racemic ketoprofen in horses. *Journal of Veterinary Pharmacology and Therapeutics* 18, 446–450.

Lees, P., Maitho, T.E. and Taylor, J.B. (1985) Pharmacokinetics of phenylbutazone in two age groups of ponies. *Veterinary Record* 116, 229–232.

Lees, P., McKellar, Q., May, S.A. and Ludwig, B. (1994) Pharmacodynamics and pharmacokinetics of carprofen in the horse. *Equine Veterinary Journal* 26, 203–208.

Liu, S.S., Carpenter, R.L., Mackey, D.C., Thirlby, R.C., Rupp, S.M., Shine, T.S. *et al.* (1995) Effects of perioperative analgesic technique on rate of recovery after colon surgery. *Anesthesiology* 83, 757–765.

Lynn, R.C., Hepler, D.I., Kelch, W.J., Bertone, J.J., Smith, B.L. and Vatistas, N.J. (2004) Double-blinded placebo-controlled clinical field trial to evaluate the safety and efficacy of topically applied 1% diclofenac liposomal cream for the relief of lameness in horses. *Veterinary Therapeutics* 5, 128–138.

MacAllister, C.G., Morgan, S.J., Borne, A.T. and Pollet, R.A. (1993) Comparison of adverse effects of phenylbutazone, flunixin meglumine, and ketoprofen in horses. *Journal of the American Veterinary Medical Association* 202, 71–77.

MacKay, R.J., French, T.W., Nguyen, H.T. and Mayhew, I.G. (1983) Effects of large doses of phenylbutazone administration to horses. *American Journal of Veterinary Research* 44, 774–780.

Malone, E., Ensink, J., Turner, T., Wilson, J., Andrews, F., Keegan, K. *et al.* (2006) Intravenous continuous infusion of lidocaine for treatment of equine ileus. *Veterinary Surgery* 35, 60–66.

Mama, K.R., Grimsrud, K., Snell, T. and Stanley, S.D. (2009) Plasma concentrations, behavioural and physiological effects following intravenous and intramuscular detomidine in horses. *Equine Veterinary Journal* 41, 772–777.

Martin, C.A., Kerr, C.L., Pearce, S.G., Lansdowne, J.L. and Boure, L.P. (2003) Outcome of epidural catheterization for delivery of analgesics in horses: 43 cases (1998–2001). *Journal of the American Veterinary Medical Association* 222, 1394–1398.

Matthews, N.S. and Lindsay, S.L. (1990) Effect of low-dose butorphanol on halothane minimum alveolar concentration in ponies. *Equine Veterinary Journal* 22, 325—327.

Maxwell, L.K., Thomasy, S.M., Slovis, N. and Kollias-Baker, C. (2003) Pharmacokinetics of fentanyl following intravenous and transdermal administration in horses. *Equine Veterinary Journal* 35, 484–490.

May, S.A. and Lees, P. (1996) Nonsteroidal anti-inflammatory drugs. In *Joint Disease in the Horse*, McIlwraith, C.W. and Trotter, G.T. (eds), pp. 223–237. W.B. Saunders, Philadelphia, PA.

McMurphy, R.M. (1998) Providing analgesia. In *Current Techniques in Equine Surgery and Lameness*, White, N.A. and Moore, J.M. (eds), pp. 2–5. W.B. Saunders, Philadelphia, PA.

Merkens, H.W. and Schamhardt, H.C. (1988) Evaluation of equine locomotion during different degrees of experimentally induced lameness. I: Lameness model and quantification of ground reaction force patterns of the limbs. *Equine Veterinary Journal (Supplement)* September, 99–106.

Miller, S.M., Short, C.E. and Ekstrom, P.M. (1995) Quantitative electroencephalographic evaluation to determine the quality of analgesia during anesthesia of horses for arthroscopic surgery. *American Journal of Veterinary Research* 56, 374–379.

Mills, P.C. and Cross, S.E. (2007) Regional differences in transdermal penetration of fentanyl through equine skin. *Research in Veterinary Science* 82, 252–256.

Mills, P.C., Ng, J.C., Kramer, H. and Auer, D.E. (1997) Stress response to chronic inflammation in the horse. *Equine Veterinary Journal* 29, 483–486.

Muir, W.W. (1998) Anaesthesia and pain management in horses. *Equine Veterinary Education* 10, 335–340.

Muir, W.W. (2005) Pain therapy in horses. *Equine Veterinary Journal* 37, 98–100.

Neges, K., Bettschart-Wolfensburger, R. and Muller, J. (2003) The isoflurane sparing effect of a medetomidine constant rate infusion in horses. *Veterinary Anaesthesia and Analgesia* 30, 93–94.

Nolan, A.M. (2000) Pharmacology of analgesic drugs. In *Pain Management in Animals*, Flecknell, P. and Waterman-Pearson, A. (eds), pp. 21–52. W.B. Saunders, Philadelphia, PA.

Orsini, J.A., Moate, P.J., Kuersten, K., Soma, L.R. and Boston, R.C. (2006) Pharmacokinetics of fentanyl delivered transdermally in healthy adult horses – variability among horses and its clinical implications. *Journal of Veterinary Pharmacology and Therapeutics* 29, 539–546.

Otto, K.A., Voight, S., Piepenbrock, S., Deegen, E. and Short, C.E. (1996) Differences in quantitated electroencephalographic variables during surgical stimulation of horses anesthetized with isoflurane. *Veterinary Surgery* 25, 249–255.

Owens, J.G., Kamerling, S.G. and Barker, S.A. (1995a) Pharmacokinetics of ketoprofen in healthy horses and horses with acute synovitis. *Journal of Veterinary Pharmacology and Therapeutics* 18, 187–195.

Owens, J.G., Kamerling, S.G., Stanton, S.R. and Keowen, M.L. (1995b) Effects of ketoprofen and phenylbutazone on chronic hoof pain and lameness in the horse. *Equine Veterinary Journal* 27, 296–300.

Owens, J.G., Kamerling, S.G., Stanton, S.R., Keowen, M.L. and Prescott-Mathews, J.S. (1996) Effects of pretreatment with ketoprofen and phenylbutazone on experimentally induced synovitis in horses. *American Journal of Veterinary Research* 57, 866–874.

Pace, S. and Burke, T.F. (1996) Intravenous morphine for early pain relief in patients with acute abdominal pain. *Academic Emergency Medicine* 3, 1086–1092.

Pascoe, P.J., Ducharme, N.G., Ducharme, G.R. and Lumsden, J.H. (1990) A computer-derived protocol using recursive partitioning to aid in estimating prognosis of horses with abdominal pain in referral hospitals. *Canadian Journal of Veterinary Research* **54**, 373–378.

Pascoe, P.J., Steffey, E.P., Black, W.D., Claxton, J.M., Jacobs, J.R. and Woliner, M.J. (1993) Evaluation of the effect of alfentanil on the minimum alveolar concentration of halothane in horses. *American Journal of Veterinary Research* **54**, 1327–1332.

Peek, S.F., Semrad, S.D. and Perkins, G.A. (2003) Clostridial myonecrosis in horses (37 cases 1985–2000). *Equine Veterinary Journal* **35**, 86–92.

Peterbauer, C., Larenza, P.M., Knobloch, M., Theurillat, R., Thormann, W., Mevissen, M. *et al.* (2008). Effects of a low dose infusion of racemic and *S*-ketamine on the nociceptive withdrawal reflex in standing ponies. *Veterinary Anaesthesia and Analgesia* **35**, 414–423.

Raekallio, M., Taylor, P.M. and Bennett, R.C. (1997a) Preliminary investigations of pain and analgesia assessment in horses administered phenylbutazone or placebo after arthroscopic surgery. *Veterinary Surgery* **26**, 150–155.

Raekallio, M., Taylor, P.M. and Bloomfield, M.A. (1997b) A comparison of methods for evaluation of pain and distress after orthopaedic surgery in horses. *Veterinary Anaesthesia and Analgesia* **24**, 17–20.

Rietmann, T.R., Stauffacher, M., Bernasconi, P., Auer, J.A. and Weishaupt, M.A. (2004) The association between heart rate, heart rate variability, endocrine and behavioural pain measures in horses suffering from laminitis. *Journal of Veterinary Medicine Series A* **51**, 218–225.

Robertson, S.A., Sanchez, L.C., Merritt, A.M. and Doherty, T.J. (2005) Effect of systemic lidocaine on visceral and somatic nociception in conscious horses. *Equine Veterinary Journal* **37**, 122–127.

Robinson, T.M., Kruse-Elliott, K.T., Markel, M.D., Pluhar, G.E., Massa, K. and Bjorling, D.E. (1999) A comparison of transdermal fentanyl versus epidural morphine for analgesia in dogs undergoing major orthopedic surgery. *Journal of the American Animal Hospital Association* **35**, 95–100.

Ross, M.W. (2003) Movement. In *Diagnosis and Management of Lameness in the Horse*, Ross, M.W. and Dyson, S.J. (eds), pp. 60–73. Saunders, St. Louis, MO.

Sanchez, L.C., Robertson, S.A., Maxwell, L.K., Zientek, K. and Cole, C. (2007) Effect of fentanyl on visceral and somatic nociception in conscious horses. *Journal of Veterinary Internal Medicine* **21**, 1067–1075.

Sandler, A.N., Baxter, A.D., Katz, J., Samson, B., Friedlander, M., Norman, P. *et al.* (1994) A double-blind, placebo-controlled trial of transdermal fentanyl after abdominal hysterectomy. Analgesic, respiratory, and pharmacokinetic effects. *Anesthesiology* **81**, 1169–1180.

Santos, L.C., de Moraes, A.N. and Saito, M.E. (2009) Effects of intraarticular ropivacaine and morphine on lipopolysaccharide-induced synovitis in horses. *Veterinary Anaesthesia and Analgesia* **36**, 280–286.

Schatzmann, U., Gugelmann, M. and Cranach, J. (1992) Visceral and peripheral pain detection models in the horse, using flunixin and carprofen. In *Animal Pain*, Short, C.E. and Poznak, A. (eds), pp. 411–420. Churchill Livingstone, Edinburgh.

Schweinitz, D.G., Deyaert, M., Joris, D., Pendeville, E. and Gouverneur, J.M. (1999) Thermographic diagnostics in equine back pain. *Equine Practice* 15, 161–177.

Sellon, D.C., Roberts, M.C., Blikslager, A.T., Ulibarri, C. and Papich, M.G. (2004) Effects of continuous rate intravenous infusion of butorphanol on physiologic and outcome variables in horses after celiotomy. *Journal of Veterinary Internal Medicine* 18, 555–563.

Singelyn, F.J., Deyaert, M., Joris, D., Pendeville, E. and Gouverneur, J.M. (1998) Effects of intravenous patient-controlled analgesia with morphine, continuous epidural analgesia, and continuous three-in-one block on postoperative pain and knee rehabilitation after unilateral total knee arthroplasty. *Anesthesia and Analgesia* 87, 88–92.

Snow, D.H., Douglas, T.A., Thompson, H., Parkins, J.J. and Holmes, P.H. (1980) Phenylbutazone toxicity in ponies. *Veterinary Record* 106, 68.

Steffey, E.P., Pascoe, P.J., Woliner, M.J. and Berryman, E.R. (2000) Effects of xylazine hydrochloride during isoflurane-induced anesthesia in horses. *American Journal of Veterinary Research* 61, 1225–1231.

Steffey, E.P., Eisele, J.H. and Baggot, J.D. (2003) Interactions of morphine and isoflurane in horses. *American Journal of Veterinary Research* 64, 166–175.

Sysel, A.M., Pleasant, R.S., Jacobson, J.D., Moll, H.D., Modransky, P.D., Warnick, L.D. *et al.* (1996) Efficacy of an epidural combination of morphine and detomidine in alleviating experimentally induced hindlimb lameness in horses. *Veterinary Surgery* 25, 511–518.

Sysel, A.M., Pleasant, R.S., Jacobson, J.D., Moll, H.D., Warnick, L.D., Sponenberg, D.P. *et al.* (1997) Systemic and local effects associated with long-term epidural catheterization and morphine-detomidine administration in horses. *Veterinary Surgery* 26, 141–149.

Taylor, P.M. (1998) Effects of surgery on endocrine and metabolic responses to anaesthesia in horses and ponies. *Research in Veterinary Science* 64, 133–140.

Taylor, P.M., Pascoe, P.J. and Mama, K.R. (2002) Diagnosing and treating pain in the horse. Where are we today? *Veterinary Clinics of North America: Equine Practice* 18, 1–19.

Thomasy, S.M., Slovis, N., Maxwell, L.K. and Kollias-Baker, C. (2004) Transdermal fentanyl combined with nonsteroidal anti-inflammatory drugs for analgesia in horses. *Journal of Veterinary Internal Medicine* 18, 550–554.

Thoren, T., Sundberg, A., Wattwil, M., Garvill, J.E. and Jurgensen, U. (1989) Effects of epidural bupivacaine and epidural morphine on bowel function and pain after hysterectomy. *Acta Anaesthesiologica Scandinavica* 33, 181–185.

Tobin, T. (1979) The non-steroidal anti-inflammatory drugs: II. Equiproxen, meclofenamic acid, flunixin and others. *Journal of Equine Medicine and Surgery* 3, 298–302.

Welsh, J.C., Lees, P., Stodulski, G., Cambridge, H. and Foster, A.P. (1992) Influence of feeding schedule on the absorption of orally administered flunixin in the horse. *Equine Veterinary Journal (Supplement)* 24(February), 62–65.

Wilcke, J.R., Crisman, M.V., Scarratt, W.K. and Sams, R.A. (1998) Pharmacokinetics of ketoprofen in healthy foals less than twenty-four hours old. *American Journal of Veterinary Research* 59, 290–292.

Willemen, M.A., Savelberg, H.H. and Barneveld, A. (1999) The effect of orthopaedic shoeing on the force exerted by the deep digital flexor tendon on the navicular bone in horses. *Equine Veterinary Journal* 31, 25–30.

Wolfe, T.M. and Muir, W.W. (2003) Local anesthetics: pharmacology and novel applications. *Compendium on Continuing Education for the Practicing Veterinarian* **25**, 916–927.

Woolf, C.J. (2004) Pain: moving from symptom control toward mechanism-specific pharmacologic management. *Annals of Internal Medicine* **140**, 441-451.

Woolf, C.J. and Chong, M.S. (1993) Preemptive analgesia – treating postoperative pain by preventing the establishment of central sensitization. *Anesthesia and Analgesia* **77**, 362–379.

Zarucco, L., Driessen, B. and Scandella, M. (2007) Continuous perineural block of the palmar nerves: a new technique for pain relief in the distal equine forelimb. *Clinical Techniques in Equine Practice* **6**, 154–164.

Euthanasia as an Equine Welfare Tool

Jay G. Merriam

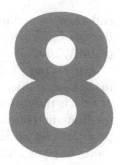

8.1 Introduction

There is no set view on the correct application and prescription for the standardized use of euthanasia in equine medical practice or as a welfare tool. The myriad situations and variety of presentations seen in equine practice have little or no counterpart in either small animal or human medicine. The Veterinarian's Oath of the USA prescribes that we 'temper pain with anesthesia,' yet did not envision the sea of possibilities seen in a complex world. Therefore, we must seek to understand that case-specific ethical reasoning is often the only guide available. As such, we will attempt to illustrate, via USA case-based reports, the current state of euthanasia as it applies to horses and today's world, realizing that there is indeed a range of views and options available. In all cases, considering the best interests of the horse will guide us down a twisting path toward doing the right thing.

The term 'euthanasia' is derived from the Greek terms *eu*, meaning 'good,' and *thanatos*, meaning 'death.' A 'good death' would be one that occurs with minimal pain and distress. Euthanasia is the act of inducing humane death in an animal. It is the responsibility of veterinarians and human beings to ensure that, if an animal's life is to be taken, it is done with the highest degree of respect, and with an emphasis on making the death as painless and distress-free as possible. Euthanasia techniques should result in rapid loss of consciousness followed by cardiac or respiratory arrest and the ultimate loss of brain function. In addition, the technique should minimize distress and anxiety experienced by the animal prior to loss of consciousness. One useful source of information on euthanasia is the guidelines produced by the American Veterinary Medical Association (AVMA, 2007). This panel recognized that the absence of pain and distress cannot always be achieved, but attempts to balance the ideal of minimal pain and distress with the reality of the many environments in which

Equine Welfare, First Edition. Edited by C. Wayne McIlwraith and Bernard E. Rollin.
© 2011 by UFAW. Published 2011 by Blackwell Publishing Ltd.

euthanasia is performed. A veterinarian with appropriate training and expertise for the species involved should be consulted to ensure that proper procedures are used (AVMA, 2007).

Veterinarians are given the right to provide finite closure to an animal suffering in the face of disease or infirmity that will not expediently end its life. The factor of time is thus inserted into the equation; we hasten to aid or abet such a process for humane reasons. And as Shakespeare's Hamlet said, 'there's the rub'! The protocols for an ideal euthanasia are well known and are, by some measures, more humane than those for capital punishment according to at least one Supreme Court of the United States! As society changes and animals become more disposable, unwanted, displaced or simply no longer useful, veterinarians are asked to intervene in cases and ways that would have been unthinkable in generations past. Consider the following cases, all based on actual clinical situations, analyze your response to them, and compare with the ethical outcomes discussed.

8.2 Some Example Cases Based on Clinical Situations

Case 1
The prized and beloved working stock horse that provided the means to support a family is becoming infirm, slow, aged, or simply unable to continue working. The family believes that feed and shelter are scarce commodities that cannot be spared for an animal that does not produce. In days past, he would have been led out to a distant pasture and shot by the owner. His carcass would have been recycled and a new colt brought into the string. Or he would have been turned out to 'winter pasture' from which he would simply not return in spring. Or, in a more common recent variant in the still rural West, he would have been trailered to a remote desert site and turned loose on Bureau of Land Management (BLM) land forever. Sometimes these horses are rounded up as 'wild' horses in gathers of real ones.

Outcome
The once needed, now infirm (or at least unnecessary), working horse is often presented as part of an equation where multiple variables are in play, including age, economics, and sometimes attachment. Though veterinarians have the right to provide the service of euthanasia, one should not feel compelled to do so in the healthy 'unwanted' horse against one's conscience in response to the future possibility of owner-mediated neglect, abandonment, or abuse. Yet, each case must be assessed individually, and it may be that offering the animal a quick, humane death is preferable to the vagaries of facing a winter of starvation or animal attack or both (AAEP, 2007; AVMA, 2007).

Case 2

The formerly loved and successful show horse of the young, urban daughter's childhood fascination with horses has suddenly become idled as his rider goes off to college. He is leased to a succession of riders while he is still owned by the original family. As economic hardship befalls the owners, the horse becomes gravely ill, requiring extensive medical treatment at a referral facility. Once stabilized, the owners take the horse to a new stable, leaving a large bill unpaid. Further medical complications arise, and, despite the recommendations of the treating veterinarian, the owner refuses euthanasia and demands that her horse be saved, despite offering no financial assistance. Humane officers are alerted, and the horse is removed to a local clinic, where euthanasia on humane grounds is recommended. However, the owner continues to prevent euthanasia of the animal, which dies several weeks later at the clinic. By all accounts, the horse's final days were painful and difficult. The owner then filed suit for malpractice against the humane organization and the referral hospital.

Outcome

Owners willfully preventing euthanasia in the face of major debilitation are often acting out of guilt and remorse. They cannot, however, force a veterinarian to provide care at their own expense and time. The only requirement of the veterinarian is to temper pain with anesthesia, and this includes euthanasia. Most states in the USA have 'good Samaritan' laws that protect the veterinarian from prosecution for ending an animal's life without the owner's consent if the situation calls for it. Few spell out just what that situation would be. The case used as an illustration is still under litigation, but in most cases the 'Samaritan' statutes apply. This does not prevent owners from filing suits, but should allow ruling in the veterinarian's favor. Once treatment has begun, it is difficult to discontinue or withhold care if the outcome is considered likely to be successful.

Case 3

In the USA, the Bureau of Land Management (BLM) routinely gathers wild, free-roaming horses from Government lands in compliance with the Wild and Free Roaming Horse and Burro Protection Act. These 'gathers' help to control the ever-growing equine populations and prevent mass starvation and resource degradation that accompanies overgrazing. The horses are evaluated and policy requires that any horses unable to fend for themselves by virtue of age, infirmity or genetic defects are humanely euthanized by the staff veterinarians. The others gathered to relieve population pressures (as determined by analysis of the land's carrying capacity) are then prepared for adoption, long-term holding, or permanent holding in government-leased sanctuaries, where all males are gelded and mares separated to prevent population growth. These herds are then managed and individuals allowed to age until they die naturally or must be destroyed. The BLM has proposed mass euthanasia of large numbers of gathered horses for reasons of overcrowding, range degradation, underfunding, and lack of open range.

Outcome

The BLM has been charged with maintaining the status of the mustang or wild horse as a symbol of the American West on Federal lands, while simultaneously not allowing its population to swell, its range to be degraded, or herds to be slaughtered, starved or preyed upon to extinction. All the while, in the face of decreasing budgets and increasing range pressure from outside, BLM agents are allowed to capture, remove, and geld or euthanize infirm, aged, 'defective' or superfluous horses. The BLM can adopt out desirable individuals as long as they are not sold for slaughter or abused. While the herds continue to grow unchecked, the population ages, and those threatened with death by severe weather events are rescued. Staff veterinarians are asked to euthanize 'genetically defective' animals, but are prevented from using birth control on herds or individuals. Current plans include large-scale euthanasia, since holding facilities and budgets are overtaxed, and slaughter for food has become illegal in the USA. Transporting the horses out of the country is also illegal if it is for slaughter for human consumption. There is an ongoing discussion about long-term solutions, but the law of unintended consequences truly plays a large part, as does the lack of political will to address the imperfections in the current laws.

Case 4

A group of horses 'rescued' by a benevolent organization are found to be in deplorable conditions of disease and malnutrition on an urban property once owned or leased by the now defunct organization. The animals are all too lame, malnourished, or ill to be easily rehabilitated, and there is no agency or group that has the resources for the project. You are called to perform euthanasia on 16 horses.

Outcome

The unintended consequence of the ban in the USA on transport for slaughter has spawned numerous well-meaning but consistently underfunded 'rescue organizations' that seek out unadoptable or malnourished, abandoned, or abused horses for rescue. The problem of feeding and maintaining large numbers of horses has been routinely underestimated, as has their potential marketability. There has been much talk about finding and confiscating such horses, but many agencies are reluctant and unable to do so. The use of euthanasia in such situations is never popular, but can be reasonably done on a case-by-case basis if there is no alternative means to provide for the animals. This is similar to the BLM's dilemma and needs to be addressed legislatively. Until then, conscience and ethics must guide us in each case. The AVMA guidelines (AVMA, 2007) permit the euthanasia of animals that are not adoptable for reasons of behavior, health or suitability.

Case 5

A rancher in the USA has sufficient land for burial and asks you, as a veterinarian, to euthanize his old, lame, but well cared-for and beloved ranch horse. He takes him to a specified place far out of sight and asks you to meet him there, perform the task humanely, and agrees to bury him with his own equipment later that day. A week later you are cited by the Federal Department of Fish and Wildlife for the deaths of two Golden Eagles that gorged themselves on the remains and died of pentobarbital toxicity.

Outcome
Once the decision to euthanize has been made, it is the veterinarian's responsibility to follow appropriate rules for use of medications in an appropriate manner, and, by extension, to control their introduction into the environment. Failure to do so is punishable under many State or Federal regulations. In this case, the veterinarian failed to assure that the end-user of the controlled substances was disposed of properly, in the same way that it is the veterinarian's responsibility to track any medical waste generated. Carcass disposal must be controlled by the veterinarian in such cases (AAEP, 2010).

Case 6
A client with a couple of well-loved ponies calls a veterinarian one winter morning because one of them cannot walk and is standing in the freezing rain, immobile. The veterinarian finds a compound, comminuted radial fracture, which, in her opinion, requires immediate euthanasia. The owner asks her to speak to her seven-year-old son about what has happened to his pony. You explain that the pony is hurt very badly, is in a lot of pain, and must be 'put to sleep.' The little boy seems to understand as you and his mother explain carefully what will happen. The euthanasia goes smoothly and the pony breathes her last easily. The little boy pats her softly, turns to you and says, 'So when will she wake up?'

Outcome
Appropriate communication is both an acquired skill and a requirement in all situations where euthanasia is to be performed. Never assume that your client understands what is about to happen. Appropriate discussion of euthanasia with a minor depends on age, level of understanding, and parental wishes (AVMA, 2007).

Case 7
The Highway Patrol calls a veterinarian late one night for assistance at a trailer rollover involving horses. The veterinarian arrives as a Life Flight rescue helicopter is leaving and hears thrashing from within the trailer. One horse is standing outside the trailer, seemingly unhurt, but the one inside the trailer is thrashing. It is apparent that femoral fracture has most likely occurred, and euthanasia is probably the only reasonable course of action. The owner's last words as he was lifted onto the helicopter were 'Tell doc to do whatever he can, these are valuable racehorses!' He is from another state, is not one of your clients, and was driving alone.

Outcome

Clearly, the USA's 'Samaritan' statute applies if the injuries are, in your best judgment, grievous enough to require euthanasia. If logistics, location of appropriate clinical facilities, or other limitations apply that would extend the animal's suffering, the veterinarian is permitted to apply his/her best judgment and perform euthanasia without fear of legal repercussions. Insurance companies will routinely accept such a decision as long as it is rendered in a fair and impartial manner.

Case 8

It is September in New England and a veterinarian is called to euthanize a 28-year-old, retired, lame show horse who, though he is healthy, is a bit unsteady on his feet from time to time, has trouble getting up and down sometimes, and that the owner would like to have euthanized before the ground freezes and it's impossible to dig. Contrast this with another scenario: it is January in New England, the wind chill is –20 degrees, and there is an elderly horse down in the paddock next to the house. The owners want to 'try something' but funds are limited as well as facilities and assistance. The local Board of Health has specifically prohibited animal burial in the aquifer region of this particular town.

Outcome

It is imperative that we all attempt to limit environmental pollution via medications dispensed or discarded. Recent work shows that the volume of human medications flushed down the drain in any city has had effects on wildlife and is traceable in many distant aquifers. The choices that clients make should be carefully weighed against such information. Before the demise of most rendering plants in the USA, residues of pentobarbital were found in the various glues and pastes made as by-products of the rendering. Most urban clients are reluctant to accept gunshot as a means of euthanasia, and the increasingly strict firearms laws will make this very humane alternative less available. The captive bolt is a very safe and effective alternative, but client acceptance is similar to euthanasia by gunshot (Blackmore, 1985; Longair et al., 1991).

Case 9

A successful, nationally ranked show horse is examined for a sub-acute lameness, which has sidelined his career. Diagnostics and initial therapy has given an indication of a back injury that will definitely prevent further showing. Bone scans and ultrasound scans confirm this. The horse is then the subject of a 'loss of use' claim. After months of rest and consultation with the insurer and referring veterinarians, it is clear that he will need to receive butazoladin daily to lead a comfortable life. A veterinarian is called to perform euthanasia on humane grounds. The horse is in excellent general health, but chronically lame (grade 2, where grade 0 is sound and grade 5 is non-weight-bearing) and seems quite bright and alert. Is humane destruction justified?

Outcome

The aging show horse covered by insurance that will soon lapse is a special case that presents many dilemmas and inherent conflicts of interest. Owners who insured their purchase with 'loss of use' insurance are often guided by business interests and an attitude that there is no room for an attachment or bond. The horse in question often could be quite happily retired to a school string or just retired, living without medication. In such cases, where there is no threat of death or chronic pain, it may be difficult to agree to euthanize. It is acceptable to recuse oneself or refuse to perform euthanasia in such circumstances. In many cases, once the owner is appraised of the situation, a negotiated settlement with the insurer is possible. AAEP guidelines (AAEP, 2010) support euthanasia in cases where the animal will be maintained on analgesic medications for life. Financial considerations should not enter into such decisions.

8.3 Resolution

Each of these scenarios is based on real cases witnessed by the author within the last three decades of life as a veterinary practitioner. The situations have been disguised to protect the various parties from recrimination, but all are factual. Let's re-examine each and look at what was done, what could have been done better, and what one might have done. More importantly, let's examine the welfare of the horses involved. Following that, add in the legal concerns that accompany the use of controlled substances and firearms. Additional factors for consideration include the involvement of humane officers, and State and Federal statutes, as well as one's own evaluation.

The challenge to develop a 'one size fits all' template is daunting in equine practice. We can draw some lessons from small-animal practice, where millions of domestic pets are euthanized yearly for lack of ownership, behavioral issues such as aggression, or simply because they are being discarded (AVMA, 2007). It can be useful also to compare approaches and methods adopted for animals used in scientific procedures and for food production. Yet we must still concern ourselves with the international slaughter industry, to which many thousands of domestic horses in the USA are being consigned, often for no other reason than those illustrated above. There are still horses being raised in feedlots in the USA, then exported alive for 'processing' in other countries. Where we stand on each of the above issues may often be somewhat at odds with our views on others. For example, we may have different views about the slaughter of purpose-raised horses sold for specialty meat overseas and about the euthanasia of wild horses that cannot be adopted. Both will be euthanized, one with a captive bolt and then processed into food, the other with an overdose of barbiturate while standing in a squeeze chute. Neither will suffer, but one may add to our toxic wastes in the environment and the other will provide a consumer with food. In the USA, veterinarians often learn basic surgical and medical skills on horses kept for the purpose, and this is governed by university Institutional Animal Care and Use Committees. Is it humane or ethical to euthanize horses strictly because they are no longer useful?

8.4 Methods of Euthanasia

A variety of physical and chemical methods for euthanasia of horses are available and approved for use (AVMA, 2007; HSA, 1999). These include dispatch using captive bolt or free-bullet firearms (HSA, 2005, 2006) and administration of anesthetic overdoses. In each case the duty is to provide a painless, humane, and, if possible, dignified end. Recent US Supreme Court rulings on capital punishment were made in response to a suit pressing for the adoption of the same standards as are provided for animals. The rulings continue to permit the use of skeletal muscle relaxants *prior* to barbiturate overdose in capital punishment, in spite of the fact that it was demonstrably painful and impaired the ability to determine actual time of death. Such use of muscle relaxants is not permitted in veterinary medicine (although, in the USA, it is accepted in extreme cases where an animal cannot be immobilized for intravenous injection). Anesthetic agents other than barbiturates have been tried, but are not routinely used.

Intravenous pentobarbital is the best choice for equine euthanasia using anesthetic overdose (AVMA, 2007). Because of the large volume needed, an intravenous catheter placed in the jugular vein will facilitate the procedure. Excitable or fractious animals may first be tranquilized using acepromazine or an alpha-2 adrenergic agonist, but these drugs may prolong the time to loss of consciousness and may result in muscular activity and agonal gasping. Opioids may further facilitate restraint (AVMA, 2007).

Captive bolt or free-bullet methods can provide excellent, humane, and instantaneous euthanasia, but both methods depend upon accurate bolt or bullet placement (HSA, 2005, 2006). Although it often kills outright, the captive bolt is used in slaughter of food animals as a stunning method and, in these animals, death prior to recovery of consciousness is ensured by blood loss through throat cutting. It is always necessary to ensure that irreversible loss of consciousness has been achieved. The use of guns may not be safe or acceptable in urban situations or not desired by owners for various reasons. However, because of their humaneness, these are often the preferred methods. Although, of course, if not performed properly, they may cause suffering and possible human endangerment.

In addition to the information sources mentioned above, recommendations and excellent interactive diagrams for the technique of captive bolt or gunshot euthanasia are also provided by Shearer and Nicoletti (2009). This features excellent anatomic illustrations and should be reviewed as a training method. Drawing an 'X' from the medial canthus of the eyes to the base of the opposite ear and shooting or penetrating just above the center is recommended. As mentioned above, it is recommended that, following use of the captive bolt, death is ensured by immediate exsanguination. This needs to be clearly explained to the client in advance.

8.5 Conclusions

There are many good reasons to employ euthanasia in the conduct of equine practice. Unfortunately, there are many gray areas associated with its use, and many veterinarians may find that their views toward euthanasia will change over the course of their careers. The ethical considerations are very complex and have only been briefly examined here. Further reading is suggested (see e.g. AAEP, 2007, 2010; AVMA, 2007). The fact that the veterinary profession in many countries has the privilege of administering euthanasia is often a source of wonder to its colleagues in human medicine, and certainly offers unique insight into the debate raging over its use in humans.

References

AAEP (2007) *Euthanasia Guidelines*. American Association of Equine Practitioners, Lexington, KY. Available at: http://www.aaep.org/euthanasia_guidelines.htm.

AAEP (2010) *Ethical and Professional Guidelines*. American Association of Equine Practitioners, Lexington, KY. Available at: http://www.aaep.org/images/files/2010EthicProfGuidelines.pdf.

AVMA (2007) *AVMA Guidelines on Euthanasia*. American Veterinary Medicine Association, Schaumburg, IL. Available at: http://www.avma.org/issues/animal_welfare/euthanasia.pdf.

Blackmore, D.K. (1985) Energy requirements for the penetration of heads of domestic stock in the development of a multiple projectile. *Veterinary Record* **116**, 36–40.

HSA (1999) *Farewell – Making the Right Decision*. Humane Slaughter Association, Wheathampstead, Herts, UK. Available at: http://www.hsa.org.uk/Resources/Publications/Farewell%20leaflet%20for%20web%20APRIL%2009.pdf.

HSA (2005) *Humane Killing of Livestock using Firearms*. Guidance Notes No. 3, 2nd edn. Humane Slaughter Association, Wheathampstead, Herts, UK. See: http://www.hsa.org.uk/Publications/Guidance%20Notes.html.

HSA (2006) *Captive Bolt Stunning of Livestock*. Guidance Notes No. 2, 4th edn. Humane Slaughter Association, Wheathampstead, Herts, UK. See: http://www.hsa.org.uk/Publications/Guidance%20Notes.html.

Longair, J.A., Finley, G.G., Lariel, M.A. *et al.* (1991) Guidelines for euthanasia of domestic animals by firearms. *Canadian Veterinary Journal* **32**, 724–726.

Shearer, J.K. and Nicoletti, P. (2009) *Procedures for Humane Euthanasia of Sick, Injured, and/or Debilitated Livestock*. University of Florida, Extension, College of Veterinary Medicine, Institute of Food and Agricultural Sciences. Available at: http://www.vetmed.ufl.edu/extension/Dairy/humaneeuthanasia/pref.htm.

Equine Welfare and Integrative Veterinary Medicine

Kevin K. Haussler

9

Integration is defined as the act of combining something into an integral whole, with the implication that the whole functions smoothly and is greater than the sum of its parts (Meeker and Mootz, 2005). Clinical integration occurs when diverse disciplines (e.g., a veterinary surgeon, physical therapist, trainer, and farrier) work together in the best interest and for the welfare of the equine patient. Human integrative medicine promotes the use of both conventional medical care and the adoption of some complementary and alternative medicine (CAM) concepts, such as prevention, diet, exercise, and emotional and spiritual health (Meeker and Mootz, 2005). Integrative medicine offers a philosophy that focuses on health and healing (instead of disease and technology), an emphasis on the central role of the patient–practitioner relationship, respect of client preferences, and intentional activation of the body's innate healing capabilities (Snyderman and Weil, 2002).

I support a broad and inclusive definition of what integrative veterinary medicine is and what it has to contribute to equine welfare. Integrative veterinary medicine is not only limited to conventional or evolving medical or surgical approaches, but also incorporates the diagnostic and therapeutic offerings of equine chiropractic, acupuncture, physical therapy, and other unconventional medical approaches that are not routinely taught within the veterinary curricula, but are widely considered encompassed under the umbrella of CAM. Many of these techniques have been borrowed from human medicine based on their perceived therapeutic effectiveness and applied to horses with the goal of achieving some of the same beneficial effects. Additional components of integrative medicine include principles and practices of equitation science and horsemanship, such as proper tack fit and use, riding techniques, working or racing surfaces, behavior, and any other field or area of interest that may directly impact a horse's health and well-being (Goodwin *et al.*, 2008). The context of this chapter is that we as a profession are obliged to investigate and objectively assess any modality or management practice that has the potential to benefit the health and well-being of horses.

9.2 What's in a Name?

Unfortunately, there are a wide variety of terms used to describe complementary and alternative therapies, some of which include 'non-traditional, unconventional, unproven, and non-evidence-based' (Rollin, 2006). Rightly or wrongly, many of the applied terms have negative connotations, which often do not accurately represent what CAM is or what it has to offer veterinary medicine. In my opinion, the term 'integrative veterinary medicine' more accurately encompasses the intent and activities of most veterinarians or sports medicine practitioners who provide complementary or alternative therapies within their equine practices. Integrative veterinary medicine provides a philosophical framework for incorporating any form of diagnostic or therapeutic modality that demonstrates some level of evidence of being both safe and effective in managing a specific disease process or improving general equine welfare. The premise of 'doing all that you reasonably can do' often requires us to expand our current knowledge base, pursue training or continuing education in new and evolving fields, consult with or refer to colleagues who have pursued specialized postgraduate training in select fields, or confer with human counterparts who are willing to participate in translational medicine or complicated and unique surgical procedures. Integrative medicine encourages the use of the scientific process to investigate novel diagnostic and therapeutic procedures and does not condone the application of untested therapies. It is critical that we validate all diagnostic procedures, therapeutic techniques, and management practices for clinical efficacy in improving well-being or managing disease processes that negatively impact equine welfare.

The National Center for Complementary and Alternative Medicine (NCCAM) defines complementary and alternative medicine[1] as 'a group of diverse medical and health care systems, practices, and products that are not presently considered to be part of conventional medicine.' CAM is represented by a very diverse collection of professions with unique philosophies, traditions, procedures, professional attributes, histories, and patients, which often do not espouse conventional pharmaceuticals or surgical techniques (Kaptchuk and Eisenberg, 2001). Therefore, it is easy for some critics of CAM to make sweeping generalizations that these non-traditional forms of medicine are non-scientific and therefore are not valid forms of diagnosis or treatment (Ramey and Ernst, 1999). However, since many CAM

[1] See: http://nccam.nih.gov/health/whatiscam/overview.htm.

practices use widely varying diagnostic or therapeutic approaches to health care, making broad generalizations about them as a whole can be difficult and outright inaccurate.

The term 'alternative medicine' implies that it can be used in place of traditional medicine and surgery. Acupuncture, as practiced by some traditional Chinese medicine (TCM) practitioners, could be considered a form of alterative therapy because in their hands acupuncture is used to treat or manage the majority of disease conditions that their patients present with. In these practices, acupuncture is often used as an alternative to Western medicine or surgery. The term 'complementary medicine' infers that the applied treatment is used together with and somehow complements traditional veterinary care. Physical therapy is an example of complementary therapy, as it is often used in conjunction with surgical recovery or for the rehabilitation of injuries to help restore full neurologic or musculoskeletal function. Complementary and alternative therapies have also been described in terms of 'proven' and 'unproven' (Fontanarosa and Lundberg, 1998). However, a more useful working definition or categorization of scientific evidence used to determine the attributes of a novel or unconventional therapy may be in defining them as 'tested' or 'untested' (or 'known' and 'unknown'). The use of the terms 'proven' and 'unproven' can be confusing, since a proven modality could be proven to be either effective or ineffective. The word 'proven' also suggests that no further work is needed in the area, since it is proven or somehow complete, and research efforts do not ever need to be directed toward that issue again. Untested diagnostic or therapeutic techniques easily fall into the category of unknown knowledge regarding their predictive value, safety, biological activity, or effectiveness. If a therapy is untested, then it is not possible to make any judgment or valid criticism regarding its perceived efficacy or safety (Ramey and Ernst, 1999).

Most practitioners tend to view information that does not readily fit into their existing knowledge base with suspicion, and rightly so. The terms 'traditional' and 'non-traditional' are used to describe techniques, procedures, or substances that are or are not taught in the typical veterinary school education. For any recent or long-ago graduate of veterinary school, it can safely be said that you did not learn from your veterinary education absolutely everything that you needed to be successful in private practice, public health, administration, practice management, or research. There continue to be a multitude of new topics and vast areas of interest that are of critical importance to the welfare of the horse, and for your success as a practitioner, but are not taught to any useful degree in veterinary schools around the world. Poor saddle fit is considered one of the leading causes of back pain in horses, yet it remains the rather exclusive domain of experienced saddlers, and the basics of 'good' versus 'bad' saddle fit are rarely taught in any veterinary school (Fruehwirth et al., 2004). The same can be said of improperly used or poor fitting saddle pads, bits, bridles, reins, draw reins, and harnesses, or the use of any restraint device that is used to overcome the horse's natural desire to avoid pain or altered gait associated with lameness (Manfredi et al., 2005; Roepstorff et al., 2002). As a profession, we agree that racing surfaces, proper shoeing, hoof care, riding ability and technique, and dental health affect athletic performance and are critical to the welfare of the horse; yet none of these topics are covered to any useful degree in most veterinary school curricula. In fact, the entire field of equine sports medicine has largely developed outside of academia within specialty practices, and only recently have a few academic institutions incorporated or offered some of the services related to a successful sports medicine practice. In the absence of an obvious, blockable lameness or conclusive diagnostic imaging findings, what does a practitioner who is limited to prescribing medications or performing surgery have to offer a client who complains of reduced performance in the elite equine athlete? We are often forced to inform clients to come back 'when the condition worsens.' This is one situation where the unique evaluation and diagnostic procedures associated with many integrative medicine approaches can make a substantial, beneficial contribution to equine welfare.

9.3 What Does Integrative Medicine Have to Offer?

Equine welfare encompasses all aspects of animal well-being. Providing welfare to the horse consists of more than reducing or preventing pain and goes far beyond providing appropriate medications or surgical procedures. We have responsibilities to provide proper housing, management, nutrition, disease prevention and treatment, responsible care, humane handling, and humane euthanasia (Tannenbaum, 1995). As human beings interested in providing similar comforts and health-care options to the animals in our lives as we currently enjoy, the boundaries of what we do with and for the horses in our lives (and what they can do for us) are constantly expanding.

Traditional veterinary medicine has primarily focused its efforts on improving equine welfare by providing pain relief. As a result, we now have a wide selection of pharmaceutical agents designed to manage acute pain, but unfortunately relatively few to effectively address chronic pain or muscle hypertonicity. Most acute soft tissue and orthopedic injuries are readily managed medically or surgically and resolve without any residual adverse effects. However, some injuries or disease processes do not completely resolve and may produce chronic pain, persistent muscle hypertonicity, stiffness, and altered gait patterns that cannot be eliminated even with aggressive or long-term medical or surgical management. Veterinary medicine lacks proven and effective methods to reverse or manage the long-term adverse effects of joint immobilization, altered proprioception, compensatory gait issues, muscle weakness or atrophy, and undefined causes of poor performance. The human fields of sports medicine, physical therapy, occupational therapy, exercise physiology, sports psychology, manual therapy, and athletic training have unique tools and approaches to address many of these similar issues in elite human athletes. Currently, we lack formal training, clinical experience, and a strong body of equine-specific scientific evidence to support the use of these novel evaluation or treatment techniques, which are used routinely in human rehabilitation, but have not been thoroughly evaluated for rehabilitating equine athletes. Borrowing from human applications, integrative veterinary medicine has the potential to provide safe and effective approaches for musculoskeletal and neurologic rehabilitation of both acute and chronic pain, proprioception, flexibility, strength, and endurance in horses. Proprioceptive rehabilitation has an important role to serve in the management of ataxic horses. Improved limb and spinal flexibility has the potential to prevent progressive joint degeneration and dysfunction (van Harreveld *et al.*, 2002). We need additional treatment options with evidence of effectiveness for maintaining or improving joint health, bone strength, tendon and ligament healing, and overall athletic performance.

Additional areas that might also influence equine welfare or quality-of-life issues include providing mental and physical stimulation, as well as meeting the emotional and social needs of horses (McBride and Hemmings, 2009). Horses need more mental stimulation than that provided by enforced stall rest or repetitive dressage movements day-in and day-out with limited or no turnout provided for months at a time. Cross-training is a technique used in human athletes that has implications for improving both physical and mental equine health. Over the millennia, horses have evolved to be highly efficient at locomotion over long distances, and yet we continue to negatively impact a horse's welfare by confining them to box stalls or small paddocks for months on end in the name of rehabilitation or preventing injuries. Confinement without appropriate mental stimulation continues to be a source of many of the behavioral issues that currently effect bored, frustrated or chronically stalled and unhandled horses (McBride and Hemmings 2009).

Practitioners are constantly faced with uncertainty. In an ideal world, all of our diagnostic tests would be 100% accurate and all proposed therapies would be 100% safe and effective, in 100% of our clients, as applied by 100% of practitioners. Unfortunately, horses sometimes have vague or unusual clinical presentations or unexpected adverse reactions to our medical or surgical treatments. One important reason why alternative and complementary therapies exist and have entered equine practice is that typical medications or procedures are not always effective or without unwanted effects. All medications have specific indications, and a single drug or surgical procedure can rarely address all of the issues associated with a disease process. The extra-label use of medications serves an important role in cases with limited therapeutic possibilities, even though a specific medication has not been tested for efficacy or safety in a particular species or for a known disease condition. Surgical procedures are often borrowed from human or small-animal applications and applied to the horse with no blinded, randomized controlled clinical evaluation. Not all musculoskeletal disorders are amendable to medical management or surgical correction. Therefore, clients and cutting-edge practitioners are always seeking novel but often untested diagnostic or treatment techniques that might show promise in the management of select conditions. Emerging medical approaches that are used effectively in human medicine for the diagnosis or management of chronic diseases should be evaluated for possible use in equine practice. Translational medicine has the potential to provide novel diagnostic and therapeutic modalities that improve the health and well-being of horses. However, what we are allowed to do in practice and what we will be permitted to do in practice in the future will be dependent upon what we can prove to be safe and effective (Haldeman, 2000). All diagnostic procedures and treatment techniques must be validated using the scientific method and evidence-based medicine principles. There is an emerging trend within integrative veterinary medicine for randomized, controlled studies to be conducted with objective outcome parameters to begin assessing the clinical efficacy of some of these therapies in horses (Haussler *et al.*, 2007; Xie *et al.*, 2005). However, debate continues about whether and how to integrate unconventional and often unproven procedures or techniques into the veterinary profession (Ramey and Rollin, 2004).

For most disease conditions, a series of therapeutic options can be provided to owners. However, if an owner rightly or wrongly perceives that they are not being provided with the best (or deemed necessary) procedure or therapy to address their horse's health and well-being, then they will likely seek information or treatment from other licensed professionals or lay practitioners. I believe that the majority of clients honestly seek out those therapies that they perceive are the best for their horses. Sometimes their motives may be misplaced, such as wanting to get a horse to perform at a level that it is not physically or mentally capable of. Unfortunately, some practitioners may choose to ignore the needs of their clients or nullify their requests for CAM by suggesting that they do not really know what is best for their horse (Ramey, 1999). Historically, human physicians have been accused of dismissing the needs or illnesses of certain patients by claiming that an illness 'was all in their heads' when they could not readily provide a specific diagnosis or effective treatment for that particular patient. It is our duty to inform and educate clients as to what we as licensed professionals perceive is the best for the horse, based on our personal experience and the existing knowledge base. However, we should also be open to any new therapies that have the potential to provide a therapeutic option that is currently lacking. Prescribing prolonged stall rest or pasture turnout with the hope that a chronic musculoskeletal injury will somehow resolve itself is no longer an acceptable method of treatment for most owners or progressive-minded veterinarians (Grant, 2003). Bed rest is now contra-indicated for most people with chronic or recurrent back problems (Waddell *et al.*, 1997). In veterinary medicine, similar studies need to be done that challenge clinical dogma or long-held traditional beliefs that have not been adequately tested.

It is certainly possible that, by providing untested CAM therapies, practitioners are depriving horses and owners of other more effective or tested therapies. However, until well-designed research studies are conducted to evaluate the efficacy of both proven and unproven therapies for specific disease conditions together in randomized, controlled trials, then there is little evidence to know one way or the other if the untested technique will provide poor-quality or ineffective treatment. That is, of course, unless a specific treatment modality or proposed nutraceutical or botanical product has no theoretical evidence for biological activity. If a modality has the potential to provide any therapeutic benefits, then, if applied inappropriately, that therapy also has to the risk of doing harm. One of the first tenets of organized medicine is 'above all, do no harm.' Unfortunately, we often induce pain or discomfort with many of the medical or surgical procedures used in equine practice. However, the induced pain or suffering is judged clinically to be worth the potential benefits gained from the procedure. With regards to CAM, a risk for inducing pain or suffering also exists, but the prevalence or severity of those risks is largely unknown since many have not been formally tested for unwanted or adverse effects in horses. Therefore, a clinically useful benefit versus risk analysis cannot be determined for many of these therapies (Ramey and Rollin, 1999). In humans, adverse effects of acupuncture, chiropractic, physical therapy, and other rehabilitative practices have been reported (Oliphant, 2004; Rubinstein et al., 2007; Taylor et al., 2005; Vas et al., 2006). Currently, we can only extrapolate and presume that similar reactions also occur to some extent in horses exposed to these same treatments.

9.4 The Scientific Method

Some critics claim that alternative or complementary therapies are not 'scientific' or scientifically based (Ramey and Jarvis, 1999). However, it is often unclear exactly what is meant, especially since review of the human acupuncture, chiropractic, and physical therapy literature clearly suggests otherwise. Numerous studies exist that have scientifically evaluated proposed mechanisms of action or the clinical efficacy of acupuncture, chiropractic, and various physical therapy modalities (Berman and Straus, 2004; Bjordal et al., 2007; Bronfort et al., 2004; Cherkin et al., 2003; Ernst, 1997; Gross et al., 2004; Maigne and Vautravers, 2003). It is no longer credible for anyone to state that 'there is no scientific basis for spinal manipulation or chiropractic treatment' (Haldeman, 2000). It is true that certain studies suggest that a particular modality may lack biological activity or is not clinically effective for managing a specific disease process, but that does not equate to a modality being labeled as 'non-scientific.' Unfortunately, bias and selective memory are innate characteristics of humans. We are constantly influencing and interpreting and reinterpreting our thoughts and the actions of those around us. Fortunately, the scientific method provides a valuable tool to limit bias and prejudice and hopefully produce valid results that we can believe in. The scientific method is a collection of techniques used to investigate phenomena, acquire new knowledge, and integrate existing knowledge. The scientific method provides a process for critical observation, objective measurement, thoughtful reassessment of ideas, and knowledge refinement, which help to differentiate scientific efforts from pseudoscience.

The scientific method consists of a series of stages that include:

(1) defining a problem or asking an interesting question,
(2) designing a method to answer the question,
(3) performing an experiment that tests a hypothesis,
(4) analyzing the data to see if our observations support or refute the hypothesis,
(5) publishing and sharing the results, and
(6) continually reassessing existing evidence and its clinical application.

The scientific method is an iterative and flexible process and is not a fixed or consecutive series of steps. New information gained from a particular experiment or published study may cause a scientist to back up, skip forward, or repeat steps at any point in the overall process in an effort to refine their scientific inquiry. Failure of the hypothesis to address the question of interest or failure of the experiment to produce the expected results causes reflection and reassessment of the experimental design. The scientific method works best in situations where the phenomena of interest can be readily isolated, extraneous factors can be measured or eliminated, and the system under study can be repeatedly tested after making limited, controlled changes to it. The scientific method can never absolutely verify (i.e., prove the truth of something); it can only falsify or disprove a hypothesis.

Most veterinary practitioners are not trained or equipped to effectively test new therapies, so they must rely on research institutions to do so (Rollin, 2006). The problem is that most traditional veterinary research institutions are not designed, by definition, to provide leading or cutting-edge information for any alternative or complementary medical systems. New discoveries related to integrative medicine often come from individual interested researchers or from practitioners seeking to help their patients or being directed by their clients as to what therapies they perceive will optimize health or maximize performance in their horses. However, CAM practitioners can no longer afford to isolate themselves from mainstream veterinary medicine through barriers resulting from unique jargon, practice patterns, philosophical basis, and lack of evidence (Kopansky-Giles et al., 2005). CAM practitioners can no longer use the excuse that a modality is not testable by scientific methods. A specific modality may not be testable using conventional research methods; however, innovative and imaginative researchers – both within and outside the field of veterinary medicine – can often provide insights on how to approach this issue. Examples of unconventional research methods include the development of an appropriate sham or simulated acupuncture treatment (Cherkin et al., 2009), the development for objective measures of back pain or stiffness in horses (Haussler and Erb, 2006; Haussler et al., 2007), investigating the clinical efficacy of a botanical medicine that has numerous pharmaceutically active ingredients (McPartland and Pruitt, 1999), or assessing the efficacy or dosage of a homeopathic remedy based on the principle of identifying detectable drug concentrations, when other mechanisms may be responsible for perceived beneficial effects (Khuda-Bukhsh, 2003; Khuda-Bukhsh et al., 2009). The search for unconventional methods or approaches to measure clinical outcomes or mechanisms of action also provides a valuable opportunity for collaboration with basic scientists and clinical researchers active in human-related fields.

A common criticism against doing CAM research is that purveyors of untested therapies or nutraceuticals state that they already know that their product 'works' based on personal experience or limited clinical research. The argument often heard is why should they (or their company) waste valuable time and resources to establish what they already know to be true. In addition, there is always the underlying risk that a modality can be shown to have little or no clinical efficacy, which would likely cause a reduction in sales or a hopeful reconsideration of continued use in clinical practice. If we are serious about advancing the health care and potential welfare of our equine patients, then we must make an active effort to determine which forms of integrative medicine have established clinical efficacy and which ones have not. If a modality shows promise of efficacy, then we need to determine how to maximize its clinical effects. We cannot afford to keep doing something because we believe that it helps when there is no evidence to support that it does. This is where the principles of evidence-based medicine can serve an important role in making informed clinical decisions in regard to integrative veterinary medicine.

9.5 Evidence-Based Veterinary Medicine

> It is not too much science, but a narrow and impoverished view of science, which handicaps contemporary medicine.
>
> Leon Eisenberg (1988)

It is easy to criticize something that we know little about. CAM is a very broad and diverse collection of therapies, such as inserting fine needles, manipulating joints beyond the end-range of their physiologic joint motion, or providing aquatic therapy for therapeutic purposes, to which most practitioners have not been exposed in their formal veterinary educations. Therefore, our perceptions are often based on personal experience or the public press, and not on an extensive review and consideration of the biological activity, mechanism of action, dosage, cost-effectiveness, clinical efficacy, or potential safety considerations. At times, both promoters and critics of CAM are equally guilty of blindly ignoring the available evidence or selectively citing literature to support their positions. Some critics argue that, if no objective evidence exists to support a therapy's safety or effectiveness, then using that modality cannot be rationally justified (Ramey and Rollin, 1999). Evidence-based medicine provides a useful framework from which we can assess and conscientiously apply both tested and untested therapies in equine practice (Bonnett, 1998). Evidence-based veterinary medicine has been defined as 'the use of current best evidence in making clinical decisions' (Shaw, 2001). This process involves integrating an individual's clinical experience with the best available clinical evidence from systematic research (Sackett *et al.*, 2000). Unfortunately, the majority of clinical decisions are rarely based on best evidence or systematic research. Decision-making is often influenced by anecdote (i.e., personal clinical experiences) and the distortion of perceived outcomes. In evidence-based medicine, reduced reliance is placed upon clinical acumen, intuition, personal experience, and expert opinion (Bonnett, 1998). When available, we need to place more emphasis on evidence from accurate recording of information and randomized controlled trials (RCTs) (Cockcroft and Holmes, 2003a). The process of evidence-based medicine includes (Cockcroft and Holmes, 2003a):

(1) transforming information into a series of questions,
(2) performing a search for the best available evidence with which to answer those questions,
(3) critically evaluating the evidence for its validity (i.e., closeness to the truth) and usefulness (i.e., clinical applicability),
(4) applying the information to clinical judgments and actions, and
(5) evaluating the outcomes of the resulting decisions and actions.

In the evidence-based medicine process, the quality of information or evidence is ranked from strongest to weakest, based on the probability that a study generates reliable conclusions and recommendations (Cockcroft and Holmes, 2003a):

- Level 1 – Meta-analyses of RCTs and systematic reviews (strongest evidence).
- Level 2 – High-quality, randomized, double-blind, placebo-controlled, clinical trials.
- Level 3 – Clinical trials using historical controls; cohort and observational studies.
- Level 4 – Uncontrolled case series.
- Level 5 – Clinical experience, expert opinion, case reports, and *in vitro* research (weakest evidence).

The purpose of evidence-based medicine is to acquire the best level of evidence available. Unfortunately, most CAM literature is not readily accessible to most practitioners or included in PubMed or other publicly available databases. A large amount of information related to CAM appears in abstracts, in conference proceedings, and in non-indexed or non-peer-reviewed publications. The most commonly available levels of evidence in both the veterinary and CAM literature are often case reports, retrospective and uncontrolled case series, and a limited number of RCTs (Bonnett, 1998). Many of these studies fail to withstand intense scientific scrutiny.

Meta-analyses of RCTs and systematic reviews provide the strongest levels of evidence and provide a foundation on which clinical guidelines and standards of care in human medicine are based (Cockcroft and Holmes, 2003c). Unfortunately, the literature base in veterinary medicine has limited depth and breadth compared to human evidence-based medicine. A physician may dismiss a single case report as mere anecdote, whereas a veterinary practitioner may be grateful to have found a single published reference on the topic of interest (Cockcroft and Holmes, 2003a). The CAM literature is often rightly criticized for a lack of high-quality studies. Most systematic reviews of the clinical efficacy of human CAM therapies are limited to a low number of RCTS that have valid and reliable diagnostic criteria or outcome measures and adequate sample sizes (Bronfort *et al.*, 2001; McNeely *et al.*, 2006). Many studies have clinical heterogeneity and poor methodological quality with short-term follow-ups, which make it difficult to draw valid conclusions.

Critics of CAM often depict RCTs as the only valid form of evidence and choose to ignore the large body of lower-level evidence available. In the absence of documented scientific evidence of treatment safety or effectiveness, clinical experience may provide the only evidence (Cockcroft and Holmes, 2003a). However subjective personal experience might be, it plays an important role in the way we practice veterinary medicine (Cockcroft and Holmes, 2003c). If a specific treatment has worked for us in the past, then that provides good evidence for us not to change our approach and to try it again. A therapeutic trial (i.e., a treat-and-see approach) is a valid methodology for treating individual patients (Cockcroft and Holmes, 2003b). In order to select the best treatment for an individual patient, a trial of different therapies may be used sequentially to assess which one works best for that patient. Clinical acumen, experience, and judgment are important, but we must also move beyond our dependence on anecdote and strive for basing our clinical decisions on higher levels of evidence (Bonnett, 1998).

A large proportion of the veterinary literature consists of case reports and case series, which serve an important role in acquiring evidence and may provide more precise estimates of therapeutic effectiveness, but do not provide strong cause-and-effect inferences. Case series may also serve as early indicators of developing diagnostic or novel treatment techniques and are useful as hypothesis generators. Observational studies dominate the surgical literature and often use inclusion and exclusion criteria to reduce variability. RCTs provide the most reliable evidence of treatment efficacy and control of bias and confounding variables. Our natural bias as veterinarians is to believe that horses get better because of our treatment, and often that may be true. However, horses certainly do improve on their own, or appear to do so, because of the natural resolution of a disease process or fluctuation in clinical signs. Well-designed RCTs provide a useful tool to assess measurable treatment effects, when compared to an appropriate control group. However, we often lack methodically performed, rigorous, large-scale clinical studies, access to established databases, and large numbers of clinical subjects.

As a profession, we should cast our net for effective treatments as widely as possible, and it is our obligation to use the best evidence available to support our clinical decisions (Cockcroft and Holmes, 2003a). It is important to consider all therapeutic possibilities (both traditional and integrative), even if we may not currently understand or are unable to fully explain the physiological basis for their perceived effects (Bonnett, 1998; Cockcroft and Holmes, 2003a). However, the scientific method and evidence-based medicine should always be actively employed to document potential therapeutic benefits and adverse effects (Shaw, 2001). Scientifically validated treatments and procedures are more likely to be safe and effective than untested ones. Therefore, known effective therapies should be the preferred option when available. Practitioners of evidence-based medicine are not cynical about unproven therapies, but they remain skeptical about all treatments (Cockcroft and Holmes, 2003a). Numerous human RCTs have evaluated the effectiveness of chiropractic for various musculoskeletal disorders, but systematic reviews still are not conclusive regarding efficacy, selecting the most appropriate form of treatment for a select disease, optimal dosages and frequency of treatments, and cost-effectiveness compared to other forms of therapy (Bronfort *et al.*, 2005). This does not imply that chiropractic methods are ineffective. It only means that conclusive evidence one way or the other has not yet been obtained. Given the large body of human CAM literature available for review, it is unlikely that we will ever attain a satisfactory level of evidence regarding objective evaluation of all the various forms of CAM used in veterinary medicine due to limited resources and capabilities. However, it would behoove us to direct our efforts and resources toward diagnostic and therapeutic techniques that show the most promise in humans and specifically evaluate those therapies for clinical use in horses.

9.6 Constraints to Obtaining Quality Evidence

The focus of most CAM institutions is on teaching and clinical duties, and much less emphasis is placed on scholarly activities (Brennan *et al.*, 1997). There is a perception that teaching future practitioners is more important than assuring that what is taught is based on information gained from scientific exploration rather than a preconceived theory. Most university faculties lack a critical mass of individuals with similar CAM research interests to provide intellectual stimulation, which is essential for productive research programs. There is also a lack of appreciation for scientific rigor, misconceptions about what constitutes scientific evidence, and misconceptions about the time, effort and resources needed to develop the evidence (Brennan *et al.*, 1997). In the past, there has been a fixation on 'proving that a specific modality works' and a lack of interest in exploring the fundamental nature of the disease process treated or the mechanisms underlying the therapeutic interventions. The argument is often made that treatments are individualized, which makes designing high-quality clinical trials difficult. In addition, few CAM colleges have the needed laboratory space or equipment for establishing strong research programs and lack adequate support staff in the technical, methodological, statistical, and grant-writing areas needed for sustained research efforts (Brennan *et al.*, 1997). Therefore, researchers often lack productive research programs and a consistent publication history in well-respected journals in their respective fields. Viable external funding sources are often limited, and there is a lack of high-quality research proposals that can successfully compete for Federal funding. Owing to resource limitations, results from one laboratory or group are rarely independently replicated, which is also a common problem in veterinary research.

Issues directly related to integrative veterinary medicine research that need to be addressed include:

(1) educate practitioners in how to conduct scientifically valid clinical research and the process of evidence-based medicine,
(2) develop collaborative research with human colleagues investigating aspects of CAM,
(3) document intra-examiner and inter-examiner reliability of CAM diagnostic procedures,
(4) conduct concordance (or agreement) studies comparing different diagnostic methods,
(5) assess both short-term and long-term treatment effects,
(6) compare the efficacy of different chiropractic techniques (or different forms of acupuncture stimulation or different physical therapy programs) for select disease conditions,
(7) compare the safety and efficacy of CAM therapies to traditional forms of medical or surgical treatment, and
(8) develop initial guidelines for CAM standards of care in veterinary medicine.

9.7 Placebo Effects in Veterinary Medicine

The word *placebo* is Latin for 'I shall please.' Placebo effects are often viewed as a nuisance in clinical trials, which need to be filtered out or removed, when in fact the placebo effect represents a powerful therapeutic ally in providing effective health care. The placebo effect is a well-recognized, but poorly understood, phenomenon, which involves a non-specific psychological or physiological therapeutic effect of a medical intervention that lacks specific activity for the condition being treated (McMillan, 1999). A beneficial effect of placebo administration has been reported in 60–90% of all human diseases (Benson and Friedman, 1996), and a placebo response rate of approximately 35% is common (Beecher, 1955). However, higher rates have been reported and are most frequently associated with diseases that have clinical signs that wax and wane, fluctuate, or spontaneously resolve (Roberts *et al.*, 1993). The power of the placebo draws upon the innate ability of the body to heal itself spontaneously (Bennet, 1999). Components of the placebo effect include characteristics of:

(1) the drug or procedure,
(2) the practitioner,
(3) the patient, and
(4) the health-care setting or environment.

The 'total drug effect' is a conceptual model whereby the overall effect that a drug has on an individual usually depends on a number of different factors in addition to (or separate from) its pharmacological action (Helman, 2001). The drug itself can have indirect effects based on its color, shape, form, brand name, and cost. Therapeutic procedures can have effects based on the discomfort or pain produced, the level of invasiveness (injection versus surgery), novelty (e.g., acupuncture), perceived high technology or sophistication (e.g., laser therapy), or unusualness (e.g., detailed and extensive history-taking in homeopathy).

The exact mode(s) of action of placebos is (are) not known (Ernst, 2001). However, potential mechanisms in humans include operant conditioning, classical conditioning, guilt reduction, transference, suggestion, persuasion, role demands, hope, faith, labeling, selective symptom monitoring, misattribution, cognitive dissonance, control theory, anxiety reduction, expectancy effects, and endorphin release (Richardson, 1994). Obviously, horse owners, riders, and trainers are susceptible to the same placebo effects reported in human patients (Kienzle et al., 2006).

The placebo response seems to require a recognition by the patient for an intention to treat (McMillan, 1999). Because it is generally presumed that animals lack certain cognitive abilities, the existence of placebo effects in animals seems counterintuitive; however, animals have been experimental subjects in studies evaluating mechanisms of placebo effects for many years (Ader and Cohen, 1982; Gorczynski, 1990; Price and Soerensen, 2002). Classical conditioning, expectancy, endogenous opiates, and the effect of human contact are the four primary theories used to explain perceived placebo effects reported in animals (McMillan, 1999). Conditioning is defined by a set of operations in which a neutral conditional stimulus is paired with a biologically significant unconditional stimulus (Siegel, 2002). Once conditional responses are established, they are very well retained, even for years. Most people who care for pets observe that animals respond to non-specific effects; however, animals do not 'know' that they are receiving a medical intervention in the same way that humans do (Ernst, 2001). In human studies, placebo effects are primarily due to expectations of an individual patient. However, in veterinary studies, the placebo response can be because of the effects on the animal, but more importantly may be a result of expectations of the pet owner regarding treatment, where owners are responsible for administration of the treatment and outcome measures are derived solely from the owner's subjective observations (Munana et al., 2010). A positive response to placebo administration, manifesting as a decrease in seizure frequency of 26–46%, has been reported in epileptic dogs (Munana et al., 2010). Similarly, significant placebo effects have been reported in dogs treated for hip dysplasia with gold bead implantation (Jaeger et al., 2005) or osteoarthritis with carprofen (Vasseur et al., 1995).

Numerous studies have demonstrated that human contact has both positive and negative measurable effects on animals (McMillan, 1999). Comfort of animals and their human caregivers has been argued to be the primary goal of veterinary medical practice, instead of the treatment and prevention of disease (McMillan, 1998).

Overlooking the importance of the veterinarian–client–patient relationship and the intricacies of human–animal interactions disregards the influence of placebo effects on owners, who are the primary caregivers and determiners of whether a patient is perceived to be 'doing better' or not after treatment (Jaeger *et al.*, 2005). The mental attitude of owners is also important for the recovery of animals: 'if the owner or the veterinarian or both believe that the pet will die of its cancer, they are right and the pet cannot be saved' (Straw and Rodney, 1996). Animals can – and often do – perceive and respond to the emotional state of humans (Feddersen-Petersen, 1994). The practitioner can provide a powerful contribution to the placebo effect or even act as a therapeutic agent themselves (Hawkins, 2001). When asked to describe the qualities that make a good doctor, human patients list attributes such as kindness, willingness to listen, sympathy, patience, tolerance, and understanding, which are all associated with greater patient satisfaction (Sachs, 1982). Collectively, these attributes are often referred to as someone's 'bedside manner' – or stall-side manner in the case of equine practitioners. Health-care providers can positively influence the perceived effectiveness of their therapies by their attitude, beliefs, self-confidence, empathy, warmth, expectations, air of authority, manner of speaking, and clothing or personal appearance (Helman, 2001). Practitioners can also negatively affect clinical outcomes or minimize placebo effects by: poor history-taking and examination; poor communication skills, including body language and no eye contact; lack of knowledge of encouraging aspects of a disease's natural history; lack of knowledge of the range of therapies available, their relative success rates, their availability, and their advantages and disadvantages; lack of familiarity with the treatment chosen, lack of clarity about what to expect from the treatment, the instructions and warnings to give, and the likely time course necessary; unawareness of the importance of giving encouragement; and personal stress and burn-out.

If a therapeutic relationship established between doctor and patient enhances treatment, then all practitioners need to be trained in how to activate and optimize these healing pathways (Hawkins, 2001). Clinicians can begin to use these effects skillfully by: speaking positively (yet truthfully) about the therapy being prescribed to help create positive expectations; providing encouragement and education to empower the patient (or client) to take positive action; developing relationships of trust, compassion, and empathy; providing reassurance to relieve anxiety and fear; learning about the individual's unique outlook, values, past experiences, and belief systems; and creating ceremony and ritual that facilitate meaning and expectancy for the patient (Barrett *et al.*, 2006). The healing process is often initiated when a physician sits down and listens to a patient's story. Providing a diagnosis and assurance that a condition will improve contributes to resolution of the disease process (Thomas, 1987). Any health provider interested in optimizing treatment efficacy should consciously maximize placebo effects (McMillan, 1999).

In human medicine, the patient contributes to the placebo effect based on their psychological state, suggestibility, trust, involvement, intelligence, personality, and their social, cultural and economic milieu (Helman, 2001). In veterinary medicine, not only do we provide care for our equine patients, but also we actively interact with owners, trainers, and farm managers of those horses. Patient (or client) factors that negatively influence the placebo effect include: lack of knowledge of encouraging aspects of a disease's natural history, or success rates achievable with therapy; previous experience of therapeutic failure; depression; doubts about the therapist; fear of the treatment's adverse effects; lack of knowledge as what to expect from the treatment and the likely time course necessary; and poor communication.

Finally, the clinical setting or physical environment in which a therapy takes place affects placebo responses (Helman, 2001). These factors include the appearance, ambience, and location of a clinic; the clinic's reputation as a likely source of help; the appearance and behavior of the staff; the organization of appointments and waiting time; the length of time spent at the clinic; and how financial considerations are handled. Ritualistic symbols often help to create an atmosphere of belief, expectation, and trust in a practitioner's healing abilities. These symbols include formal dress (i.e., white-coat syndrome), elaborate diplomas on the wall, rows of large textbooks on the shelves, shiny or elaborate instruments in the treatment room or surgical suite, advertisements for pharmaceutical products, uniformed and deferential assistants, and faint smells of disinfectant (or, conversely, urine and manure). The placebo effect is a summation of all of the above effects, but without the pharmacological presence of any drug. Even if a treatment has a physical basis (e.g., surgery or radiotherapy), there is always likely to be some element of placebo effect present.

It is possible that integrative veterinary medicine may provide more opportunities to maximize placebo effects in both our equine patients and clients. A common complaint of clients and an obvious concern for most practitioners is the amount of time spent with each patient. The least amount of time spent with each patient provides an opportunity to see an increased number of patients in a day, but at the risk of providing less effective doctor–patient interactions. Integrative medicine practitioners often devote an increased amount of time to examination or treatment procedures; their approach is slow, calm, and relaxed; time is spent addressing all of client's concerns and questions; repeated and frequent follow-up visits may be provided; a calm and relaxed environment is provided, and treats may be offered to patients to assess passive spinal flexibility; and most therapies are noninvasive. Pain, fear, and heavy restraint is counterproductive to the application of most integrative therapies. Since sedation is not used for most procedures, then full patient and owner cooperation is required during the patient–doctor interaction.

9.8 Objective Outcome Measures

To better address equine welfare issues and to produce quality CAM research, we need valid and reliable diagnostic criteria and objective outcome measures to assess the functional aspects of neurologic and musculoskeletal disorders. Without measurable outcome parameters, we are hampered in our goal of identifying potential biological effects or the treatment efficacy of any modality. Currently, we lack valid and accurate tests for acute and chronic pain, proprioception, flexibility, muscle hypertonicity, strength, and endurance. Subjective assessment of spinal stiffness in humans has poor inter-examiner repeatability (Kawchuk and Herzog, 1995; Mootz *et al.*, 1989). To address this potential shortcoming in horses, an objective measure of thoracolumbar stiffness has been developed and used to assess the effect of chiropractic treatment in an experimental model of acute back pain (Haussler *et al.*, 2007). Recently, pressure algometry has been used to assess mechanical nociceptive thresholds in both acute and chronic pain syndromes in horses (Haussler and Erb, 2006; Varcoe-Cocks *et al.*, 2006). More evidence is needed before we can confidently incorporate pressure algometry use into clinical practice, but it is only one of many tools that have the potential to objectively assess parameters related to musculoskeletal dysfunction, integrative medicine, and equine health and well-being.

9.9 Evidence for Equine Integrative Medicine

Most alternative and complementary therapies have not been evaluated in a systematic manner for efficacy or safety in horses. Despite this, many practitioners still espouse their use and continue to apply unproven therapies in their daily practices. We should obviously use proven safe and effective therapies if they are available for the condition of interest that our patients present with (Rollin, 2006). Unfortunately, in clinical practice, we often have limited diagnostic and therapeutic tools available to us, and some of these techniques have only the lowest levels of evidence for efficacy. Chronic back pain is a certain welfare issue in horses; however, there are few medical or surgical approaches with any documented level of evidence for either safety or effectiveness. In two RCTs, chiropractic treatment and acupuncture have both demonstrated higher levels of efficacy for reducing signs of back pain than phenylbutazone (Sullivan *et al.*, 2008; Xie *et al.*, 2005). However, the standard practice for many veterinarians continues to be prescribing phenylbutazone for chronic back pain in horses. Unproven therapies absolutely need to be tested with the most appropriate research methods available; however, it must be remembered that an untested modality is not synonymous with a non-functional or ineffective modality (Rollin, 2006). When evaluating CAM research, it should be remembered that a lack of evidence is not a proof of ineffectiveness (Bonnett, 1998). The specific modality may be untested, and the scientific method and evidence-based medicine principles need to be applied until new evidence is accumulated to judge the modality effective or ineffective.

Until new knowledge is published, one could say that it does not exist nor can it be readily expanded upon. Although human chiropractors have been treating animals for decades, there is unfortunately only limited published evidence that chiropractic techniques are effective in horses. There are no descriptions of spinal examination procedures, no descriptions of indications for treating horses, no technique manuals describing what methods to use for which specific conditions, and only a few case reports describing vague musculoskeletal disorders that presumably responded to a single treatment or a series of chiropractic treatments. Anecdotal evidence, undisputed belief, and sharing information by word of mouth provide only the lowest levels of evidence-based medicine. For CAM to continue to develop, higher levels of evidence need to be obtained and integrated into the knowledge base. Historically, there has been a paucity of evidence available for CAM use in animals due mostly to a lack of qualified clinicians capable of applying scientific methods to investigate the myriad of untested therapies, the absence of researchers in academia with interest or clinical training in the diagnostic or therapeutic techniques of interest, and no funding sources for this type of research (Brennan et al., 1997). To the author's knowledge, there is currently only a single active academic researcher in each of the areas of equine chiropractic, acupuncture, and physical therapy in North America. We desperately need more resources directed toward focused research in these areas to make any worthwhile progress in evaluating the safety, potential mechanisms of action, and clinical efficacy of these therapies, and their potential contributions to equine welfare.

9.9.1 Equine chiropractic

Some veterinarians have stated that they do not have a problem with chiropractic techniques applied to horses, but they do have concerns about some of the individuals delivering those services. Many individuals providing 'chiropractic care' have no professional training, others are licensed human chiropractors but lack appropriate equine experience, some do not collaborate with the veterinarians responsible for a horse's care, and some entrepreneurial professionals practice beyond their human scope of practice and provide injections or are involved in other unethical activities. Unfortunately, these individuals do little to advance the equine chiropractic profession and are often a distraction to providing high-quality integrative veterinary medicine and interest in pursuing equine chiropractic research.

The focus of recent equine manual therapy research has been on assessing the clinical effects of chiropractic techniques in pain relief, improving flexibility, reducing muscle hypertonicity, and restoring spinal motion symmetry. Obvious criticism has been directed at the physical ability to even induce movement in the horse's back. Pilot work has demonstrated that manually applied forces associated with chiropractic techniques are able to produce substantial segmental spinal motion (Haussler et al., 1999). Two randomized, controlled clinical trials have utilized pressure algometry to assess mechanical nociceptive thresholds (MNTs) in the thoracolumbar region of horses, and demonstrated that chiropractic treatment can reduce back pain (or increase MNTs) (Haussler and Erb, 2003; Sullivan et al., 2008). Additional studies have assessed the effects of equine chiropractic techniques on increasing passive spinal mobility (i.e., flexibility) and reducing longissimus muscle tone (Haussler *et al.*, 2007; Wakeling *et al.*, 2006). The effect of chiropractic treatment on asymmetrical spinal movement patterns in horses with documented back pain suggests that chiropractic treatment elicits slight but significant changes in thoracolumbar and pelvic kinematics, and that some of these changes are likely to be beneficial (Faber *et al.*, 2003; Gómez Alvarez *et al.*, 2008).

Additional studies are needed to determine how long the clinical effects of chiropractic treatment persist in horses and to ascertain whether this modality can enhance athletic performance. We lack a valid animal model for studying the effects of spinal manipulation, which would allow characterization of the anatomic, biomechanical, neurophysiologic, pathophysiologic, cellular, and biochemical changes associated with joint mobilization or high-velocity thrusts (Brennan *et al.*, 1997; Vernon, 1995). Further understanding of the local and systemic effects of manipulation on pain reduction and tissue healing is also needed. Controlled trials using different forms of manual therapy (e.g., manual thrusts versus instrument-assisted thrusts versus manipulation under anesthesia) need to be done to determine which method is most effective for treating specific disease processes. Directed research is also needed to evaluate the potential sources of back pain in horses, which include: impinged dorsal spinous processes; synovitis or osteoarthritis of the dorsal synovial articulations of the vertebral column; thoracolumbar myositis; desmitis of the spinal or sacroiliac ligaments; cellular and biochemical changes to structures within and adjacent to the intervertebral foramen; mechanisms of peripheral and central sensitization of the spinal cord and peripheral nerves; pathophysiology of articular innervation; and altered neurophysiology of the local autonomic nervous system.

9.9.2 Equine acupuncture

The most common equine welfare-related issue for using acupuncture is pain relief. A single systematic review of acupuncture use in veterinary medicine has been conducted to assess the existing clinical evidence, which included 14 randomized controlled trials and 17 non-randomized controlled trails in several species (Habacher *et al.*, 2006). Overall, the methodological quality of veterinary acupuncture studies is low, but encouraging evidence exists for altering cutaneous pain in horses, which warrants further investigation in rigorous trials. In a series of studies, a large number of horses ($n = 350$) presenting with a chief complaint of poor performance, presumably due to primary back pain, were treated with several different forms of acupuncture stimulation, and pain alleviation varied from 53% to 87% (Martin and Klide, 2001). Unfortunately, there were no control groups in these studies, so neither the natural course of back pain resolution nor the true effectiveness of acupuncture treatment could be determined. Needle acupuncture and electro-acupuncture both provide cutaneous analgesia in horses, compared to a control group of no needle placement (Skarda *et al.*, 2002). However, electro-acupuncture is more effective than needle acupuncture for activating the release of β-endorphins into the cerebrospinal fluid (Skarda *et al.*, 2002). Needle acupuncture appears to be slightly more effective than low-level laser stimulation (laser acupuncture) or sterile isotonic saline injection (aquapuncture) for reducing pain (Martin and Klide, 2001).

In a randomized controlled study evaluating treatment efficacy for chronic thoracolumbar pain, electro-acupuncture was compared to phenylbutazone and control (i.e., oral saline) groups (Xie *et al.*, 2005). Electro-acupuncture produced significant decreases in thoracolumbar pain scores after three treatments, which remained reduced 14 days after the last treatment, compared to the other two treatment groups. Electro-acupuncture using local acupuncture points and high-frequency (80–120 Hz) stimulation may be more effective in relieving local pain, whereas distant points and low-frequency (20 Hz) stimulation may produce more generalized analgesia (Xie *et al.*, 2001). It is suggested that a minimum of three electro-acupuncture treatments are required for effective treatment of chronic thoracolumbar pain in horses (Xie *et al.*, 2005). Using needle acupuncture, it is recommended that horses receive weekly treatments for eight weeks, and most horses improve after five to eight treatments (Martin and Klide, 2001).

Acupuncture diagnosis consists of identifying an exaggerated response to superficial stimuli, which may be a useful component to an integrated pre-purchase examination for lameness in sport horses (McCormick, 2006). However, electro-acupuncture has variable effectiveness for reducing pain associated with either experimentally induced or naturally occurring lameness (Steiss *et al.*, 1989; Xie *et al.*, 2001). It has been hypothesized that intra-articular pathologies activate acupuncture channels and extra-articular pathologies (e.g., foot abscess, splints, tendonitis, and subchondral bone disease) do not, but little scientific evidence in the form of blinded, controlled studies exist to support this theory (McCormick, 1996, 1997, 1998, 2006). Electro-acupuncture also has mixed effectiveness for providing analgesia associated with experimental models of small intestine or rectal distension in horses (Merritt *et al.*, 2002; Skarda and Muir, 2003). Further studies are needed to determine the effectiveness of acupuncture in clinical cases of documented colic.

To provide stronger evidence, high-quality studies with appropriate control groups are needed to assess the efficacy of acupuncture for treating various acute and chronic visceral and somatic pain syndromes. Small sample sizes, inadequate statistical power, clinical heterogeneity, and the lack of appropriate control groups (i.e., other than needling at non-acupuncture sites) prevent the development of rigorous acupuncture studies. Future studies require validated, clinically oriented outcome parameters to assess the efficacy of acupuncture stimulation for various lameness or pain syndromes. Studies are also needed to determine the specificity and sensitivity of acupuncture point reactivity in the diagnoses of known local visceral, soft tissue, osseous or articular pathology, and under what circumstances acupuncture points are activated. Additional studies are required to determine whether the analgesic effect produced by needle acupuncture and electro-acupuncture stimulation in horses varies if the stimulation is provided at specific acupuncture points or at non-specific points (Xie *et al.*, 2005). Appropriate animal models need to be developed to assess the clinical effects and safety of acupuncture in a controlled and systematic manner. Finally, a standard for high-quality acupuncture needs to be based on the consensus of experts and evidence for appropriate selection of acupuncture points, dosage (i.e., frequency and duration), and type of acupuncture stimulation shown to be most effective for select musculoskeletal or visceral disorders (Habacher *et al.*, 2006).

9.9.3 Equine physical therapy and rehabilitation

Over the history of veterinary medicine, various forms of physical therapy and rehabilitation have been applied to horses and are currently regularly applied by most veterinarians or equine physiotherapists; however, the unfortunate fact is that we have very little scientific evidence from well-designed studies that any of these treatment techniques are effective in horses (Buchner and Schildboeck, 2006; McGowan *et al.*, 2007). A major contributing factor to the lack of evidence is that the field of physical therapy encompasses such a wide variety of diagnostic and treatment approaches, which include manual techniques (e.g., soft tissue and articular mobilization, and stretching), therapeutic modalities (e.g., electrical muscle stimulation, therapeutic ultrasound, and hot and cold therapies), and innumerable forms of exercise (e.g., continuous passive motion, assisting weight-bearing, proprioceptive challenges, swimming, strengthening, and endurance). Additional therapies that are not traditionally considered within the realm of physical therapy include therapeutic massage, extracorporeal shock-wave therapy, hyperbaric oxygen therapy, and orthotics and prosthetics. Equine rehabilitation also often incorporates therapeutic and corrective hoof care and shoeing, different working surfaces, corrective dental care, proper nutrition and energy content of the diet, training devices, and basic ground work (Ridgway and Harman, 1999). All of the above treatment techniques have potential clinical applications in equine welfare, but there is a substantial need for an increased number of high-quality, focused research projects.

It is beyond the scope of this chapter to review the physical therapy and rehabilitation literature for all aspects of physical and physiological mechanisms of action, treatment modalities, or specific clinical applications. Basic science research is needed on the biological activity of the various therapies. Much of this information does exist for humans, laboratory animals or dogs, but has rarely been evaluated in horses (McGowan *et al.*, 2007). Prolonged or repeated exposure to ice–water baths does have therapeutic benefits in the distal limb of horses, but has not been evaluated for the management of neck or back pain. RCTs are needed to document specific healing mechanisms and possible preventive effects for both cryotherapy and heating modalities (Buchner and Schildboeck, 2006). Hydrotherapy (i.e., exercise in an underwater treadmill or swimming pool) is commonly recommended post-surgery to improve muscle strength, cardiovascular fitness, and joint range of motion during reduced or non-weight-bearing exercise (Geytenbeek, 2002; Misumi *et al.*, 1993; Nankervis and Williams, 2006). Further studies are needed to assess specific physiologic and biomechanical effects of all physical therapy techniques for specific disease conditions or within a validated equine model of musculoskeletal dysfunction (e.g., carpal osteochondral fragment model) (Frisbie *et al.*, 1998).

Exercise is one of the most common rehabilitative prescriptions for musculoskeletal, neurologic, cardiovascular, and respiratory disorders. There is good evidence to suggest that exercise is effective for a wide range of chronic disorders in humans (Smidt *et al.*, 2005); however, most therapeutic exercise programs for horses are based mainly on intuition, anecdotal evidence, and tradition (Grant, 2003). RCTs investigating the efficacy of mild, moderate, and strenuous exercise (in its various forms) on pain, proprioception, joint range of motion, and neuromotor control are needed. Additional studies are required to assess changes in and healing of muscle, bone, cartilage, tendon, and ligament, as well as the prevention of musculoskeletal injuries due to compensatory lameness. The evaluation of most electrotherapy, magnetic field therapy, therapeutic ultrasound, and low-level laser therapy modalities is hampered by the lack of well-designed studies, poorly defined indications and dosages, and the absence of validated treatment protocols (i.e., intensity, duration, and frequency) (Buchner and Schildboeck, 2006). Many of these therapies have some level of clinical evidence in humans, and have the potential for effective use in the rehabilitation of horses; however, the biological activity of all of these treatment modalities needs to be evaluated in defined musculoskeletal lesions and assessed with objective outcome parameters. Equine skin and the overlying hair coat may block deep tissue effects of low-level laser therapy and therapeutic ultrasound (Esnouf *et al.*, 2007; Steiss and Adams, 1999). The results of basic science studies need to be synthesized into focused clinical research that develops and validates effective treatment protocols for clearly defined clinical issues using objective assessments.

9.9.4 Other equine integrative medicine approaches

Nutraceuticals, botanical medicine, and homeopathy also may play some role in equine welfare or pain management, but unfortunately they suffer similarly from the absence of well-designed, high-quality evidence in horses (Wynn and Schoen, 1998). Focused research into plausible mechanisms of action, active ingredients, biological activity, toxicity, specific case selection, objective outcome parameters, use of control groups and blinding, and adequate follow-up are needed to develop a firm foundation on which future clinical studies can begin to provide reliable evidence for or against the continued use of these controversial therapies in equine practice (Bone 2007).

9.10 Licensed Professionals and Lay Practitioners

One of the primary reasons why complementary and alternative approaches exist and persist is that we as veterinarians are not meeting, and often cannot meet, all of our client's needs. If clients ask us to reset their horse's shoes and we do not have a full-time farrier on staff, then they will need to go to someone else that offers that service. If we cannot provide an experienced rider or arena to assess if a vague lameness or back problem is aggravated by additional weight in the saddle or not, then owners will go somewhere else or we will treat the horse without having a full clinical assessment. If a horse has an unexpected vaccine reaction and we cannot remember if it is better to apply an ice pack or a hot pack over the site of heat and swelling, then owners will ask someone who can provide the requested information. If clients want to know why their horse has reduced neck flexibility only in left lateral bending and we are not able to identify any structural disorder with any of our diagnostic imaging capabilities or alter the severity of the stiffness with any non-steroidal anti-inflammatory drug (NSAID) or intra-articular corticosteroid injections, then they will investigate other therapies that offer some promise of efficacy. It is our responsibility as licensed professionals to refer clients to colleagues or other licensed professionals outside the veterinary profession that have specific expertise or can provide services that we are not capable of providing.

It has been suggested that no particular scientific or veterinary expertise may be necessary for the application of CAM and that lay people should be providing these therapies (Ramey and Rollin, 2004). Unfortunately, this argument ignores the large body of evidence available within the fields of acupuncture, chiropractic, physical therapy, and other related fields that describe the advanced diagnostic or therapeutic skills needed and the safety implications of unskilled personnel providing these therapies. It is likely that untrained or unlicensed practitioners are much more apt than trained or certified practitioners to cause injury or misapply a therapy based on the horse's presenting complaints (Ramey and Ernst, 1999). An obvious contraindication to cervical manipulation would be if a foal had a cervical fracture. However, if the lay practitioner or licensed human professional treating the foal is unaware of the untoward clinical or neurologic signs, then they would likely treat a foal with neck pain and chronic 'popping' sounds produced every time the neck was moved side-to-side. Common sense and basic veterinary training provide a valuable foundation and knowledge base from which to judge if an untested modality might be indicated or contra-indicated in a particular case and the clinical skills needed to monitor potential treatment effects or adverse reactions. Licensed professionals have a duty to keep abreast of the most recent literature and latest clinical developments to determine what services or therapies to provide their clients. Lay practitioners do not have a similar duty and have only limited abilities to expand their knowledge base of new or untested therapies with the scientific method or evidence-based medicine processes. The majority of State veterinary practice Acts in the USA now state that providing CAM therapies is considered the practice of veterinary medicine and needs to be provided by or overseen by veterinarians. In human medicine, it is clear that physicians are in a position to take charge of integrative medicine, which may or may not exclude CAM practitioners and lay practitioners (Snyderman and Weil, 2002). The veterinary profession needs to make a similar commitment and decide how collaborative efforts with licensed human CAM practitioners with interests in horse health and welfare can work alongside or in conjunction with veterinarians to form interdisciplinary or multidisciplinary practices. This clinical model would ensure that patients receive the best of what integrative medicine has to offer, and that services would be provided by individuals with appropriate training and expertise (Meeker and Mootz, 2005).

In summary, the following four actions have been proposed to evaluate how integrative therapies may further contribute to equine welfare (Ramey and Ernst, 1999).

(1) Practitioners need to get beyond their bias and prejudices regarding alternative or complementary therapies. CAM practitioners cannot continue to blindly provide untested therapies without any consideration of the scientific method or use of objective outcome parameters. Critics of these untested therapies risk losing credibility if they continue to make generalized statements about avoiding unscientific and ineffective therapies when there is indeed a scientific basis for the proposed therapy and some level of evidence for therapeutic efficacy. Unfortunately, we will never have all of the proof needed to convince everyone within the profession that integrative veterinary medicine is valid or has an important role to serve.

(2) We need to be aware of what has been tested and what has not been tested. It is easy to fall into the trap of repeatedly quoting a single source that supports our biased position regarding the perceived benefit or harm of a specific CAM modality. Science is based on a collection of knowledge from very disparate sources. The information that we consider critical to the practice of veterinary medicine is only a small part of that body of knowledge. We need to be able to review all of the information available in an objective and evidence-based manner to make the best decisions possible regarding the use of equine integrative therapies.

(3) Many more studies and better-quality research are needed. If we are to advance as a profession, then we cannot continue to rely on hearsay, clinical experience, expert opinion, and case reports to direct our future clinical decision-making. We need well-designed research studies that objectively answer our questions of safety, mechanism of action, efficacy, and cost-effectiveness of each of the currently untested therapies that we use or would like to consider using in our practices.

(4) Research funds need to be made available and directed toward investigating the use of integrative therapies for improving equine health and welfare. The current availability of monies for research in this area is almost non-existent. Researchers have to be creative in seeking private funding or be very driven to extract research monies from current funding mechanisms. Fortunately, a few well-designed studies can provide much needed evidence and initiate a scientific foundation on which to assess an untested modality.

Integrative veterinary medicine is an exciting field and has the potential to offer measurable benefits to the well-being of the horse and owner. A growing body of evidence and increased public demand for services continue to support the integration of these (yet to be fully tested) diagnostic and therapeutic approaches into mainstream veterinary medicine practices and academia. It is up to us as a profession to decide how integrative veterinary medicine will contribute to equine welfare in the future.

References

Ader, R. and Cohen, N. (1982) Behaviorally conditioned immunosuppression and murine systemic lupus erythematosus. *Science* **215**, 1534–1536.

Barrett, B., Muller, D., Rakel, D., Rabago, D., Marchand, L. and Scheder, J. (2006) Placebo, meaning, and health. *Perspectives in Biology and Medicine* **49**, 178–198.

Beecher, H.K. (1955) The powerful placebo. *Journal of the American Medical Association* **159**, 1602–1606.

Bennet, P. (1999) Placebo and healing. In *Textbook of Natural Medicine*, Pizzorno, J.E. and Murray, M.T. (eds). Churchill Livingstone, Edinburgh.

Benson, H. and Friedman, R. (1996) Harnessing the power of the placebo effect and renaming it 'remembered wellness'. *Annual Review of Medicine* **47**, 193–199.

Berman, J.D. and Straus, S.E. (2004) Implementing a research agenda for complementary and alternative medicine. *Annual Review of Medicine* **55**, 239–254.

Bjordal, J.M., Johnson, M.I., Lopes-Martins, R.A., Bogen, B., Chow, R. and Ljunggren, A.E. (2007) Short-term efficacy of physical interventions in osteoarthritic knee pain. A systematic review and meta-analysis of randomised placebo-controlled trials. *BMC Musculoskeletal Disorders* **8**, 51.

Bone, K.M. (2007) Evaluating, designing, and accessing herbal medicine research. In *Veterinary Herbal Medicine*, Wynn, S.G. and Fougère, B.J. (eds), pp. 87–97. Mosby Elsevier, St. Louis, MO.

Bonnett, B. (1998) Evidence-based medicine: critical evaluation of new and existing therapies. In *Complementary and Alternative Veterinary Medicine: Principles and Practice*, Schoen, A.M. and Wynn, S.G. (eds), pp. 15–20. Mosby, St. Louis, MO.

Brennan, P.C., Cramer, G.D., Kirstukas, S.J. and Cullum, M.E. (1997) Basic science research in chiropractic: the state of the art and recommendations for a research agenda. *Journal of Manipulative and Physiological Therapeutics* **20**, 150–168.

Bronfort, G., Assendelft, W.J., Evans, R., Haas, M. and Bouter, L. (2001) Efficacy of spinal manipulation for chronic headache: a systematic review. *Journal of Manipulative and Physiological Therapeutics* **24**, 457–466.

Bronfort, G., Haas, M., Evans, R.L. and Bouter, L.M. (2004) Efficacy of spinal manipulation and mobilization for low back pain and neck pain: a systematic review and best evidence synthesis. *Spine Journal* **4**, 335–356.

Bronfort, G., Haas, M. and Evans, R. (2005) The clinical effectiveness of spinal manipulation for musculoskeletal conditions. In *Principles and Practice of Chiropractic*, Haldeman, S. (ed.), 3rd edn, pp. 147–166. McGraw-Hill, New York.

Buchner, H.H. and Schildboeck, U. (2006) Physiotherapy applied to the horse: a review. *Equine Veterinary Journal* **38**, 574–580.

Cherkin, D.C., Sherman, K.J., Deyo, R.A. and Shekelle, P.G. (2003) A review of the evidence for the effectiveness, safety, and cost of acupuncture, massage therapy, and spinal manipulation for back pain. *Annals of Internal Medicine* **138**, 898–906.

Cherkin, D.C., Sherman, K.J., Avins, A.L., Erro, J.H., Ichikawa, L., Barlow, W.E., Delancy, K., Hawkes, R., Hamilton, L., Pressman, A., Khalsa, P.S. and Deyo, R.A. (2009) A randomized trial comparing acupuncture, simulated acupuncture, and usual care for chronic low back pain. *Archives of Internal Medicine* **169**, 858–866.

Cockcroft, P.D. and Holmes, M.A. (2003a) Introduction. In *Handbook of Evidence-Based Veterinary Medicine*, Cockcroft, P.D. and Holmes, M.A. (eds), pp. 1–21. Blackwell Publishing, Oxford.

Cockcroft, P.D. and Holmes, M.A. (2003b) Research studies. In *Handbook of Evidence-Based Veterinary Medicine*, Cockcroft, P.D. and Holmes, M.A. (eds), pp. 67–83. Blackwell Publishing, Oxford.

Cockcroft, P.D. and Holmes, M.A. (2003c) Sources of information. In *Handbook of Evidence-Based Veterinary Medicine*, Cockcroft, P.D. and Holmes, M.A. (eds), pp. 34–54. Blackwell Publishing, Oxford.

Ernst, E. (1997) Acupuncture as a symptomatic treatment of osteoarthritis: a systematic review. *Scandinavian Journal of Rheumatology* **26**, 444–447.

Ernst, E. (2001) Towards a scientific understanding of placebo effects. In *Understanding the Placebo Effect in Complementary Medicine: Theory, Practice and Research*, Peters, D. (ed.), pp. 17–29. Churchill Livingstone, St. Louis, MO.

Esnouf, A., Wright, P.A., Moore, J.C. and Ahmed, S. (2007) Depth of penetration of an 850 nm wavelength low level laser in human skin. *Acupuncture and Electro-Therapeutics Research* **32**, 81–86.

Faber, M.J., van Weeren, P.R., Schepers, M. and Barneveld, A. (2003) Long-term follow-up of manipulative treatment in a horse with back problems. *Journal of Veterinary Medicine Series A* **50**, 241–245.

Feddersen-Petersen, D. (1994) Some interactive aspects between dogs and their owners: are there reciprocal influences between both inter- and intraspecific communication? *Applied Animal Behaviour Science* **40**, 78–84.

Fontanarosa, P.B. and Lundberg, G.D. (1998) Alternative medicine meets science. *Journal of the American Medical Association* **280**, 1618–1619.

Frisbie, D.D., Kawcak, C.E., Baxter, G.M., Trotter, G.W., Powers, B.E., Lassen, E.D. and McIlwraith, C.W. (1998) Effects of 6α-methylprednisolone acetate on an equine osteochondral fragment exercise model. *American Journal of Veterinary Research* **59**, 1619–1628.

Fruehwirth, B., Peham, C., Scheidl, M. and Schobesberger, H. (2004) Evaluation of pressure distribution under an English saddle at walk, trot and canter. *Equine Veterinary Journal* **36**, 754–757.

Geytenbeek, J. (2002) Evidence for effective hydrotherapy. *Physiotherapy* **88**, 514–529.

Gómez Alvarez, C.B., L'Ami, J.J., Moffat, D., Back, W. and van Weeren, P.R. (2008) Effect of chiropractic manipulations on the kinematics of back and limbs in horses with clinically diagnosed back problems. *Equine Veterinary Journal* **40**, 153–159.

Goodwin, D., McGreevy, P.D., Heleski, C., Randle, H. and Waran, N. (2008) Equitation science: the application of science in equitation. *Journal of Applied Animal Welfare Science* **11**, 185–190.

Gorczynski, R.M. (1990) Conditioned enhancement of skin allografts in mice. *Brain, Behavior, and Immunity* **4**, 85–92.

Grant, B.D. (2003) Rest and rehabilitation. In *Diagnosis and Management of Lameness in the Horse*, Ross, M.W. and Dyson, S.J. (eds), pp. 788–791. Saunders, Philadelphia, PA.

Gross, A.R., Hoving, J.L., Haines, T.A., Goldsmith, C.H., Kay, T., Aker, P. and Bronfort, G. (2004) A Cochrane review of manipulation and mobilization for mechanical neck disorders. *Spine* **29**, 1541–1548.

Habacher, G., Pittler, M.H. and Ernst, E. (2006) Effectiveness of acupuncture in veterinary medicine: systematic review. *Journal of Veterinary Internal Medicine* **20**, 480–488.

Haldeman, S. (2000) The evolution of chiropractic – science and theory. In *International Conference on Spinal Manipulation*, Northwestern Health Sciences University, Bloomington, MN, September.

Haussler, K.K. and Erb, H.N. (2003) Pressure algometry: objective assessment of back pain and effects of chiropractic treatment. *Proceedings of the American Association of Equine Practitioners* **49**, 66–70.

Haussler, K.K. and Erb, H.N. (2006) Pressure algometry for the detection of induced back pain in horses: a preliminary study. *Equine Veterinary Journal* **38**, 76–81.

Haussler, K.K., Bertram, J.E.A. and Gellman, K. (1999) *In-vivo* segmental kinematics of the thoracolumbar spinal region in horses and effects of chiropractic manipulations. *Proceedings of the American Association of Equine Practitioners* **45**, 327–329.

Haussler, K.K., Hill, A.E., Puttlitz, C.M. and McIlwraith, C.W. (2007) Effects of vertebral mobilization and manipulation on kinematics of the thoracolumbar region. *American Journal of Veterinary Research* **68**, 508–516.

Hawkins, J. (2001) How can we optimize non-specific effects? In *Understanding the Placebo Effect in Complementary Medicine: Theory, Practice and Research*, Peters, D. (ed.), pp. 69–88. Churchill Livingstone, St. Louis, MO.

Helman, C.G. (2001) Placebos and nocebos: the cultural construction of belief. In *Understanding the Placebo Effect in Complementary Medicine: Theory, Practice and Research*, Peters, D. (ed.), pp. 3–16. Churchill Livingstone, St. Louis, MO.

Jaeger, G.T., Larsen, S. and Moe, L. (2005) Stratification, blinding and placebo effect in a randomized, double blind placebo-controlled clinical trial of gold bead implantation in dogs with hip dysplasia. *Acta Veterinaria Scandinavica* **46**, 57–68.

Kaptchuk, T.J. and Eisenberg, D.M. (2001) Varieties of healing. 1. Medical pluralism in the United States. *Annals of Internal Medicine* **135**, 189–195.

Kawchuk, G. and Herzog, W. (1995) The reliability and accuracy of a standard method of tissue compliance assessment. *Journal of Manipulative and Physiological Therapeutics* **18**, 298–301.

Khuda-Bukhsh, A.R. (2003) Towards understanding molecular mechanisms of action of homeopathic drugs: an overview. *Molecular and Cellular Biochemistry* **253**, 339–345.

Khuda-Bukhsh, A.R., Bhattacharyya, S.S., Paul, S., Dutta, S., Boujedaini, N. and Belon, P. (2009) Modulation of signal proteins: a plausible mechanism to explain how a potentized drug Secale Cor 30C diluted beyond Avogadro's limit combats skin papilloma in mice. *Evidence-Based Complementary and Alternative Medicine.* doi:10.1093/ecam/nep084.

Kienzle, E., Freismuth, A. and Reusch, A. (2006) Double-blind placebo-controlled vitamin E or selenium supplementation of sport horses with unspecified muscle problems. An example of the potential of placebos. *Journal of Nutrition (Supplement)* 136, 2045S–2047S.

Kopansky-Giles, D., Walker, B. and Borges, S. (2005) Integration of chiropractic into multidisciplinary and hospital-based settings. In *Principles and Practice of Chiropractic,* Haldeman, S. (ed.), 3rd edn, pp. 1165–1179. McGraw-Hill, New York.

Maigne, J.Y. and Vautravers, P. (2003) Mechanism of action of spinal manipulative therapy. *Joint Bone Spine* 70, 336–341.

Manfredi, J., Clayton, H.M. and Rosenstein, D. (2005) Radiographic study of bit position within the horse's oral cavity. *Equine and Comparative Exercise Physiology* 2, 195–201.

Martin, B.B., Jr. and Klide, A.M. (2001) Acupuncture for treatment of chronic back pain in horses. In *Veterinary Acupuncture: Ancient Art to Modern Medicine,* Schoen, A.M. (ed.), pp. 467–473. Mosby, St. Louis, MO.

McBride, S. and Hemmings, A. (2009) A neurologic perspective of equine stereotypy. *Journal of Equine Veterinary Science* 29, 10–16.

McCormick, W.H. (1996) Traditional Chinese channel diagnosis, myofascial pain syndrome and metacarpophalangeal joint trauma in the horse. *Journal of Equine Veterinary Science* 16, 562–567.

McCormick, W.H. (1997) Oriental channel diagnosis in foot lameness of the equine forelimb. *Journal of Equine Veterinary Science* 17, 315–321.

McCormick, W.H. (1998) The origins of acupuncture channel imbalance in pain of the equine hindlimb. *Journal of Equine Veterinary Science* 18, 528–534.

McCormick, W.H. (2006) The incidence and significance of excess acupuncture channel imbalance in the equine sport horse purchase examination, 1999–2004. *Journal of Equine Veterinary Science* 26, 322–325.

McGowan, C.M., Stubbs, N.C. and Jull, G.A. (2007) Equine physiotherapy: a comparative view of the science underlying the profession. *Equine Veterinary Journal* 39, 90–94.

McMillan, F.D. (1998) Comfort as the primary goal in veterinary medical practice. *Journal of the American Veterinary Medical Association* 212, 1370–1374.

McMillan, F.D. (1999) The placebo effect in animals. *Journal of the American Veterinary Medical Association* 215, 1999.

McNeely, M.L., Armijo Olivo, S. and Magee, D.J. (2006) A systematic review of the effectiveness of physical therapy interventions for temporomandibular disorders. *Physical Therapy* 86, 710–725.

McPartland, J.M. and Pruitt, P.L. (1999) Side effects of pharmaceuticals not elicited by comparable herbal medicines: the case of tetrahydrocannabinol and marijuana. *Alternative Therapies in Health and Medicine* 5, 57–62.

Meeker, W.C. and Mootz, R.D. (2005) Integration of chiropractic in health care. In *Principles and Practice of Chiropractic*, Haldeman, S. (ed.), 3rd edn, pp. 135–146. McGraw-Hill, New York.

Merritt, A.M., Xie, H., Lester, G.D., Burrow, J.A., Lorenzo-Figueras, M. and Mahfoud, Z. (2002) Evaluation of a method to experimentally induce colic in horses and the effects of acupuncture applied at the Guan-yuan-shu (similar to BL-21) acupoint. *American Journal of Veterinary Research* 63, 1006–1011.

Misumi, K., Sakamoto, H. and Shimizu, R. (1993) The validity of swimming training for two-year-old Thoroughbreds. *Journal of Veterinary Medical Science* 56, 217–222.

Mootz, R.D., Keating, J.C., Jr., Kontz, H.P., Milus, T.B. and Jacobs, G.E. (1989) Intra- and interobserver reliability of passive motion palpation of the lumbar spine. *Journal of Manipulative and Physiological Therapeutics* 12, 440–445.

Munana, K.R., Zhang, D. and Patterson, E.E. (2010) Placebo effect in canine epilepsy trials. *Journal of Veterinary Internal Medicine* 24, 166–170.

Nankervis, K.J. and Williams, R.J. (2006) Heart rate responses during acclimation of horses to water treadmill exercise. *Equine Veterinary Journal (Supplement)* 38(S36), 110–112.

Oliphant, D. (2004) Safety of spinal manipulation in the treatment of lumbar disk herniations: a systematic review and risk assessment. *Journal of Manipulative and Physiological Therapeutics* 27, 197–210.

Price, D.D. and Soerensen, L.V. (2002) Endogenous opioid and non-opioid pathways as mediators of placebo analgesia. In *The Science of the Placebo: Toward an Interdisciplinary Research Agenda*, Guess, H.A., Kleinman, A., Kusek, J.W. and Engel, L.W. (eds), pp. 183–206. BMJ Books, London.

Ramey, D. (1999) Afterword. In *Consumer's Guide to Alternative Therapies in the Horse*, Ramey, D. (ed.), pp. 201–204. Howell Book House, Foster City, CA.

Ramey, D. and Ernst, E. (1999) Common misconceptions about alternative medicine. In *Consumer's Guide to Alternative Therapies in the Horse*, Ramey, D. (ed.), pp. 35–42. Howell Book House, Foster City, CA.

Ramey, D. and Jarvis, W.T. (1999) Scientific versus unscientific thinking. In *Consumer's Guide to Alternative Therapies in the Horse*, Ramey, D. (ed.), pp. 25–34. Howell Book House, Foster City, CA.

Ramey, D. and Rollin, B.E. (1999) The ethics of providing therapy. In *Consumer's Guide to Alternative Therapies in the Horse*, Ramey, D. (ed.), pp. 43–54. Howell Book House, Foster City, CA.

Ramey, D. and Rollin, B.E. (2004) Regulatory considerations. In *Complementary and Alternative Veterinary Medicine Considered*, Ramey, D. and Rollin, B.E. (eds), pp. 179–195. Iowa State University Press, Ames, IA.

Richardson, P.H. (1994) Placebo effects in pain management. *Pain Reviews* 1, 15–32.

Ridgway, K. and Harman, J. (1999) Equine back rehabilitation. *Veterinary Clinics of North America: Equine Practice* 15, 263–280.

Roberts, A.H., Kewman, D.G., Mercier, L. and Hovell, M. (1993) The power of nonspecific effects in healing: implications for psychological and biological treatments. *Clinical Psychology Review* 13, 375–391.

Roepstorff, L., Johnston, C., Drevemo, S. and Gustas, P. (2002) Influence of draw reins on ground reaction forces at the trot. *Equine Veterinary Journal (Supplement)* **34**(S34), 349–352.

Rollin, B.E. (2006) The ethics of alternative veterinary medicine. In *An Introduction to Veterinary Medical Ethics; Theory and Cases*, 2nd edn, Rollin, B.E. (ed.), pp. 93–101. Blackwell Publishing, Ames, IA.

Rubinstein, S.M., Leboeuf-Yde, C., Knol, D.L., de Koekkoek, T.E., Pfeifle, C.E. and van Tulder, M.W. (2007) The benefits outweigh the risks for patients undergoing chiropractic care for neck pain: a prospective, multicenter, cohort study. *Journal of Manipulative and Physiological Therapeutics* **30**, 408–418.

Sachs, H. (1982) Can patients influence health decisions? *Journal of the Royal College of General Practitioners* **32**, 691–694.

Sackett, D.L., Straus, S.E., Richardson, S.W. and Rosenberg, W. (2000) *Evidence-Based Medicine: How to Practice and Teach EBM*. Churchill Livingstone, Edinburgh.

Shaw, D. (2001) Veterinary medicine is science-based: an absolute or an option? *Canadian Veterinary Journal* **42**, 333–334.

Siegel, S. (2002) Explanatory mechanism for placebo effects: Pavlovian conditioning. In *The Science of the Placebo: Toward an Interdisciplinary Research Agenda*, Guess, H.A., Kleinman, A., Kusek, J.W. and Engel, L.W. (eds), pp. 133–157. BMJ Books, London.

Skarda, R.T. and Muir, W.W., III (2003) Comparison of electroacupuncture and butorphanol on respiratory and cardiovascular effects and rectal pain threshold after controlled rectal distention in mares. *American Journal of Veterinary Research* **64**, 137–144.

Skarda, R.T., Tejwani, G.A. and Muir, W.W., III (2002) Cutaneous analgesia, hemodynamic and respiratory effects, and beta-endorphin concentration in spinal fluid and plasma of horses after acupuncture and electroacupuncture. *American Journal of Veterinary Research* **63**, 1435–1442.

Smidt, N., de Vet, H.C.W., Bouter, L.M. and Dekker, J. (2005) Effectiveness of exercise therapy: a best-evidence summary of systematic reviews. *Australian Journal of Physiotherapy* **51**, 71–85.

Snyderman, R. and Weil, A.T. (2002) Integrative medicine. Bringing medicine back to its roots. *Archives of Internal Medicine* **162**, 395–397.

Steiss, J.E. and Adams, C.C. (1999) Effect of coat on rate of temperature increase in muscle during ultrasound treatment of dogs. *American Journal of Veterinary Research* **60**, 76–80.

Steiss, J.E., White, N.A. and Bowen, J.M. (1989) Electroacupuncture in the treatment of chronic lameness in horses and ponies: a controlled clinical trial. *Canadian Journal of Veterinary Research* **53**, 239–243.

Straw, R.C. and Rodney, C. (1996) Why treat cancer in pets? In *Oregon Veterinary Medical Association Summer Meeting*, pp. 8–9.

Sullivan, K.A., Hill, A.E. and Haussler, K.K. (2008) The effects of chiropractic, massage and phenylbutazone on spinal mechanical nociceptive thresholds in horses without clinical signs. *Equine Veterinary Journal* **40**, 14–20.

Tannenbaum, J. (1995) What is animal welfare? In *Veterinary Ethics: Animal Welfare, Client Relations, Competition and Collegiality*, 2nd edn, Tannenbaum, J. (ed.), pp. 150–175. Mosby-Yearbook, St. Louis, MO.

Taylor, N.F., Dodd, K.J. and Damiano, D.L. (2005) Progressive resistance exercise in physical therapy: a summary of systematic reviews. *Physical Therapy* **85**, 1208–1223.

Thomas, K.B. (1987) General practice consultation: is there a point in being positive? *British Medical Journal (Clinical Research Edition)* **294**, 1200–1202.

van Harreveld, P.D., Lillich, J.D., Kawcak, C.E., Turner, A.S. and Norrdin, R.W. (2002) Effects of immobilization followed by remobilization on mineral density, histomorphometric features, and formation of the bones of the metacarpophalangeal joint in horses. *American Journal of Veterinary Research* **63**, 276–281.

Varcoe-Cocks, K., Sagar, K.N., Jeffcott, L.B. and McGowan, C.M. (2006) Pressure algometry to quantify muscle pain in racehorses with suspected sacroiliac dysfunction. *Equine Veterinary Journal* **38**, 558–562.

Vas, J., Perea-Milla, E., Mendez, C., Sanchez Navarro, C., Leon Rubio, J.M., Brioso, M. and Garcia Obrero, I. (2006) Efficacy and safety of acupuncture for chronic uncomplicated neck pain: a randomised controlled study. *Pain* **126**, 245–255.

Vasseur, P.B., Johnson, A.L., Budsberg, S.C., Lincoln, J.D., Toombs, J.P., Whitehair, J.G. and Lentz, E.L. (1995) Randomized, controlled trial of the efficacy of carprofen, a nonsteroidal anti-inflammatory drug, in the treatment of osteoarthritis in dogs. *Journal of the American Veterinary Medical Association* **206**, 807–811.

Vernon, H. (1995) Basic scientific evidence for chiropractic subluxation. In *Foundations for Chiropractic: Subluxation*, Gatterman, M.I. (ed.), pp. 105–122. Mosby-Yearbook, St. Louis, MO.

Waddell, G., Feder, G. and Lewis, M. (1997) Systematic reviews of bedrest and advice to stay active for acute low back pain. *British Journal of General Practice* **47**, 647–652.

Wakeling, J.M., Barnett, K., Price, S. and Nankervis, K. (2006) Effects of manipulative therapy on the longissimus dorsi in the equine back. *Equine and Comparative Exercise Physiology* **3**, 153–160.

Wynn, S.G. and Schoen, A.M. (1998) Fundamentals of complementary and alternative veterinary medicine. In *Complementary and Alternative Veterinary Medicine; Principles and Practice*, Schoen, A.M. and Wynn, S.G. (eds), pp. 3–13. Mosby, St. Louis, MO.

Xie, H., Colahan, P. and Ott, E.A. (2005) Evaluation of electroacupuncture treatment of horses with signs of chronic thoracolumbar pain. *Journal of the American Veterinary Medical Association* **227**, 281–286.

Xie, H., Ott, E.A., Harkins, J.D., Tobin, T., Colahan, P.T. and Johnson, M. (2001) Influence of electro-acupuncture on pain threshold in horses and its mode of action. *Journal of Equine Veterinary Science* **21**, 591–600.

Alternative Medicine and Equine Welfare – Challenging the Science

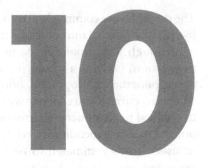

David W. Ramey

The late twentieth century saw the rebirth of diverse and unrelated approaches to medicine known by various names, including 'alternative,' 'complementary,' or 'integrative,' or, as historian of medicine James Whorton has wryly noted, 'vernacular' medicine (Whorton, 2002). It is virtually impossible to define what is meant by such terminology; there are literally thousands of such approaches, from the relatively well known, for example, acupuncture or chiropractic, to the almost unknown, for example, craniosacral therapy (Raso, 1994). In its broadest applications, the term 'alternative' has even been used to include interventions such as the routine administration of vitamin supplements or the use of nutraceutical products.

'Alternative' approaches to medicine, many of which were on the verge of becoming historical curiosities, have been received with some enthusiasm, supported by largely glowing – and largely uncritical – reports of 'success' from lay publications and anecdotal testimony from horse owners and practitioners, practitioners who range from graduate veterinarians, to non-veterinarians 'certified' by private organizations, to individuals who have no formal training whatsoever. Magazines devoted to various aspects of horsemanship regularly run features extolling the virtues of the various approaches. Myriad websites offer a variety of generally unverifiable claims.

Equine Welfare, First Edition. Edited by C. Wayne McIlwraith and Bernard E. Rollin.
© 2011 by UFAW. Published 2011 by Blackwell Publishing Ltd.

The therapies are commonly presented as almost without risk, occasionally bulwarked by (usually false) claims of longevity, and almost certainly as worth a try.

Although individual approaches are employed by a significant minority of the population, taken as a whole, in human medicine, expenditures on treatments such as acupuncture, chiropractic, homeopathy, nutritional supplements, herbal medicine, etc., currently are on par with those spent on 'non-alternative' medicine (visits to medical practitioners, pharmaceuticals, etc.). In 2005, it was estimated that total out-of-pocket expenditures relating to 'alternative' therapies in the USA were 'conservatively' estimated to be \$27.0 billion. This figure was comparable to the projected out-of-pocket expenditures for all US physician services (Institute of Medicine, 2005). While the level of use of such modalities in veterinary medicine is largely unknown, there is unquestionably a vocal minority of practitioners who advocate a particular approach, albeit in the absence of supporting scientific data, a number of horse owners who employ (and pay for) them, and a good bit of commerce going on around them.

It is curious, at least to those who hold that therapies should be demonstrated to be effective by scientific evaluation prior to their implementation, that such success as there is from 'alternative' approaches to medicine exists in the virtual absence of scientific support showing that they actually do any good for the horse; indeed, there is an obvious disconnect between the glowing assertions and the scientific reality. Whereas claims of effectiveness abound, those claims are largely unsupported by any unbiased evidence of effectiveness when evaluated under controlled conditions (evidence collected under controlled conditions is the generally accepted standard for scientific evidence of effectiveness). Still, the lack of scientific support for 'alternative' practices has apparently not done much to dissuade interest in them.

Regardless, most 'alternative' approaches to medicine are certainly at odds with the majority view of medicine, and that view of how medicine should be evaluated and practiced, regardless of who is applying them. While challenging the majority view is often worthwhile – and often critical for progress – it is also evident that the lack of scientific support is of little concern to the people who choose to employ such therapies. Nor does it appear to be a major concern to horse owners that unlicensed and unregulated individuals are applying therapies to their horses. Given such questions, it seems reasonable to ask: 'Are "alternative" therapies beneficial to horses?'

10.2 Risks and Benefits

By definition, welfare is something that promotes well-being. It would seem virtually indisputable that anyone who is interested in the welfare of horses is also likely to be interested in providing good care for them. Such care would certainly include good food, safe housing, regular exercise, and proper hoof care: that is, the things that horses need in order to maintain themselves in healthy condition. It that same vein, it would seem obvious that the medical interventions chosen to help horses when they are afflicted by disease, or those interventions that are promoted to maintain health, should be more likely than not to benefit the horse. If there were no benefit to the horse, an intervention would be, at best, a waste of time and money, and, at worst, harmful. Conversely, there would seem to be little purpose or reason in providing poor-quality care for horses; quite simply, poor-quality care, either intentionally or unintentionally, is harmful to horses. No one advocates giving poor-quality care to horses. But what of therapies or interventions that have no obvious value, but also carry little risk of obvious harm?

There would seem to be little purpose in providing care that is of no value to horses. That is, if no measurable improvement in the quality of a horse's life resulted from the care provided to it, there would seem to be no reason for it to be given to the horse. An intervention that has no therapeutic value is, at its foundation, a waste of time and money for the horse owner. Complicating such discussions are the effects of treatments on owners; sometimes an owner may feel that an intervention is important, and may feel better for having provided it, even if the horse is not directly helped. Still, if the welfare of the horse is the foremost consideration, it is difficult to make a reasoned argument that valueless therapies should be provided to horses just so that the owner or provider of the therapy can feel better.

In addition to being wasteful, providing valueless therapies or interventions may put horses at risk of harm. Subjecting horses to the stress of unnecessary handling and treatment is certainly not in their best interest, and various therapeutic maneuvers, medications, and nutritional supplements have the potential risk for direct harm. For example, horses and their handlers have been occasionally injured by interventions such as electro-acupuncture (somewhat understandably, horses may not like to have electric currents run through their bodies); and 'natural' treatments such as tea tree oil can provoke inflammatory reactions when applied to the skin of sensitive horses. Thus, if horse welfare is the foremost consideration in providing treatment, minimizing the risk of harm from an intervention should be important.

Of course, there are risks and benefits that accompany just about every activity. As part of daily living, most people make risk–benefit assessments, and react accordingly. Many such assessments are made emotionally. For example, a person might think that the risk of a bungee cord breaking may not be worth the exhilarating benefit of plunging off a bridge, and choose to avoid such activity. Others might find the benefit large and the risk small (as evidenced by a successful business, appropriate insurance, etc.), and go ahead and leap off into space.

However, rational risk–benefit assessments are greatly assisted by data. So, for example, if one were assessing the safety of bungee jumping, one might want to know the total number of people who have tried the activity, and then look at the number of people who were injured, killed (or even just scared to death) before deciding whether to take the jump. One might also look for indicators that a particular bungee jumping operation is safe: for example, choosing a provider of the jumping services with a long history of safety, avoiding frayed cords, appropriate insurance, etc. Risks and benefits surround horse-related activities as well. Riding a horse has some risk; for example, when assessing risks and benefits, an inexperienced rider may choose not to ride a horse that is difficult to control, simply because the risk of injury to the rider (and horse) outweighs any potential benefit of a good ride.

The point is that, for rational risk–benefit assessments to be conducted, data must be available. Surgery for an intestinal problem can save a horse's life; unfortunately, some horses do not recover. Over time, data has been collected on the chances of recovery after surgery from particular problems. This information is critically important for horse owners, who want to know the likelihood of a successful outcome prior to spending money on surgery. Unfortunately, when it comes to 'alternative' therapies in horses, such data is essentially non-existent. That is, there is very little data – even after decades of use and promotion – that can be used to guide people interested in such practices.

If an intervention or product has no demonstrable value, then there is no reason to assume even the slightest amount of risk. Risk is not warranted if no benefit can be expected. Further, if a valueless intervention were to result in detrimental changes, there would be no reason whatsoever to perform it. So, for example, garlic, which may be fed to horses in an effort to control stable flies, is not merely harmless; horses fed garlic at more than 0.2 g/kg per day developed Heinz body anemia (Pearson *et al.*, 2005).

Of course, there is also the matter of cost. Horses do not pay their way; their owners do. The cost of employing 'alternative' medicine in equine care has apparently never been studied. But while the cost of 'alternative' procedures is certain, the benefit has *not* been established. It certainly does not seem to be in anyone's interest to spend money on needless services, even if there is no direct risk to the horse.

Thus, it would seem incumbent on those interested in equine welfare to make sure that the interventions that they provide to horses carry both the likelihood of benefit, as well as an acceptable risk–benefit profile. And even though such studies are few, the good-quality studies that have been done in horses routinely fail to show that 'alternative' procedures provide relevant clinical benefits. For example, a single acupuncture treatment did not help horses with severe recurrent airway obstruction (Wilson *et al.*, 2004). No studies have been published that show that chiropractic maneuvers have clinically relevant benefits. Most herbal and nutraceutical products have not been scientifically tested in horses, and very few studies have investigated safe, effective doses (Williams and Lamprecht, 2008).

In the interest of the well-being of horses, things that people do to horses should be more likely to cause benefit than harm. Furthermore, if there is a possibility of harm, there should be a likelihood of benefit to the horses that would justify the risk. Finally, to be able to make rational decisions about whether there is risk, benefit, or harm associated with a procedure, someone has to be keeping track. Otherwise, it is not possible to make an informed decision.

10.3 Making Decisions

Complicating discussions about equine welfare is the fact that horses do not make decisions on their welfare for themselves. That is, domesticated horses are kept in circumstances that are chosen for them, according to the preferences of the individual horse owner. They do not make important decisions about health care for themselves. Instead, there are literally millions of people who are interested in looking after horses, and many of these people are presumably interested in information that would help them make decisions about the best way to take care of their horses.

In a perfect world, one could envision a scenario whereby health-care decisions would be relatively straightforward for horse owners. Conditions could be identified, and various treatments could be described. Those treatments could be tested, and found to be more or less likely to be effective. As new treatments came along, they could be tested, and take their place in the therapeutic armamentarium. Ineffective therapies could be discarded along the way. Treatments would progress; time and money would be saved by horse owners; horses would benefit from better care.

If only it were so easy!

When making health-care decisions for their horses, horse owners do not necessarily have easy access to unbiased information. Scientific information is usually couched in professional vernacular, and somewhat hidden in professional journals, to which most people do not subscribe. Even that information may not necessarily be good: scientific information can itself be corrupted, as it is a human endeavor. Furthermore, many people do not use scientific information to make health-care decisions anyway, instead relying on more convenient, and even more compelling (to them), sources of information. Finally, other factors can mitigate medical decisions: for example, a horse with a surgical colic might be euthanized due to the owner's financial circumstances, even if the likelihood of a successful outcome is good.

As a result, people looking to make decisions on their horse's welfare are often deprived of access to, or may not even be interested in, the most current and relevant information by which to make a rational risk–benefit assessment. Instead, they may choose other, often less reliable, information sources, including magazines (supported by advertising), internet websites (often with products or services to sell), or practitioners of particular approaches (who have their own vested interest in performing their services). Relying on less-than-reliable information sources that may be provided by people who have a financial or emotional stake in a therapy makes it more likely that choices made based on such information will not be sound. Indeed, by manipulating such sources of information – and, make no mistake, such manipulation occurs, with alarming regularity – interventions and services that are of questionable benefit can be easily put into an attractive light.

10.4 Health Belief Models

The thought processes pertaining to making decisions in human medicine have been thoroughly studied. It is perhaps useful to look at those reasons, and see if some parallels can be drawn in discussions about veterinary medical care and equine welfare.

Human health-care decision-making models typically view health-care behaviors as a product of the rational assessment of the balance between the barriers to a certain action and the possible benefits to be received from it. Important relevant variables in the decision-making process include the perceived seriousness of, and susceptibility to, a particular disease or condition; these perceptions also influence perceptions of the effectiveness of treatment, in addition to other factors such as demographics, and socio-psychological variables, e.g., the horse owner's personal ethos (Redding *et al.*, 2000).

From a veterinary perspective, it is generally assumed that horses are passive recipients of the veterinarian's ministrations (not always accepting when applied, of course, but certainly passive when it comes to the decisions being made). Disease and health are considered to have an underlying biomedical cause. When health is interrupted, there is also a cause, for example, a virus, bacteria, internal parasite, or a cancer cell; treatment is focused on removing such intruders from the horse's body, using interventions such as injections or surgery. Further, health is also maintained by making sure that certain biomedical principles are followed, for example, making sure that horses have access to clean water for hydration, or good-quality food for vitamins, minerals, and protein.

However, while perhaps sound mechanistically, fulfilling the horse's needs is not the only variable in the equation. Considering only the horse's needs or welfare, which certainly should have primacy, ignores the horse owner's perspective of their horse's illness (WHO, 2003), psycho-social influences (Blackwell, 1992), as well as the aforementioned impact of the owner's financial circumstances. Otherwise stated, when considering equine welfare, horse owners are usually *active* decision-makers, and do not merely receive and follow the instructions given to them by their veterinarians, and may not even be particularly interested in the evidence supporting or negating various treatment options. But, as noted previously, without accurate information, such active decision-making is not necessarily *good* decision-making.

The first health belief model was developed in 1966 by the late Professor Irwin Rosenstock, of the University of Michigan, School of Public Health (Rosenstock, 1966). Rosenstock proposed a psychological model for studying and promoting the uptake of social psychology services. This model has been refined over subsequent decades to adapt to evolving and emerging evidence about how knowledge and perceptions influence personal responsibility (Glanz *et al.*, 2002). While the model was originally intended to predict the response to treatment from acute or chronically ill human patients, more recently the model has been expanded, and is now used in an effort to predict health behaviors in general (Ogden, 2007).

The original health belief model stated that people engage in health-care behaviors primarily due to one of four factors. These factors were identified as follows:

(1) *Perceived susceptibility.* If a person believes that there is a risk for a problem to develop, they may change their behavior; conversely, if there is no perceived risk, there is little reason to make a change. So, for example, if a horse owner believes – or can be made to believe – that there is a risk to their horse, that owner may be more likely to engage in therapy to prevent or treat that risk.

(2) *Perceived severity.* If a person believes that a consequence can be avoided by changing a behavior, that person may change the behavior. The likelihood of change happening is directly related to how seriously the consequence is perceived. So, for example, a particular feed change may be provoked if it is perceived that the feed may cause colic; a particular drug may be avoided because of a perceived threat of risk (e.g., therapeutic doses of phenylbutazone may be eschewed because of excessive concerns about gastric ulceration); a particularly vaccination may not be chosen if there is a perceived threat to the horse. Clearly, these perceptions can be influenced, for example, by broad generalizations such as 'drugs are bad,' or condemnation of a particular treatment as being 'not natural.'

(3) *Perceived benefits.* If some intervention is perceived as being helpful to the horse, a person may elect to do it. Conversely, if an intervention is perceived as being harmful, that person may avoid it. So, for example, if a product is promoted to 'assist digestion,' it may be perceived as being good, even if there is no evidence that a particular horse's digestive processes need boosting. The perceptions of the seriousness of, or susceptibility to, a problem with a horse's health are themselves influenced by other factors. These factors may stimulate a response on the part of the horse owner to do something for the horse (presumably, in the best interests of the horse). These factors are of one of two broad types.

    (a) *Internal.* That is, the factors come directly from the horse, causing the horse owner to believe that something is wrong. Examples of internal factors that cause people to take action on behalf of their horses include objective variables, such as a measurable fever, loss of appetite by the horse, lameness, etc. These internal factors are the sorts of things that can be measured, or at least assessed, by attending personnel. However, internal factors that influence perception can also by quite subjective. For example, complaints such as 'poor performance' are not necessarily measurable, and may not even be medical. That is, a horse that is not performing up to its anticipated capabilities may do so for a variety of reasons that have nothing to do with the horse's health (e.g., tack, poor riding, unsuitability of the horse to the task for which it has been chosen, etc.).

    (b) *External.* External factors come from outside sources, such as information obtained from veterinarians, lay horse publications, the internet, or

other horse owners. Such information is easily available and highly persuasive, but also subject to manipulation, for example, from advertisers
who may be interested in selling their product or service regardless of the
scientific information supporting or negating it.

(4) *Perceived barriers.* An intervention may be difficult to perform, either
     because it is physically demanding, because there are social barriers (e.g.,
     it may be difficult, or even against the law, to perform veterinary proce-
     dures without a veterinary license), or because it is expensive. In the face
     of such barriers, an intervention is less likely to be performed. Accordingly,
     if a therapy is easy to do, say, for example, placing a magnetic boot on an
     injured leg, it will be more likely to be performed by a horse owner than
     a surgery that requires general anesthesia.

Of course, none of these four factors that help predict health-care behavior exist
in a vacuum. Other things influence what actually causes someone to take a health-
related action. Thus, human health-care models have been revised to add mediating
factors that connect the various perceptions with the health behavior. Such mediating
factors include the following:

- Demographic variables such as age, gender, ethnicity, and occupation.
- Socio-psychological variables such as social economic status, personality, and
  coping strategies.
- Self-efficacy, that is, an individual's belief in his or her ability to produce effects (this
  concept was not added to the health belief model until 1988). Otherwise stated, if a
  person thinks that he or she can succeed, he or she will be likely to give something
  a try; if that person thinks that failure is likely, failure is likely to follow.
- Cues to action. Cues to action come from outside of the individual. They are
  external influences that prompt desires to make a change, or give something a
  try. So, for example, a horse owner may be persuaded to use an 'alternative'
  therapy after having read an uncritical article in a lay horse publication or news-
  paper, after having seen a brochure or website produced by someone who is
  promoting a good or service, or after having heard of a horse that was allegedly
  'helped' by an intervention. Cues to action prompt people to stop thinking
  about doing something, and actually doing it.
- Health motivation, that is, whether an individual is driven to stick to a given
  health goal.
- Perceived control (which is one measure of level of self-efficacy), whereby a
  person may undertake an intervention feeling that it gives some control over a
  problem.
- Perceived threat, that is, whether the danger caused by *not* engaging in a certain
  recommended intervention is great; for example, the risk of a horse contracting
  West Nile virus can be mitigated by effective vaccination, and this prompts
  horse owners to vaccinate against the disease.

- Openness. Openness is a psychological quality, the characteristics of which include appreciation for art, emotion, adventure, unusual ideas, imagination, curiosity, and a variety of experience. These sorts of people are likely to be easily persuaded to try 'something new.' Indeed, studies have indicated that the quality of openness is strongly predictive of the use of 'alternative' medicine (Wheeler and Hyland, 2008).

All of the factors and perceptions listed above may be seen as independent predictors of health-care behavior. However, the relationships between these variables have not been explicitly detailed (Stroebe and de Wit, 1996), and each individual component has not been clearly defined. Furthermore, it is not clear what happens when factors are combined (Armitage and Connor, 2000), although it seems likely that there is some sort of an additive effect.

Regardless, it seems inarguable that all of those factors and perceptions could be relatively easily influenced. Indeed, appealing to such influences and perceptions appears to be one of the strengths of 'alternative' medicine. So, for example, discussing therapies in terms of whether or not they are 'natural' or 'gentle' or 'healing' may add to a perception of benefit, but obscures questions as to whether the therapies have any inherent value. Furthermore, since 'alternative' medicine is, almost by definition, conducted outside the realm of science (as an 'alternative' to it), and science may not necessarily be viewed favorably by some, characterizing a therapy as outside of the realm of science may actually be a selling point; it follows that decisions to use 'alternative' medicine may be made without concern to the scientific constraints that have been developed in an effort to provide unbiased information about health care. Indeed, many 'alternative' approaches to medicine regularly ignore science, and may even misstate facts (e.g., equine acupuncture is demonstrably *not* thousands of years old). However, such problems often appear not to be particular concerns to either consumers or purveyors of 'alternative' medicine.

People who use 'alternative' medical approaches appear to be particular targets for the unsupported – albeit attractive – claims of 'alternative' medicine. In addition to the qualities of openness, those who are less inclined to use 'alternative' medicine are less inclined to use rational scientific assessments in their decision-making processes (Wheeler and Hyland, 2008). They also tend to be more anxious about health in general, and somewhat more depressed than the general population (Dilhuydy, 2003). Purveyors of 'alternative' medicine such as chiropractic regularly make unsupported and unscientific statements (Grod *et al.*, 2001). Such statements are likely to appeal to people who are anxious about their horse's health. These appeals would pose ethical problems if they were to be used to encourage unwarranted fears in susceptible individuals so as to sell a product or service.

It is perhaps paradoxical that discussions about how people chose health care for their horses may overlook the horse itself. Horses simply do not need to receive products or services that have no value; if effective products or services are avoided due to irrational fears, horses may even be at risk of harm. If horse owners choose health services for their horses based on their perceptions, rather than hard data, they put themselves at risk for manipulation, and accordingly at risk for wrong and wasteful decisions. That would certainly not seem to be necessarily in the horse's best interest, at least if it is in the horse's best interest to provide it with treatments that are likely to work, and to avoid those treatments that are not.

10.5 Expectations and False Promises

As was previously noted, when it comes to choosing therapeutic interventions, there is usually some measurable benefit to compare against risk. But in addition, there is, or at least there should be, one other consideration. There should be objective evidence that the condition exists, or that the treatment has a chance of working. So, if one pays to jump off a bridge, or to ride a horse, there is a virtual certainty that the activity will happen. That is, barring extreme extenuating circumstances, one will certainly fall, or certainly be on the back of the horse, after paying money to have done so.

One certainly does not engage in activities such as horseback riding or bungee jumping because of the hope or promise that the activity will follow. Presumably, one would not be happy to find that the promised jump off a bridge was merely a garden step, or that the promised ride on the horse was merely an opportunity to hop up on a mannequin for a photo opportunity. Under such circumstances, that person would be justifiably outraged to find that his or her money had been wasted on a false representation.

In medicine, as well, interventions are provided with a certain expectation. Therapies are generally provided based on an expected benefit or a demonstrated action. So, for example, if a horse has an infection, and that infection is caused by bacteria, one can reasonably expect that an antibiotic will be a useful intervention. Even though there's no *guarantee* that the antibiotic will cure the infection, even if antibiotics are overused or abused, antibiotics have been tested, they do kill bacteria, and they often help to reverse the course of infectious disease. (Antibiotics do carry a certain risk of harm; for example, certain antibiotics can cause diarrhea, but that risk is generally known, as well.)

Fundamental to these expectations and perceptions of benefit is that the provider of the therapy is telling the truth. In the above example, it's true that antibiotics kill bacteria. To use other examples, certain vaccinations are effective at preventing certain diseases. Anthelmintics are fairly effective at removing internal parasites from the horse's intestines, etc. There is a reasonable expectation to go with the therapy. The fact is that such therapies *usually* work, and have been shown to work, so there is a reasonable expectation of a result.

Unfortunately, in the area of truth, 'alternative' medicine often diverges dramatically from scientific, mainstream medicine. 'Alternative' medicine offers horse owners much in the way of promises, but little in the way of demonstrated effectiveness. In addition, much of the information provided to promote the use of 'alternative' medicine simply isn't true. There are numerous examples. For example, acupuncture practitioners may talk about acupuncture points, channels ('meridians'), and mysterious energies ('Qi'). In fact, such things have never been shown to exist as discrete structures in a living organism (Ramey, 2005). Otherwise stated, there is no such thing as an acupuncture point, any more than there is a big red dot somewhere in Cincinnati, Ohio, that corresponds to the big red dot on the map. They may assert that veterinary acupuncture is thousands of years old, by way of inferring that, if it's been around so long, it must be good; in fact, there's nothing remotely resembling the modern practice of acupuncture in the historical veterinary literature of China. The current application of fine needles dates back to the late 1960s. Prior to that, 'needles' were large awls, used to puncture the skin of animals and pounded in with hammers, a practice that was decried as inhumane in the 1820s (Ramey and Buell, 2004).

Similarly, whereas chiropractic promises relief from spinal vertebrae that are out of place ('subluxations'), legs that are too long, or ribs that have sprung from their locations – all diagnoses that have been made in clinical settings – in fact, such things have never been demonstrated in any species. In fact, the concepts of chiropractic are not based on solid science, and its therapeutic value has not been demonstrated beyond reasonable doubt (Ernst, 2008). Homeopathy practitioners fail to divulge that their remedies are made with essentially infinite dilutions that fail to leave a single molecule of the active substance in solution (Weissmann, 2006). Instead, they rely on 'energies' and vibrations of their nostrums, energies that are apparently powerful enough to modify biological processes, yet too discrete to be measured. They also fail to note that the best evidence indicates that such remedies are merely placebos, with no demonstrable therapeutic effect (Rijnberk and Ramey, 2007).

Still, in spite of the lack of scientific evidence, and the false claims, 'alternative' approaches certainly do not lack promise, even if some may lack any rational expectation of effectiveness. However, horse owners interested in such approaches are simply not told such things. Instead, they may be told of the promise, and of the mystery. They may be informed that medications may be unacceptably dangerous due to their side-effects, and that medications should be avoided. They may be told that their horses have problems or conditions, even if those problems or conditions cannot be demonstrated by any reliable method. Alternatively, non-existent problems may be 'demonstrated' by unreliable methods (e.g., applied kinesiology). They may be persuaded that the therapies 'might' help, that they can be 'integrated' with effective therapies so as to do 'everything you can,' that veterinarians 'don't want people to know,' etc. In short, when it comes to 'alternative' approaches – and this would also include many nutritional concoctions, as well as nutraceuticals – horse owners are being sold products and services by appealing to the things that are most likely to make them choose a therapy, with barely a nod towards the truth, or to scientific evidence.

Here's a theoretical example. One could easily sell a rock, allegedly full of subtle 'energies,' that could be rubbed over a horse's abdomen to cure colic. The rock may have been a treatment in ancient Mongolia. It certainly couldn't directly harm the horse (although, by delaying treatment, there could certainly be some indirect harm). Under such circumstances, would the rock also be worth a try? The promise would be great. The cost to the purchaser of the rock would be assured. The person buying the rock would have done so with the best of intentions, albeit while being anxious, and perhaps even depressed about the horse's condition. But, most importantly, the benefit to the horse would be zero. If the welfare of the horse is the foremost consideration, there would be no reason to use or buy the rock.

10.6 Getting Answers

If the horse's welfare is best served when interventions are provided that are likely to provide benefit (even if there is some risk of harm), then it would seem to behoove people who are looking after the horse's welfare to go to some lengths to try to assure that such interventions are provided. Can such questions be answered?

The scientific point of view not only takes the position that questions can be answered, but also offers a method for answering them. Of course, disputes as to whether or not a specific therapy or intervention is effective are not limited to 'alternative' approaches to medicine; indeed, they are the lifeblood of scientific debate. Under such a scientific framework, ideas are proposed, evidence is gathered, and, ultimately, conclusions are drawn. This process, though somewhat tedious, and often time-consuming, is generally productive, and it has resulted in many advances in medicine, albeit not as quickly as anyone would like (even scientists). It is the framework under which 'evidence-based medicine' is practiced, according to the Centre for Evidence-Based Medicine.[1]

However, with science, as with every other human endeavor, there are varying degrees of excellence. Even the best orchestra can be difficult to listen to if it is conducted poorly; in that same manner, a poorly conducted scientific study can lead to results that are inaccurate, leading to erroneous conclusions. Certainly, there have been many studies on various 'alternative' modalities; however, they are of varying quality. As a result, there is no scientific consensus that any 'alternative' approach is effective for any condition, in any species, beyond effects that could be expected from giving placebos.

Even when single studies on 'alternative' modalities show initial promise, they usually cannot be replicated. For example, in 1998, it was reported that a microdose of prostaglandin at the putative 'bai hui' acupuncture point offered advantages over typical intramuscular injections for luteolysis, ovulatory intervals, and systemic responses in mares (Alvarenga et al., 1998). However, subsequent work indicated that, while a lower dose than had previously been used *was* effective for the studied parameters, there was no difference in effect when the injection was

---

[1] See http://www.cebm.net/.

given at other sites that were *not* acupuncture points (Nie *et al.*, 2001). The failure to replicate studies – even studies conducted in good faith, on conventional therapies, under the best of conditions – usually means that the initial study came to erroneous conclusions.

The quality of studies on 'alternative' medicine is also at frequent issue. That is, if one doesn't do good work designing and conducting a study, the results are likely to be spurious. So, for example, in one critical appraisal of human acupuncture studies conducted in China between 2000 and 2006, out of 686 randomized controlled trials conducted, the methodological quality was lower than the international standard *in every single paper* and only *one* paper described the trial technological process used during the study (Geng *et al.*, 2008). The phrase 'garbage in, garbage out' applies to *all* scientific trials.

However, when it comes to getting answers, the scientific point of view is certainly not unchallenged. There are, in fact, myriad ways that people get answers – for example, based on a satisfactory personal experience. But if there are many ways to answer the questions pertaining to therapeutic effectiveness, accordingly there is likely to be much dispute over which particular intervention is of benefit. That is, while (hopefully) most interventions are applied with the best of intentions, and with the horse's best interest in mind, some people may genuinely feel that those interventions are effective, while others may feel – equally as genuinely – that they are simply a waste of time (and money), depending on the framework from which the questions are answered.

Some people understandably feel that *they* are the ones who can best decide if an intervention is of benefit, or if it is likely to produce more good than harm. People are routinely persuaded that an intervention is beneficial because of the improvement that they perceive in their horse following a treatment. The *post hoc, ergo propter hoc* ('after this, therefore because of this') fallacy is based upon the mistaken idea that, merely simply because one thing follows another, the first event was a cause of the second event. As such, these people are often not persuaded by evidence, or feel that their particular circumstance is 'special,' and that somehow the rules do not apply to them (Dawes *et al.*, 1989). Indeed, some people have suggested that 'science' and 'objectivity' are themselves merely arbitrary social constructs, and, as a result, anecdote, testimony, and clinical (personal) experience should be given equal weight to scientific lines of evidence, which only *claim* to be more objective (Wyllys, 2003).

As was previously noted, people make decisions based on all sorts of criteria, e.g., emotions, their particular world-view, fear, their religious foundations, based on unbiased testing, etc. While unbiased scientific testing may be the medical 'gold standard,' and it represents the pinnacle of a rational approach to problem-solving, some people may not feel that it is necessary to make their own personal decisions about their horse's health care using such criteria. That is, they may feel that they can appropriately make such decisions for themselves. However, if a rational process is not used to make decisions regarding horse welfare (and, if one follows the human example, clearly, the process is not always rational), and if the decision-making process can be influenced, it follows that the door will be open to all sorts of therapeutic assertions, and all sorts of psychological manipulation.

10.7 Challenging Science

Without question, 'alternative' approaches to medicine challenge the scientific framework that has been the foundation of veterinary medicine. That veterinary medicine considers itself based in science is hardly debatable; the first line of the Veterinarian's Oath commits a veterinarian 'to use my *scientific* [emphasis added] knowledge and skills for the benefit of society.' However, the distinction between scientific and 'alternative' medicine is not always clear; what is currently known as 'alternative' medicine may ultimately include some useful therapies that are consistent with modern science. Still, for example, many plants contain pharmacologically active ingredients, not all plants have been evaluated, and it is within reason to think that there are as-yet-undiscovered pharmacologically active ingredients in some plants, somewhere, and it is certainly important to investigate promising leads.

However, 'alternative' medicine also includes other therapies that have no apparent value, as well as therapies that, if they were of value, would challenge the basic assumptions of science, e.g., homeopathy. Paradoxes abound: on the one hand, hundreds of scientific studies (of varying quality) of myriad modalities exist; on the other, it may be claimed that scientific methodology is inadequate for the study of 'alternative' medicine (Mathie, 2003), or that scientific study is unnecessary since certain therapies are alleged to have had a long history of use. That said, in human medicine, a huge number of 'alternative' approaches have been investigated over several decades of study, and virtually all of them have been unable to demonstrate consistent utility for any condition (Marcus and Grollman, 2006).

Whatever the method of evaluation, clearly science is not the driving force behind the interest in 'alternative' medicine and the welfare of horse. Veterinary colleges may include classes or continuing education symposiums on 'alternative' medicine for horses because of purported public interest in the field; nevertheless, these classes are not included because proven science demands that they be there.

Successful interventions usually also carry some reward, at least emotionally, and occasionally financially. Providing products and services to horses is the economic backbone of a multi-billion-dollar equine industry. Anyone who can be perceived as providing important services for equine welfare can be potentially rewarded. Thus, there is an incentive to provide services or products, even if evidence for their effectiveness is lacking.

Providing services in the absence of evidence is not necessarily fraudulent, or even a bad thing. Hopefully, most therapies are provided with good intentions. However, in some cases, people may advance their particular approach by making comparisons with scientific medicine that are unfavorable to it, e.g., by advancing their approach as 'less invasive' or 'less toxic.' Even blatantly false information may be provided. So, for example, while there is no evidence for the practice of fine-needle acupuncture in animals prior to the mid-twentieth century, proponents may assert that it has been practiced for thousands of years.[2] While such misinformation has nothing to do with the effectiveness of acupuncture, or its usefulness in promoting equine welfare, one can hardly support the provision of misinformation to promote a practice.

'Alternative' approaches to veterinary medicine challenge the foundations of what constitutes the practice of veterinary medicine, as well as who is qualified to provide such approaches. Certainly, it does not appear that some horse owners are particularly concerned about who is applying such therapies; they may be more concerned about their 'right' to employ any therapy of their own choosing than they are about the horse's 'right' to receive an effective therapy. But 'alternative' approaches are not only promoted and advocated by some veterinarians, they are also commonly applied by non-veterinarians, who operate outside of the educational and legal framework that has been established for the development and control of people who want to take care of animals. As non-veterinarians claim to be able to provide necessary services to horses with the same level of competency, and as public demand increases (in fact, or in perception), legislatures are being pressured to relax laws defining the practice of veterinary medicine. For example, in 2008, a Maryland woman filed a suit against the Maryland Board of Chiropractic and Massage Therapy Examiners (MBCMTE) claiming the State of Maryland was keeping her from massaging horses (Syeed, 2008). In a few states, veterinary practice acts have been modified to allow the practice of some modalities, with or without veterinary supervision. For example, in the State of Maryland, one does not need a veterinary license to provide acupuncture services to horses. Such assaults on the practice of veterinary medicine have been predicted (Ramey, 2003). Whether there will be harm to horses as a result of relaxing the standards of care to allow anyone to treat horses is unknown.

'Alternative' therapies may challenge veterinary science, but they do not come close to overthrowing it. Meanwhile, the question of whether such approaches are truly beneficial to horses remains largely unanswered. That is not to say it is unstudied; indeed, literally thousands of studies have been conducted on myriad 'alternative' therapies over the past decades. So far, no clear consensus of effectiveness for any condition has emerged. Ordinarily, humans are relatively quickly able to determine if

---

[2] For example (http://www.acupuncture.com/animals/dog.htm), it has been stated that 'Acupuncture was first discovered in China between 2696 BC and 2598 BC by Huang Di, "The Yellow Emperor," who was the third great emperor of China. Acupuncture was initiated and discovered during the Yellow Emperor's reign, and the surviving document is the "Yellow Emperor's Classic of Internal Medicine," translation by Ilza Veith, University of California Press, Berkeley, Calif. 1993. This Yellow Emperor's classic text is the basis for acupuncture and was the current book of medical care in the 2600s BC.' The only true statement here is that the book *was* translated, although even the title, as translated, is incorrect.

something is actually effective. As the years pass, it becomes less likely that any such effectiveness will *ever* be demonstrated (Turpin, 1993).

10.8 The Limits of Medicine

Whether in response to false claims, out of eager curiosity, or simply in an earnest attempt to exhaust all treatment options, it is clear that horse owners turn to 'alternative' approaches for a variety of evocative reasons. They may be persuaded that these approaches are more 'natural' than the pharmaceuticals and surgeries typically provided by professional veterinarians. They may want to do 'everything that they can' to help a horse. Other people may turn to 'alternative' approaches because their horse has a condition that cannot be cured, or even much helped, by scientific medicine (say, a chronic, degenerative arthritic condition of the horse's elbow). Or they may be told that their horse has a condition that can best be described as imaginary, such as a 'rib out of place,' or an 'energy blockage.' For such people, the value of alternative medicine most likely exists in their own minds, allowing for a bit of hope to mitigate the concern for their horse.

The search for new therapies is perfectly understandable, and even rational. In truth, scientific medicine has little effect on the outcome of many – even most – cases seen by equine veterinarians; horses often recover on their own, continue to be afflicted by chronic disease, or fail to overcome the disease process, all this in spite of treatment. So, if veterinary science has definite limits, and if veterinarians and their treatments have little effect in most cases, why shouldn't horse owners pursue alternative, non-scientific modalities? Indeed, most 'alternative' remedies are at least harmless, and, as such, they are not likely to influence the condition being treated (unless, of course, the condition is imagined). Furthermore, most clients in human medicine use 'alternative' approaches in conjunction with scientific medicine and not as a substitute. So, under such circumstances, can 'alternative' medicine be said to be in the best interest of the welfare of the horse?

Not necessarily – based on the current scientific evidence, to the extent that 'alternative' approaches to medicine produce an effect, it is likely to be on the client, *not* the horse. That is, even if such approaches produce no measurable effect on the horse, they may make the owner feel better (assuming that the owner is receptive to the promises made). Indeed, such approaches typically appeal to the very things that people use to make health-care choices. Moreover, by employing 'everything' to treat their horses, horse owners may find ways to allay their own anxiety over their horse, or at least make their horse's pain and distress seem more understandable, albeit in an unscientific way. Since alternative medicine is largely not confined by the limits of science, that is, by the constraints of rational or testable knowledge, it is virtually limitless in its powers of explanation, and horse owners can leave the therapeutic encounter with an 'alternative' therapist with a new, and often hopeful, understanding of their horse's problem.

When a horse owner asks 'Why did this happen to my horse?' or 'Why did this happen?', scientific medicine has relatively few answers. It can give a descriptive, physical explanation, but no other sense of larger purpose. On the other hand, the 'alternative' approach has persuasive dreams, innovative mechanisms of action, and even historical legends at its disposal. It can tell horse owners, as per some acupuncture 'theories,' that their horse's energy needs to be adjusted, that unidentified 'toxins' need to be pulled out their systems, or, as per some chiropractic 'theories,' that their vertebrae have popped out of place, and are simply waiting to be put back in. Many purveyors of 'alternative' medicine have a tremendous ability to put difficult situations in a new light, and to provide a sense of purpose. This makes it very powerful and alluring, especially to people who are anxious about their horse's health.

10.9 Does Science Matter?

The fact is that the value of various 'alternative' approaches to equine medicine remains almost totally unproven in scientific clinical trials. Indeed, when good-quality trials exist in horses (as well as in humans), on virtually every modality, in virtually every circumstance, the results are negative, that is, they show no useful therapeutic effect on the disease being studied. Yet the fact that these approaches remain unproven, and are still discussed, also sustains people's hopes, leaving open a medical world of almost limitless possibilities.

Scientific medicine operates within a completely different framework than does 'alternative' medicine. Scientific medicine has defined end-points. It encourages an almost endless process of hypothesis, debate, refutation, and repetition in order to prove a therapy's value; meanwhile, the person with a horse that needs treatment may not have the time or patience to wait. While this process makes scientific medicine more intellectually honest than alternative medicine, and has obviously produced more useful results in the long run, in the short term, a scientific approach may crowd out the hopes and dreams in the mind of a horse owner hoping to take care of his or her horse in the 'best' way – or in any way. Furthermore, the rational approach of scientific medicine may be shocking to horse owners, confronting them with the unvarnished truth about their horse's condition, and with little apparent concern about the feelings of the horse owner. (But note that scientific medicine *can* be delivered with compassion – compassion is part of what is known as the 'art' of medicine.)

On the other hand, 'alternative' approaches to medicine embrace mystery, and revel in hope. Patients who imagine that their horse's problem is caused by a rib out of place, or by a blockage of 'energy,' or that it can be cured by an essentially infinite dilution of a substance, can be shielded from the harsh light of scientific reality by taking solace in a particular 'alternative' approach. They may not necessarily understand the scientific debates pertaining to alternative medicine, they may not care about the history of such practices, and they may not be concerned about the lack of evidence in support of them, but they do *believe* in them. Those beliefs can likely help some horse owners cope with the feelings of helplessness and despair that can accompany the responsibility of caring for a sick or injured animal.

From the aspect of the practitioner, a lack of evidence may also be a mere inconvenience. Individuals practicing on the front lines of medicine are asked to do something to intervene in a horse's life. Unfortunately, they are also quickly confronted with the fact that some conditions simply cannot be cured. For one trained to heal, such a reality can be frustrating, even debilitating, and new avenues of treatment, even if untested, offer new challenges, and new opportunities. Happily for such individuals, 'alternative' approaches to equine medicine may consider an almost limitless number of factors in deciding which approach, or combination of approaches, is best suited for the diagnosis and treatment of the patient. While this process may be exhilarating, and provide new treatment options, the fact remains that a huge body of research exists to show that such individualistic judgments cannot compete with a more objective process that involves evaluating a small number of relevant variables, including judgment used in the differential diagnosis and prognosis of medical conditions (Dawes *et al.*, 1993). There is, in fact, no indication that 'alternative' approaches offer any diagnostic or therapeutic advantage over science-based approaches, and there is every reason to believe that no such advantages exist or will be forthcoming, given the long history of their use and concomitant lack of supporting evidence.

10.10 What About the Horses?

While the reasons for the use of 'alternative' medicines are perhaps understandable, somewhat lost in the preceding discussions is the welfare of the horse. Therapies that are dispensed merely to make the horse *owner* feel better are not necessarily consistent with the best interest of the horse's health. Whereas one might argue that, if the person were being treated, that patient is entitled to any therapy he or she chooses, this does not also mean that the person should have free rein to choose any therapy for their horse. A horse cannot choose which therapy it receives. The primary obligation of the horse owner, as well as the therapy provider, should be to the horse. As such, those individuals should logically pursue only therapies that have been scientifically validated, or at least to make sure that the therapies that are being employed are also being evaluated so that they may ultimately be adopted or discarded, as would occur in scientific trials (Ramey and Rollin, 2001). In human medicine, the right to receive an effective treatment has been supported in courts. Even those who cannot rationally choose their therapy, such as children, may be given a treatment even when such treatment is against parental wishes, such as when members of religious sects do not wish to have their children given life-saving transfusions, medicines, or surgery. Conversely, criminal charges can be and have been brought against parents who deny effective treatments to their children.

The same obligations are true for those who care for horses. As Plato[3] said of horsemanship, 'Nor does the art of horsemanship consider the interests of the art of horsemanship, but the interests of the horse.' Horse owners and those who care for horses are obliged to put the concerns of the horse above their own needs and desires. Thus, it is impossible to defend a person who is willing to allow a horse to suffer while pursuing endless 'alternatives' in the face of a chronic, incurable, painful condition, even if that person feels good about doing 'everything' possible. It is also impossible to defend people who are willing to promote their goods and services to susceptible individuals based on false and/or inaccurate information.

Even if a therapy is of no value, and does no harm to a horse, it is still not right to promote it in the absence of evidence (or, worse, by using false information). Concerns about the efficacy of therapies do not appear to be foremost among those promoting products and services for profit, nor does there seem to be much oversight in preventing false claims. As a result, horse owners face a bewildering array of unsupported claims, and almost limitless choices to assist in the maintenance of health, or the prevention and treatment of disease. While it is generally not directly harmful to the horse to provide such products and services, there is a direct cost to the credulous individual. Indeed, if people were asked, 'Do you want to do everything that you can to help your horse?', the answer would undoubtedly be 'Yes.' But if the question were phrased differently, if one asked, 'Do you want to waste time and money chasing after therapies that will be of no benefit to your horse?', the answer would likely be quite different.

10.11 Conclusions

The fact that some people may ask for 'alternative' therapies for their horses, or that others may promote them as viable medical treatments, does not mean that such therapies should be provided in the absence of good evidence for their effectiveness. The role of those who look after the welfare of horses is to promote health, relieve suffering, and, when possible, to cure disease. The door should certainly not be closed too quickly on therapies that show some promise; that said, those therapies should be evaluated in controlled conditions so that useful information can be obtained, and ineffective therapies discarded. Still, therapies that are backed by sound science, and are in accordance with sound biological principles, are those that are most likely to work, and that should accordingly be provided to horses. It is not enough for a therapy to appeal to the anxieties or desires of horse owners, or to the world-view of its purveyors. To ignore scientific evidence, as is routinely done in the field of 'alternative' medicine, is to turn a blind eye to the truth, is certainly wasteful, and puts the welfare of the horse at risk.

---

[3] Plato, *Republic*, Book 1.

References

Alvarenga, M.A., Ferreira, J.P.C., Meira, C. *et al.* (1998) Induction of luteolysis in mares utilizing a microdose of prostaglandin $F_{2\alpha}$ in the sacral lumbar space. *Journal of Equine Veterinary Science* **18**, 167–168.

Armitage, C.J. and Connor, M. (2000) Social cognition models and health behaviour: a structured review. *Psychology and Health* **15**, 173–189.

Blackwell, B. (1992) Compliance. *Psychotherapy and Psychosomatics* **58**, 161–169.

Dawes, R.M., Faust, D. and Meehl, P.E. (1989) Clinical judgment versus actuarial judgment. *Science* **243**, 1668–1674.

Dawes, R.M., Faust, D. and Meehl, P.E. (1993) Statistical prediction versus clinical prediction: improving what works. In *Handbook for Data Analysis in the Behavioral Sciences: Methodological Issues*, Keren, G. and Lewis, C. (eds), pp. 351–367. Erlbaum, Hillsdale, NJ.

Dilhuydy, J.M. (2003) Patients' propensity for complementary and alternative medicine (CAM): a reality which physicians can neither ignore nor deny. *Bulletin du Cancer* **90**(7), 623–628 (in French).

Ernst, E. (2008) Chiropractic: a critical evaluation. *Journal of Pain and Symptom Management* **35**(5), 544–562.

Geng, L.L., Lin, R.S., Sun, X.Y. *et al.* (2008) Critical appraisal of randomized clinical trials in Chinese acupuncture and moxibustion from 2000 to 2006. *Zhongguo Zhen Jiu* **28**(6), 439–443 (in Chinese).

Glanz, K.K., Lewis, F.M. and Rimer, B.K. (2002) *Health Behavior and Health Education.* John Wiley & Sons, San Francisco, CA.

Grod, J.P., Sikorski, D. and Keating, J.C., Jr. (2001) Unsubstantiated claims in patient brochures from the largest state, provincial, and national chiropractic associations and research agencies. *Journal of Manipulative and Physiological Therapeutics* **24**(8), 514.

Institute of Medicine (2005) [Committee on the Use of Complementary and Alternative Medicine by the American Public, and Board on Health Promotion and Disease Prevention] *Complementary and Alternative Medicine in the United States.* National Academies Press, Washington, DC.

Marcus, D. and Grollman, A. (2006) Review for NCCAM is overdue. *Science* **313**, 301–302.

Mathie, R.T. (2003) The research evidence base for homeopathy: a fresh assessment of the literature. *Homeopathy* **92**(2), 84–91.

Nie, G., Gooden, A.N., Braden, T.D. *et al.* (2001) Luteal and clinical response following administration of dinoprost tromethamine or cloprostenol at standard intramuscular sites or at the lumbosacral acupuncture point in mares. *American Journal of Veterinary Research* **62**(8), 1285–1289.

Ogden, J. (2007) *Health Psychology*, 4th edn. Open University Press, McGraw-Hill Education, Maidenhead, UK.

Pearson, W., Boermans, H.J., Bettger, W.J. *et al.* (2005) Association of maximum voluntary dietary intake of freeze-dried garlic with Heinz body anemia in horses. *American Journal of Veterinary Research* **66**(3), 457–465.

Ramey, D.W. (2003) Regulatory aspects of complementary and alternative veterinary medicine. *Journal of the American Veterinary Medical Association* 222(12) 1679–1682.

Ramey, D.W. (2005) Acupuncture and 'traditional Chinese medicine' in the horse. Part 2: a scientific overview. *Equine Veterinary Education* 7(2), 136–144.

Ramey, D.W. and Buell, P.D. (2004) Acupuncture and 'traditional Chinese medicine' in the horse. Part 1: a historical overview. *Equine Veterinary Education* 6(4), 218–224.

Ramey, D.W. and Rollin, B.E. (2001) Ethical aspects of proof and 'alternative' therapies. *Journal of the American Veterinary Medical Association* 218(3), 343–346.

Raso, J. (1994) *'Alternative' Health Care: A Comprehensive Guide.* Prometheus Books, Amherst, NY.

Redding, C.A., Rossi, J.S., Rossi, S.R. *et al.* (2000) Health behaviour models. *International Electronic Journal of Health Education* 3, 180–193.

Rijnberk, A. and Ramey, D.W. (2007) The end of veterinary homeopathy. *Australian Veterinary Journal* 85(12), 513–516.

Rosenstock, I.M. (1966) Why people use health services. *Milbank Memorial Fund Quarterly (Supplement)* 44(3), 94–127.

Stroebe, W. and de Wit, J. (1996) Health impairing behaviours. In *Applied Social Psychology*, Semin, G.R. and Fiedler, K. (eds), pp. 113–143. Sage Publishing, London.

Syeed, N. (2008) *Woman Sues Maryland for Right to Massage Horses.* CNSnews.com, August 11, 2008. Associated Press. Available at: http://www.cnsnews.com/news/article/33931.

Turpin, R. (1993) *Characterization of Quack Theories.* University of Texas, Austin, TX. Available at: http://tc.eserver.org/18375.html.

Weissmann, G. (2006) Homeopathy: Holmes, Hogwarts, and the Prince of Wales. *FASEB Journal* 20(11), 1755–1758.

Wheeler, P. and Hyland, M.E. (2008) Dispositional predictors of complementary medicine and vitamin use in students. *Journal of Health Psychology* 13, 516–519.

WHO (2003) *Adherence to Long-Term Therapies: Evidence for Action.* World Health Organization, Geneva, Switzerland.

Whorton, J. (2002) *Nature Cures: The History of Alternative Medicine in America.* Oxford University Press, New York.

Williams, C.A. and Lamprecht, E.D. (2008) Some commonly fed herbs and other functional foods in equine nutrition: a review. *Veterinary Journal* 178(1), 21–31.

Wilson, D.V., Berney, C.E., Peroni, D.L. *et al.* (2004) The effects of a single acupuncture treatment in horses with severe recurrent airway obstruction. *Equine Veterinary Journal* 36(6), 489–494.

Wyllys, R.E. (2003) *Science as a Social Construct.* School of Information, University of Texas, Austin, TX. Available at: http://www.ischool.utexas.edu/~l38613dw/website_spring_03/readings/ScienceSocialConstruct.html.

Part II

Human Uses and Abuses – Welfare Issues

Welfare Issues in Horse Racing

Rick M. Arthur

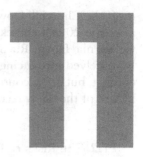

11.1 Introduction

Horse racing is a minefield for horses. There are enormous financial rewards, with horses competing near the limit of their physical ability. There is little margin of safety with a horse racing at full speed. Structural failure of bones and ligaments during racing can be, and frequently is, catastrophic for horse and rider. Estimates put fatality rates for running races in the USA at 0.12–0.50% when reported as fatalities as a percentage of starts (Hernandez *et al.*, 2001; Stover and Murray, 2008). Harness racing, both trotters and pacers, have much lower fatality rates. Harness horses race at slower speeds and have two legs on the ground at all times; this is not so with Thoroughbreds and Quarter Horses. With few exceptions, horse racing's business model and management practices do not favor the horse. The racetracks need to fill races; trainers need to keep horses in the barn; owners need to earn purses; and breeders need to sell horses to keep the horse racing industry going.

In recent years, the racing industry has begun addressing fundamental equine safety and welfare issues through a number of groups, sometimes working together and sometimes not. The Grayson/Jockey Club Research Foundation's Welfare and Safety of the Racehorse Summit began seriously identifying issues in 2006. The Racing Medication and Testing Consortium began looking at medication and drug testing issues in 2001. The National Thoroughbred Racing Association Safety Alliance and the Jockey Club Safety Committee began in 2008 in the aftermath of the Barbaro and Eight Belles injuries and subsequent fatalities in their respective Triple Crown races. Barbaro was injured in the 2007 Preakness Stakes. A three-year-old colt, Barbaro was euthanized after months of intensive care at the University of Pennsylvania's New Bolton Center from laminitis complications after multiple surgeries to repair fractures in his right hind leg. Eight Belles never made

Equine Welfare, First Edition. Edited by C. Wayne McIlwraith and Bernard E. Rollin.
© 2011 by UFAW. Published 2011 by Blackwell Publishing Ltd.

it off the Churchill Downs racetrack and was euthanized on the track immediately after the 2008 Kentucky Derby. Several racing regulatory agencies, especially the California Horse Racing Board, individuals, organizations, and even Congress have delved into racing safety and equine welfare issues. These efforts are late in coming, but are encouraging. It is too early in the process to evaluate the success or failure of the many recommendations to improve horse welfare and safety.

11.2 The Risks of Racing – the Data Available

Horse racing is an extremely competitive sport and a particularly dangerous one for both horses and riders. California has the most comprehensive racing fatality statistics in the USA (Stover and Murray, 2008). In California, in the 2008 fiscal year, 137 horses died as a direct result of racing (CHRB, 2008). That translates into 0.26% of all starts resulting in a fatality for the running breeds in California in 2008. Another 100 horses died during training at California Horse Racing Board regulated racetracks during the same 12-month period.

The California Horse Racing Board requires necropsies on all horses dying within racing and training enclosures under its jurisdiction by law and regulation. The California necropsy program was established in the early 1990s to monitor and study racing fatalities. The results are transparent, verifiable, and well accepted by all racing participants. The necropsies are performed by pathologists at the California Animal Health and Food Safety (CAHFS) laboratories, operated by the School of Veterinary Medicine at the University of California, Davis. There are three laboratories in the system within reasonably close proximity to California racetracks; all but one racetrack is within two hours of a CAHFS laboratory by motor vehicle. No other state in the USA has such an effective and in-depth program. There are no national standards to monitor racing injuries or fatalities. Fatality data is simply not rigorously monitored in most states. Reporting is haphazard, unofficial, reported by interested parties, and generally unverifiable. Training fatalities, which constitute roughly a third of all fatalities in horse racing, are usually not monitored and are rarely reported. The same is true of non-racing or non-training fatalities, which can exceed well over 20% of all fatalities for horses in training. The tendency is clearly to under-report fatalities and injuries; this has been the case for many years. Even in California, racing fatalities were not well kept at all until the last 20 years. Racing fatalities and injuries were just an accepted part of the cost of doing business. They were not thought to be important and better left unmentioned. Today, there is no question they are important, but the attitude is that they are still better left unmentioned.

National fatality data has been non-existent. The occasional reports or studies provided estimates, but no one knew for sure what the true national fatality rate was. Certainly, no State except California went to any effort to monitor fatalities, ensure accurate reporting, or publish their fatality information. Even the unrealistically optimistic estimates pointed to a much higher fatality rate in the USA as compared to what was being reported overseas (Boden *et al.*, 2007; Parkin *et al.*, 2005).

In 2006 the American Jockey Club initiated a national effort in an attempt to understand the true scope of the problem. A national database was one of the recommendations of the Grayson/Jockey Club Research Foundation's Welfare and Safety of the Racehorse Summit. The Jockey Club instructed their InCompass Solutions subsidiary, an information services company for racetracks, to develop a reporting program to gather injury and fatality information. The result was a welcome innovation, the Equine Injury Database program. To obtain cooperation from tracks and horsemen for this national program, agreements were necessary to keep all identifying information, such as the specific track, trainer, breeding information, owner, and other indentifying information, confidential. Regardless, very early in the rollout of the Equine Injury Database, even as a voluntary effort, the data quickly indicated that the national fatality rate was closer to 0.20% of starts rather than the long-stated estimate of 0.12% of starts. Even then, the Equine Injury Database did not include a number of high-risk racetracks that were reluctant to cooperate in the process.

Discussing fatalities as a percentage of starts is a useful approach for standardized reporting to compare relative fatality rates, but what is the risk to any individual horse? Here the data is not so clear. Expanding the 'fatalities per start' approach to the individual horse puts an entirely different perspective on the issue. The Jockey Club put the lifetime starts for each starter to be about 20 starts for foals of 1995, the most recent group of horses that have completed their racing careers (Jockey Club, 2010). With 20 lifetime starts and at a 0.20% fatality rate, this means the average horse has a 4% chance (20 starts × 0.20% starts = 4%) of sustaining a fatal injury during his or her racing career.

One of the goals of the Equine Injury Database is to help identify horses at greater risk of injury and to develop strategies to reduce the risk and improve safety. There are factors that have been associated with increased fatality risk. Most are related to horse management practices, such as shoeing and training intensity (Kane *et al.*, 1996, 1998; Anthenill *et al.*, 2007; Hernandez *et al.*, 2001). Relationships have also been found between pre-race examination findings – suspensory branch desmitis, for example – and subsequent racing or training injury (Cohen *et al.*, 1999; Hill *et al.*, 2001). Furthermore, certain trainers simply have higher fatality rates than others. This has been long recognized in horse racing, with little repercussion on the trainer because the relevant information is not readily available to the public.

11.3 Track Surfaces

Over the last few years, track surfaces have come under greater scrutiny as a factor in racing injuries. Turfway Park, a racetrack in northern Kentucky just across the Ohio River from Cincinnati, had experienced a high incidence of fatalities for several years. In 2005, Turfway installed a synthetic racing surface and saw an 85% decrease in racing fatalities with the new surface (Rogers Beasley, pers. comm.). There are several manufacturers of synthetic surfaces, and the components are similar for all of them. The synthetic surfaces are primarily sand coated with a wax or polymer mixed with various fiber materials. Soon after the Turfway success, the California Horse Racing Board mandated the new synthetic surfaces for their major race meets. There had been a 40% increase in racing and training fatalities over the previous three years (CHRB, 2003, 2006), and the Board wanted a quick solution. Racing fatalities have decreased at California tracks with the new surfaces by about one-third. There were a number of other regulatory changes made simultaneously, so it is unclear whether or not the decrease can be attributed entirely to the new surfaces. But, in spite of spending millions for the new surfaces, synthetic surfaces have not been the panacea some had hoped. Training fatalities have not decreased, and the surfaces, developed for international racing, have been very difficult to maintain with the heavy training traffic typical at US racetracks. Anyone who had seriously examined the high racing injury rate in US racing recognized track surfaces as just one of many contributing factors. Regardless, the preliminary results are encouraging.

11.4 The California Necropsy Program – Looking for Answers

Since 1992, all horses dying or euthanized within a racing enclosure under the jurisdiction of the California Horse Racing Board have been necropsied. From 1992 through 2008, over 5000 horses have been necropsied from California racetracks. Roughly half of those are a direct result of racing, another 30% are training fatalities, and the rest are non-racing or training deaths such as colic, laminitis, pneumonia, equine protozoal myeloencephalitis (EPM), and non-racing or training accidents. The California Horse Racing Board averaged 15 tracks operating under their jurisdiction each year during this period. California runs two Thoroughbred circuits simultaneously, one in southern California and another in northern California, year-round Quarter Horse racing in the Los Angeles area, and year-round harness racing in Sacramento. Including training centers, there will be between 5000 and 8000 horses under CHRB jurisdiction at any one time.

The necropsy program has changed the way racing and training injuries are viewed by trainers and practicing veterinarians in California. Susan Stover, Director of the J.D. Wheat Orthopedic Research Laboratory, School of Veterinary Medicine, University of California, Davis, has studied many aspects of fatal musculoskeletal racing injuries. One of the first fatal musculoskeletal racing injuries that Stover examined in depth when she first started her investigation was humeral fractures, an injury called a 'fractured shoulder' (Stover et al., 1992). Stover clearly demonstrated that the fractures were in fact progression of previously existing humeral stress fractures with evidence of pre-existing stress remodeling. Oftentimes the stress remodeling was extensive, with a large periosteal callus indicating that an injury had been present for some time. This is a recurring theme in almost all fatal racing and training injuries. Stover (pers. comm.) estimates that 90% or more of all racing or training fatalities from the California necropsy program show some evidence of pre-existing pathology at the site of the fatal injury. That is not to say the pre-existing pathology would have been detectable by current diagnostic techniques; some of the findings are microscopic, but many pre-existing injuries could have been recognized and diagnosed with the appropriate effort. The questions that horse racing and veterinary practitioners need to answer are 'Why are these injuries being missed?' and 'Are signs being ignored or are the clinical signs too obscure to be recognized?' These are fair questions and the answers are not clear.

Stover's early research led to the installation of a nuclear scintigraphy facility at Santa Anita Park, the premier racetrack in California. From the mid-1990s, when the Dolly Green Nuclear Imaging Facility was installed, through 2008, over 8000 horses have undergone nuclear scintigraphic examinations. Nuclear scintigraphy is an exceptionally sensitive diagnostic imaging tool to identify stress fractures in the horse. Humeral stress fractures provide an example of the benefits of better diagnostic capabilities. Humeral fractures are almost always fatal in adult horses, but when stress fracturing or remodeling is identified with nuclear scintigraphy or other means before a horse sustains a complete fracture, the prognosis for a full recovery is excellent. A number of potentially catastrophic injuries have similar clinical scenarios. Kotashan and Tiznow were each selected Horse of the Year in their respective champion seasons. Both horses recovered from tibial stress fractures early in their careers to go on to their champion success. Similar to the humerus, complete fractures of the tibia in the adult racehorse are almost always fatal.

11.5 Wastage Attributable to Non-fatal Racing and Training Injuries

A fatality provides a clear end-point, a bright-line inclusion criterion. What is a larger issue, not only for horse welfare but also for the economic health of horse racing, is the attrition or wastage rate for racehorses for all reasons. There are a number of ways to estimate horse attrition rates in horse racing. Field size is critically important for the size of wagering pools. Wagering is where horse racing derives purse monies and where racetracks derive most of their operating income. Field size has been decreasing for many years and is a critical industry issue. To better understand the issue, all the horses starting on May 2, 2001, at Aqueduct in New York and Hollywood Park in California were followed for two years. The attrition rate, the rate at which those horses ended their participation in *pari-mutuel* racing in the USA, was about 3% per month. Using a different approach and a larger sample – the foals of 1995 from the Jockey Club database – the average starter had made less than 20 starts and had raced for slightly less than three years. The years raced had decreased only slightly in 30 years, but the number of starts per horse had dropped by 40% in the same time. The average horse racing for three years again approximates an attrition rate of roughly 3%. In 2008, 72 638 Thoroughbred horses participated in *pari-mutuel* racing in the USA (Jockey Club, 2010). Using a 3% attrition rate and 72 638 Thoroughbred horses participating means that slightly more than 2100 horses leave horse racing each month never to race again. To be clear, the 3% are not all fatalities or non-fatal injuries. Many would be retirement to breeding and other equine endeavors, but a large percentage would be leaving because injuries ended their racing career. Horse racing is not unique with such a high athletic attrition rate. Professional football has a similarly high attrition rate, and most of those are from debilitating injuries (Halchin, 2008).

The financial cost of horse wastage in racing is enormous. As an illustration of the magnitude of the cost, the average yearling sold for $51 489 in 2008, down from the $57 107 high in 2006. The average yearling sales price times the monthly attrition of roughly 2100 horses per month puts the cost at over $100 million per month or over $1.2 billion per year. This simplistic approach provides an estimate of the total cost of wastage. This is a conservative estimate and only addresses the cost of replacing horses. In reality, the total annual attrition or wastage cost would include all operating expenses. When training, veterinary services, farriers, boarding, vanning, and all the other costs are added, the total cost would be in the billions of dollars. Putting an economic cost to racing injuries provides an opportunity to make changes in the otherwise conservative and traditional sport of horse racing. Improving horse safety is easier to accomplish when doing so provides an economic benefit.

11.6 Regulation and Effects on Equine Welfare

Horse racing is one of the most regulated sports in the world, and many of the regulations affect equine welfare. Regulations intended to protect jockeys or the integrity of a race usually protect horses indirectly. Race riding is a dangerous profession. As recently as December, 2008, jockey Sam Thompson was killed when his mount fractured her left front leg while pulling up in a 300-yard Quarter Horse race at Los Alamitos in California. His mount, Harem's Dynasty, was making her first start. Ron Turcotte, the jockey who rode Secretariat in the Triple Crown, is paralyzed from his waist down from a racing accident. In 2009, two jockeys, popular journeyman Rene Douglas and 23-year-old apprentice Michael Straight, were both paralyzed in racing accidents at Arlington Park within months of each other.

Most, but not all, racing jurisdictions require some level of pre-race examination of horses prior to racing. An examination is really overstating the process; the examinations should really be called inspections. Often, one veterinarian has as many as 100 horses to examine in a few hours before the races begin. Trainers have the horses in as good condition at the time of the pre-race examination as they will ever be. Everyone involved knows the horse must pass the pre-race examination to compete. Trainers understand the process and will often take whatever steps are necessary for the horse to pass the pre-race examination step. If a horse has heat in a tendon or joint, the horses may be iced before the examining veterinarian arrives. If an ankle has filling, the horse may have received medication to reduce any inflammation. If a horse is stiff right out of his stall, he may be walked until the examining veterinarian arrives. Getting a horse into peak condition to race is not necessarily bad. In fact, that is what a good trainer is all about. The problem arises when the true soundness condition of a horse is masked from the examining veterinarian by these efforts. There is growing concern among examining racing regulatory veterinarians about whether current medication regulations, especially non-steroidal anti-inflammatory drugs and steroidal anti-inflammatory glucocorticosteroids, compromise pre-race examinations (David, 2009).

When horses are found to be unfit or infirm, they are placed on the Veterinarian's List and are ineligible to race. Before they can race, the horse must pass a racing regulatory veterinary examination to satisfy the Horse Racing Board veterinarian that the horse is fit to race. The criterion for fitness varies from jurisdiction to jurisdiction, and even within some jurisdictions. There are many reasons horses can be placed on the Veterinarian's List. These include unsound, lame, sick, injured, and a number of other health-related categories. Sometimes there are simple procedural health issues such as submission of paperwork for Coggins test results for equine infectious anemia or vaccination records. Horses that have had health or soundness issue are required to meet specific examinations protocols. Horses on the Veterinarian's List at Thoroughbred tracks in southern California listed as lame or unsound must run five furlongs in 1 min 03 s or faster. The horse is examined by the racing regulatory veterinarian before the workout, observed by the veterinarian during the workout, and examined again by the veterinarian after the workout. Finally, a post-work sample is taken for drug testing. The horse must be sound at all steps and pass the post-workout drug test before it can be removed from the Veterinarian's List. Until that time, the horse is not allowed to race.

This system is not perfect. Until just recently there were no specific restrictions on training once a horse was placed on the Veterinarian's List – the restriction only covers racing. There have been a number of instances where the racing regulatory veterinarian has examined a horse, found the horse to be lame, and the trainer works the horse anyway, with fatal consequences for the horse.

The owner theoretically controls the care of his horses by the people he employs, but in reality few owners know what kind of care their horses are receiving. Most assume the trainer, a Racing Board-licensed professional horseman, knows how to care for horses. Information such as wins, earnings, and win percentage, typically found in the trainer standings in the *Daily Racing Form* or track program, is available. Hiring a trainer is not dissimilar to hiring any other professional. Word of mouth, reputation, and personal impression are the normal criteria. Statistics such as the number of horses a trainer has that fail to finish a race (did not finish, DNF) or did not finish in the official race charts, or horses dying under a trainer's care, are kept – they just aren't published.

Gary Lavin is a long-time racetrack practitioner. His father was a racing secretary and he was raised on the racetrack; Lavin (1987) described the American racing press as presenting the 'peaches and cream' side of racing. For years, horse racing swept the dark side of racing out of the public eye. Racing fatalities seldom made the press, and only then when a high-profile horse was involved. Only recently, after dramatic racing fatalities – such as Go For Wand in the Breeder's Cup Distaff, Barbaro in the Preakness, and Eight Belles in the Kentucky Derby – did the public begin paying attention to racing fatalities. And the public doesn't like what they see. A national poll shortly after the Eight Belles death reportedly found 38% of the public would support a ban on horse racing (Newport, 2008). A year later, without a high-profile death, an internal racing industry poll found the number had dropped to 12%.

11.7 Veterinary Medical Care in Horse Racing

Veterinary medical care in racing is very different from most other veterinary practices. The quality of care can be exceptional, especially at the higher levels of the sport. The Dubai Equine Hospital is arguably the best-equipped equine hospital in the world. Santa Anita, Hollywood Park, and Golden Gate Fields in California all have non-profit equine hospitals on-site; Belmont has several private practice equine hospitals nearby or on the track grounds. As with all veterinary services with any animal, the less valuable animals do not have as good access to medical care, but this is not so different from human health care.

The problem with veterinary medical care in horse racing lies in the unusual relationship between the trainer, owner, and veterinarian. Where the horse's welfare fits into the picture is murky. The interests of the trainer, owner, veterinarian, and horse are not always in concert, and the horse can be left without an advocate if no one assumes the role.

Medication regulations were primarily promulgated to protect the integrity of the race rather than to protect the welfare of the horse. There are a few exceptions. Furosemide to treat exercise-induced pulmonary hemorrhage (EIPH) is the best example. Furosemide is best known by the brand name Lasix; this is the origin of the 'L' in racing programs in the USA denoting that a horse is receiving furosemide. Exercise-induced pulmonary hemorrhage is hemorrhage originating in the lung during intense exercise. There are a number of studies that indicate that EIPH occurs in almost all horses undergoing intense bursts of speed (Pascoe *et al.*, 1981; Birks *et al.*, 2002). There is some debate as to whether EIPH is a diseases or normal equine exercise physiology. Regardless, furosemide has been used to control EIPH since the early 1960s. The late Alex Harthill claimed he administered furosemide to the great Northern Dancer in the 1963 Kentucky Derby well before the medication became accepted by the racing industry and regulatory agencies (Hovdey, 2009). For many years, trainers and racetrack veterinarians in the USA believed furosemide reduces EIPH and, therefore, is good for the racehorse. More recently, furosemide as a treatment for EIPH has come under greater scrutiny, but a well-designed study under racing conditions performed in South Africa has clearly shown furosemide reduces EIPH (Hinchcliff *et al.*, 2009). Horses race in most international racing jurisdictions outside the USA without furosemide and are able to compete quite well without negative consequences to equine health. Which approach is best for animal welfare, to treat equine competitors prophylactically with furosemide to reduce EIPH as in North America, or to prohibit any medication on race day as under International Federation of Horseracing Authorities (IFHA) rules?

A re-evaluation is underway for the non-steroidal anti-inflammatory drugs (NSAIDs) permitted in US racing. NSAIDs are a group of drugs with anti-inflammatory and analgesic, or pain-killing, activity. Aspirin and ibuprofen are popular NSAIDs for humans. The Racing Medication and Testing Consortium and the Association of Racing Commissioners International both have model rules allowing the use of just one of three NSAIDs at specific blood threshold levels. Like furosemide, NSAIDs are prohibited by the IFHA rules in effect in most international racing.

Another major therapeutic medication issue is the use of corticosteroids in racing. Corticosteroids are steroidal anti-inflammatories – as compared to NSAIDs, which are non-steroidal anti-inflammatories. Corticosteroids are potent drugs and can be used very effectively and properly to treat specific health and soundness problems. However, corticosteroids are heavily used both systemically and intra-articularly as joint injections. Horses entered to race have been documented as having received four different corticosteroids two days before racing and within current regulations on top of multiple intra-articular corticosteroid injections a few days earlier. There are long-term health concerns with repeated use of corticosteroids both systemically in general and on musculoskeletal structures when combined with hard training and racing. The long-term effects of corticosteroid use have not been well documented in the horse but, in my experience, racetrack practitioners generally agree that repeated corticosteroid injections in the face of significant underlying musculoskeletal pathology is detrimental to the horse.

Firing and blistering are veterinary procedures that cause endless debate. The theory behind firing and blistering is to increase blood supply to the fired or blistered area, thereby promoting healing. Whether they are effective or not, both procedures are fading out of common practice. In some parts of the world, pin-firing is banned outright as inhumane. Veterinarians seldom blister horses any more, as in the days of potent red mercury blisters. If blistering is done, it is done by trainers, stable hands or farm hands. Thirty years ago virtually every horse had pin-fired shins; today there is less than a handful at any track. Younger veterinarians shun both procedures as barbaric. Many horse owners and the public would agree. Other techniques causing local inflammation – such as cryosurgical, percutaneous freeze-firing or periosteal scraping – are less objectionable. The modern terminology for firing is percutaneous thermocautery, but the procedure hasn't changed. A hot instrument, most often a firing iron, is used to burn the skin. The procedure is done under local anesthesia and, in spite of the perception and if done properly, in my experience there is little or no discomfort to the horse. That is not the case with blistering. A hard blister is much more painful to the horse than firing.

There are constant conflicts between regulators and veterinary practitioners over drug testing. There is very little doubt that drug rules affect veterinary medical care. The best example is the drug procaine penicillin. Penicillin is still one of the best antibiotics for equine infections. The most common preparation is procaine penicillin G for intramuscular administration. Procaine penicillin G is safe, cheap, and effective. Procaine is better known by its generic name novocaine or its brand name Novocain, and there is more procaine in procaine penicillin than in most novacaine preparations. Local anesthetics are a major concern for horse racing because of their ability to desensitize or 'block' pain, allowing the injured horse to compete, a very dangerous scenario for horse and jockey. There is reluctance on the part of practitioners to use procaine penicillin G because of the drug testing problems with procaine even though procaine penicillin G is such an excellent antibiotic for horses. There are other drugs where there are no ambiguities. Erythropoietin and other blood doping agents are good examples. These drugs have been used by the unscrupulous in horse racing even though there are well-documented health risks to the horse.

11.8 Claiming and its Relationship to Equine Welfare

Racing has a number of structural flaws that unintentionally impact horse welfare. The best example is the claiming race. A claiming race is a race in which the horse is offered for sale at a specified value, the claiming price. Purses and racetrack operating commissions are funded from a percentage of *pari-mutuel* handle, the amount of money wagered on the race. Nearly all purse monies, the amount of money available to distribute among the horses in a race, derive from *pari-mutuel* handle. Competitive races have more money wagered on the race than non-competitive races. The concept of the claiming race is that horses of the same value should have the same ability. The result is an attractive wagering race for gamblers. A horse worth $100 000 ordinarily is not entered in a $50 000 claiming race. But the claiming aspect of horse racing is very much like poker. The poker equivalents of bluffing and sandbagging are allowed and some trainers are very good at it. To claim a horse, the money and claim form must be submitted before the horses come on to the racetrack. There are no pre-claim examinations as in a private purchase; in fact, the prospective owner or trainer cannot even touch the horse. The purchase through claiming is finalized, depending on the racing jurisdiction, as soon as the horse steps on to the racetrack or when the starting gate is opened. The person claiming the horse owns the horse whether the horse ends up winning by 10 lengths or is struck and killed by lightning.

Hall of Fame trainer Richard Mandella uses the analogy of claiming to the games of Hot Potato or Old Maid. There is a real incentive to racehorses in a claiming race when they have begun developing unsoundness problems. Horses that would not pass a pre-purchase examination in a private sale are often claimed. The person claiming a horse has to decide: is the trainer entering a horse in a claiming race playing poker and bluffing, or is the trainer playing Old Maid? The opportunity to mask injuries with medication is a real issue. If a horse with a superficial flexor tendonitis is claimed and runs last, the previous owner will often receive more money than if the horse had won the race and wasn't claimed. There is the added benefit of no longer owning a horse with a superficial flexor tendonitis. The new owner has no sense of responsibility for the damaged goods he has purchased and the process moves on with the horse the ultimate loser.

11.9 The Role of the Jockey

All successful jockeys are fiercely competitive; otherwise, they would not be successful. Russell Baze is a Hall of Fame jockey, the perennial leading rider on the northern California Thoroughbred circuit, and holder of the record for most wins by a jockey in the world.[1] On August 23, 2007, Baze was riding Imperial Eyes in a cheap maiden claiming race at the old Bay Meadows racetrack. Imperial Eyes was an odds-on favorite with a seven-length lead when he broke down nearing the finish line. Baze steadied Imperial Eyes and hit him twice, hard, with his whip, after the horse was clearly injured, to hang on to finish second in the race. Imperial Eyes had fractured his distal cannon bone and both proximal sesamoid bones and was euthanized shortly after the race. Baze received a 15-day suspension and a $2500 fine. There were calls from both within and outside of horse racing for a lifetime ban. Baze, a well-liked, congenial, and usually very professional rider, was contrite (Shinar, 2007): 'I am not going to defend what I did. There is no way to defend it. I made a bad decision in the heat of the moment, and I am truly sorry.'

This is not a unique situation. Just four days after the Imperial Eyes incident in California, jockey Javier Castalano repeatedly whipped his mount Indian Flare in the Ballerina Stake at Saratoga, New York, as the filly struggled to finish with a fractured pelvis. The following year, one-time Eclipse Award-winning apprentice jockey Jeremy Rose was suspended for six months following a stewards' hearing the morning of June 24, for whipping his mount, Appeal to the City, in the face during the third race at Delaware Park on June 23. In the official ruling, Delaware Park stewards contended that Rose 'engaged in extreme misuse of the whip during

---

[1] On August 14, 2010, Baze became the first jockey to reach 11 000 wins in a career.

the stretch run while on the horse Appeal to the City' (Marr, 2008). The injury to Appeal to the City required treatment at the University of Pennsylvania's famed New Bolton Center after the race. In the end, Appeal to the City recovered, but for a time there was concern whether the eye could be saved.

11.10 Whips

Spurs and war-bridles have been banned from racing for many years, but the whip is still considered an integral part of horse racing. The use of the whip is highly controversial. There is something incongruous about whipping a horse, while claiming that horses love to race. California-based horseman Monty Roberts, an internationally acclaimed horse trainer and horse behavior expert, claimed in an Australian interview (see Horsetalk, 2008):[2] 'A whip has no place in horsemanship at all. It's medieval for horses.' He also points out that a horse that wants to win, that has that competitive spirit and natural will to win, is always going to be a far better racing prospect than the one that has to be whipped for half of the race. Analysis of whip use during racing has shown that the horses hit the most frequently do not win.

Jockeys are not required to carry whips, but they usually do so. Jockeys claim whips are needed to control some horses. There is some validity to the claim, but there are just as many instances where whips have caused major accidents. At Hollywood Park in 1992, trainer Ted West instructed jockey Patrick Valenzuela not to hit his mount Interwit with the whip, and to be sure to hold the whip in his left hand (West, pers. comm.). In his races Interwit tended both to lug-in and to run away from the whip. 'Lug-in' means to drift toward the inside rail and, not surprisingly, horses often run away from the whip. A horse will typically drift right when hit left-handed and left when hit right-handed. In this instance Interwit went into the lead a hundred yards from the finish line. Shortly after pulling clear of the rest of the field, Valenzuela hit Interwit right-handed. The horse ducked hard to the left and into the rail, sustaining major injuries. After hitting the inside rail, Interwit bounced back and fell onto the track, at which point a trailing horse tripped and fell over Interwit. Both horses were euthanized as a result of their injuries.

British whipping rules are among the most comprehensive in racing, short of an outright ban. Their rules recognize three legitimate uses of the whip: safety, correction, and encouragement. *Safety* is use of the whip to avoid a dangerous situation. An example would be a horse that is out of control, where the whip could be used to keep the horse in check. *Correction* is similar to safety – using the whip either by showing or striking a horse to keep a proper running lane. *Encouragement* is allowed to try to obtain a better effort out of the horse. The use of the whip for

---

[2] Also see http://www.montyroberts.com/press-releases/monty-roberts-advocates-for-the-horse-in-horse-racing/.

encouragement is permitted only on a limited basis. The rider must show the horse the whip first and give the horse time to respond. Next the rider is allowed a backhand strike, and again the horse must be given a chance to respond before the horse is put under the whip. Thereafter, if a horse is then to be whipped, a whole series of conditions come into play, including how the whip is held, how the horse is responding, whether the horse is in contention, and even the number of times the horse is hit. More importantly, there are specifically prohibited uses of the whip even for encouragement beyond the number of hits. Horses cannot be hit, except in unusual circumstances for safety or correction, except on the hindquarters or the shoulder with the whip held for a backhanded strike. Hitting horses that are clearly winning, out of contention, past the finish line, or showing no response to the whip is prohibited. Any physical injury to the horse resulting in welts or if blood is drawn will result in fines or suspensions except in rare circumstances.

California regulations prohibit jockeys from whipping a horse on the head, flanks, or on any part of its body other than the shoulders or hindquarters. The horse cannot be whipped during the post-parade except when necessary to control the horse. More subjectively, a horse cannot be whipped when the horse is clearly out of the race, has obtained its maximum placing, or is showing no response to the whip. These regulations are rarely enforced. Excessive or brutal whipping causing welts or breaks in the skin are also prohibited. As a practical matter, whip marks on flanks are easy to find. The skin is thinner on the flanks and is more apt to welt, cut, bleed, or otherwise show whip marks. These rules can be enforced when an effort is made to do so, and they are in many racing jurisdictions. California official veterinarians are provided cameras to record evidence of whipping rule violations and file complaints against jockeys when appropriate.

Trevor Denman is the track announcer at Santa Anita and Del Mar racetracks. He is one of the keenest observers of how races are run in the world. He is an outspoken critic of how the whip is used in the USA (Denman, pers. comm.): 'Watch any race in progress down the back stretch and you will see a field of racehorses doing what they have been bred to do for the last three hundred years; running willingly and at fast speeds without any whips involved. However, when the horses reach the home stretch the whips come out. It is particularly saddening when one has to watch a horse that is obviously exhausted and has no chance of improving his position, being whipped incessantly. One also often sees a rider in a close finish start flailing away with the whip like a mad man. The closer to the wire they come, the faster and more times they whip the horse.' Denman believes the English solution offers the best compromise between the intense competitiveness of the horse race and the welfare of the horse. 'Over a decade ago British racing implemented rules that have changed the whipping rules dramatically and for the better. Two of those rules that we should implement in the US as soon as possible are that a jockey cannot raise the whip above the shoulder and a jockey must give the horse time to respond before hitting him again. The whips themselves need changing too. America's whips are the most brutal of the civilized racing world. There are new whips now available that are much more humane than the old ones. It seems like a no-brainer that these new whips should be made mandatory right away.' He is referring to the riding crop the Jockey Club Safety Committee has recommended be required as a uniform national requirement. Already many racetracks have taken the initiative without waiting for racing regulatory agencies to act and have required riders to use the padded whips on their courses. More restrictive regulations governing whipping in horse racing is inevitable.

11.11   Horse Slaughter and the Racehorse

Horse racing was front and center in the horse slaughter issue, but not because so many racehorses end up slaughtered – that is not the case. The reason is that, of all the equine sports, horse racing has the highest public profile. They were the obvious target of choice for anti-slaughter activists. Horse racing's primary audience and market is the non-horse-owning general public. In addition, several high-profile leaders in racing were major supporters of the anti-horse-slaughter movement. Prominent horse racing organizations – such as the National Thoroughbred Racing Association and the Breeder's Cup – publicly opposed horse slaughter. Horse slaughter was never a significant commercial issue for racing, which has tried to distance itself from the controversy. Other horse-related organizations with a broader horse exposure than just racing – such as the American Association of Equine Practitioners, the American Quarter Horse Association, and the American Veterinary Medical Association – recognized the potential unintended consequences of abandonment and neglect, and either opposed the anti-slaughter movement or refused to offer support.

The horse slaughter controversy had the beneficial effect for racing of focusing attention on retired racehorses. There are many more retirement, rehabilitation, and retraining programs for former racehorses today than ever before. Though funding for these efforts falls well short of what is needed, several States and racing organizations have begun experimenting with statutory or mandated funding mechanisms to augment charitable support.

Horse racing is beginning to understand that the public cares about horses. The horse is what is special about horse racing. Horse racing isn't auto racing; no one goes to a horse race to see a wreck. There is a realization that society may not tolerate horse racing much longer unless racing becomes safer and kinder to the horse. Horse racing must change to survive. The horse will be the winner.

References

Anthenill, L.A., Stover, S.M., Gardner, I.A. *et al.* (2007) Risk factors for proximal sesamoid bone fractures associated with exercise history and horseshoe characteristics in Thoroughbred racehorses. *American Journal of Veterinary Research* **68**, 760–771.

Birks, E.K., Shuler, K.M., Soma, L.R. *et al.* (2002) EIPH: postrace endoscopic evaluation of Standardbreds and Thoroughbreds. *Equine Veterinary Journal (Supplement)* 34(S34), 375–378.

Boden, L.A., Anderson, G.A., Charles, J.A., Morgan, K.L., Morton, J.M., Parkin, T.D., Clarke, A.F. and Slocombe, R.F. (2007) Risk factors for Thoroughbred racehorse fatality in flat starts in Victoria, Australia (1989–2004). *Equine Veterinary Journal* 39(5), 430–437.

CHRB (2003) *Thirty-Third Annual Report of the California Horse Racing Board.* California Horse Racing Board, Sacramento, CA. Available at: www.chrb.ca.gov.

CHRB (2006) *Thirty-Sixth Annual Report of the California Horse Racing Board.* California Horse Racing Board, Sacramento, CA. Available at: www.chrb.ca.gov.

CHRB (2008) *Thirty-Eighth Annual Report of the California Horse Racing Board.* California Horse Racing Board, Sacramento, CA. Available at: www.chrb.ca.gov.

Cohen, N.D., Mundy, G.D., Peloso, J.G. *et al.* (1999) Results of physical inspection before races and race-related characteristics and their association with musculoskeletal injuries in Thoroughbreds during races. *Journal of the American Veterinary Medical Association* 215, 654–661.

David, T. (2009) Report of the ARCI Regulatory Veterinarian Committee to the RMTC. Available at: www.rmtcnet.com/resources/NSAID_IA_Cort_Statement.

Halchin, L.E. (2008) *Former NFL Players: Disabilities, Benefits, and Related Issues,* CRS Report for Congress, pp. 5–18. Congressional Research Service, Washington, DC. Available at: http://www.policyarchive.org/handle/10207/18851.

Hernandez, J., Hawkins, D.L., Scollay, M.C. (2001) Race-start characteristics and risk of catastrophic musculoskeletal injury in Thoroughbred racehorses. *Journal of the American Veterinary Medical Association* 218, 83–86.

Hill, A.E., Stover, S.M., Gardner, I.A. *et al.* (2001) Risk factors for and outcomes of non-catastrophic suspensory apparatus injury in Thoroughbred racehorses. *Journal of the American Veterinary Medical Association* 218, 1136–1144.

Hinchcliff, K.W., Morley, P.S. and Guthrie, A.J. (2009) Efficacy of furosemide for prevention of exercise-induced pulmonary hemorrhage in Thoroughbred racehorses. *Journal of the American Veterinary Medical Association* 235, 76–82.

Horsetalk (2008) Whipping is horse racing's sore point. *Horsetalk.* Available at: www.horsetalk.co.nz/features/whipping-137.shtml.

Hovdey, J. (2009) Call him Doctor Derby. *Daily Racing Form.* April 28.

Jockey Club (2010) *Jockey Club Online Fact Book.* Available at: www.jockeyclub.com/factbook.asp.

Kane, A.J., Stover, S.M., Gardner, I.A. *et al.* (1996) Horseshoe characteristics as possible risk factors for fatal musculoskeletal injury of Thoroughbred racehorses. *American Journal of Veterinary Research* 57, 1147–1152.

Kane, A.J., Stover, S.M., Gardner, I.A. *et al.* (1998) Hoof size, shape, and balance as possible risk factors for catastrophic musculoskeletal injury of Thoroughbred racehorses. *American Journal of Veterinary Research* 59, 1545–1552.

Lavin, A.G. (1987) The image of the racetrack practitioner and AAEP ethics. In *Proceedings of the 33rd Annual Convention of the AAEP,* pp. 855–858.

Marr, E. (2008) *Update: Rose Responds to Whip Incident.* Bloodhorse.com. Available at: www.bloodhorse.com/horse-racing/articles/45859/update-rose-responds-to-whip-incident.

Newport, F. (2008) *Post-Derby Tragedy, 38% Support Banning Animal Racing.* Gallup poll. Available at: www.gallup.com/poll/107293/PostDerby-Tragedy-38-Support-Banning-Animal-Racing.aspx.

Parkin, T.D.H., Clegg, P.D., French, N.P., Proudman, C.J., Riggs, C.M., Singer, E.R., Webbon, P.M. and Morgan, K.L. (2005) Risk factors for fatal lateral condylar fracture of the third metacarpus/metatarsus in UK racing. *Equine Veterinary Journal* **37**, 192–199.

Pascoe, J.R., Ferraro, G.L., Cannon, J., Arthur, R.M. and Wheat, J.D. (1981) Exercise-induced pulmonary hemorrhage in racing Thoroughbreds: a preliminary study. *American Journal of Veterinary Research* **42**, 703–707.

Shinar, J. (2007) 'Contrite' Baze Accepts 15-Day Whip Penalty, Fine. Bloodhorse.com. Available at: www.bloodhorse.com/horse-racing/articles/40457/contrite-baze-accepts-15-day-whip-penalty-fine.

Stover, S.M., Johnson, B.J., Daft, B.M. *et al.* (1992) An association between complete and incomplete stress fractures of the humerus in racehorses. *Equine Veterinary Journal* **24**, 260–263.

Stover, S.M. and Murray, A. (2008) The California Postmortem Program: leading the way. *Veterinary Clinics of North America: Equine Practice* **24**, 21–36.

Abusive Treatment and Subsequent Policy Development within Various Breeds of Show Horses in the USA

12

Jim Heird

12.1 Introduction

Walking Horse Finale Canceled

Federal regulators had been warning Tennessee Walking Horse owners and trainers for months that too many show horses showed signs of being sored, according to e-mails and documents detailing these talks. US Department of Agriculture inspectors disqualified six out of approximately 10 horses they inspected Aug. 25 …

The World Grand Championship contest at the Tennessee Walking Horse industry's biggest showcase was canceled Saturday night, over fallout from several horse disqualifications.

The Tennessean, September 3, 2006

These headlines (Schrade, 2006; Reeves, 2006) are a vivid example of the extent to which inhumane treatment has become a part of the show horse industry in the USA. Developed originally to showcase the beauty, quality, and athleticism of the

Equine Welfare, First Edition. Edited by C. Wayne McIlwraith and Bernard E. Rollin.
© 2011 by UFAW. Published 2011 by Blackwell Publishing Ltd.

various breeds, shows in almost every breed have developed into a competition among owners and trainers to see who can obtain desired results, with at times little regard for the effect that their training methods may have on the horses they are training. Perhaps even worse, these practices have now been carried out for a long enough period of time that new generations of trainers are accepting the practices as normal. The general public would find many of these practices to be offensive, if not inhumane. Yet in some breeds these practices are not only accepted but actually defended by industry leaders, trainers, and owners.

Habituation occurs when a being is exposed to distasteful or unpleasant circumstances for a length of time until those circumstances are ignored and accepted as normal. Often, today's trainers have been exposed to inhumane practices for so long that they no longer feel empathy for the pain and/or suffering that the animal is forced to endure as it goes through a training program. Some practices have gone on for many generations, and many of today's trainers have developed their skills in a system that uses practices that they would probably have found to be distasteful when exposed to them for the first time. In short, trainers have become habituated to inhumane practice and no longer find them unpleasant, let alone inhumane.

In the author's opinion, no breed or show group is free of practices that the general public would find distasteful or unacceptable. However, many breed associations and supervisory groups are starting to police inhumane practices within their own breeds. Some of these new efforts are due to the negative publicity received concerning these practices, and some are a proactive response by the organizations to the increased awareness the public has of inhumane practices.

12.2 Common Practices Used by Various Exhibitor Groups

12.2.1 Soring in the Tennessee Walking Horse industry

Soring is the process of applying a substance or mechanical device that will result in enough pain that the horse will exaggerate its gait to relieve the pain it feels on the affected leg/legs. In the Tennessee Walking Horse shown at the highest levels, an exaggerated long stride behind and a high-action step in front are desirable. A horse sore in front will rock its weight back on the hind legs and lengthen its stride behind while leaving its front feet on the ground for short periods of time.

A common product used to sore Tennessee Walking Horses is mustard oil, a caustic product that burns the skin and leaves the horse sore enough to increase the desired high action in front and the deep reaching gait behind that characterizes the 'big lick' wanted in the show ring. Other ways to sore a horse include pressure shoeing, quicking during foot trimming, and road foundering. All basically have the same effect. The horse will quicken the lifting of the fore feet and try to shift its weight to the hindquarters.

It is important to note that, within the Tennessee Walking Horse breed, this practice is done only on the show horse. The natural non-sored Tennessee Walking

Horse still has the characteristic smooth running walk and gentle disposition for which the breed was developed.

12.2.2 Gingering and whip training of the Arabian conformation horse

Gingering is the act of placing ginger, a mild chemical irritant, in the anus of the horse to encourage it to hold its tail in a higher arch. *Whip training* is when the horse, in training, is struck with a whip until it poises and flexes its neck with its ears forward. Then when threatened in the show ring with a whip, it will poise with its ears forward and display a stretched and arched neck. The high tail carriage, the arching neck, and the alert look are desirable characteristics of the Arabian horse.

Gingering is sometimes practiced in the American Saddlebred breed to get the same tail response. Again, in this breed, a high tail setting is a desirable characteristic. In the United States Equestrian Federation rule book (2010), which includes guidelines for the judging of Arabian horses shown in conformation classes, judges are told to dismiss from the class any horse that has any whelps or visible whip marks.

12.3 Inhumane Practice Found in Various Events of the Stock Horse Breeds

12.3.1 Western pleasure horse

It is desirable for a Western pleasure horse to be quiet, calm, and obedient. Good Western pleasure horses do this naturally. However, not all horses go slow and stay quiet in novel environments. A variety of practices have been used through the years to achieve the desired look and action. In the author's own experience, a few years ago it was not uncommon to bleed a Western pleasure horse so that it would be lifeless and quiet when it went into the show ring. Marijuana was also used to mellow the horse before an event. Tying the horse's head high in the stall for several hours before competition also resulted in the desired low head carriage wanted in the show ring. Placing a block of wood in the horse's mouth for a long period before entering the show ring made the horse want to keep its mouth closed during the competition. Excessive exercise also results in the calm, quiet appearance desired.

12.3.2 Reining and working the cow horse

Both of these events are judged on the horse's ability to stop, turn, and change leads. Many horses start anticipating these maneuvers, so a common practice is to *fence* the horses. This is a training practice commonly used in training to teach the horse to stop with its hind legs under it and to listen to the cues of the trainer. The process involves loping with speed into a wall or fence until the horse listens to either the verbal or weight shift cues given by the trainer. At shows, trainers will sometimes do this for extended periods of time. The horse becomes tired and thus is abused when this practice is used to extremes. Spinning excessively as a part of the warm-up period immediately prior to the competition is a common practice.

Although spinning is a normal part of the event, it is the number and duration of the practice that makes it inhumane.

12.3.3 Trail horses, jumping horses and hunter horses

The practice common to each of these events is *poling*. Poling is when the horse's legs are struck with a 'pole' of some type as it either jumps, or is crossing a log or jumps used in the events. The pole can be anything from a light bamboo pole to a heavy metal pole. The horse picks up its feet or legs to prevent it from being struck during the practice. Like all training practices, when taken to extremes, it can and does become abusive. Another practice used in hunter and jumper training is to jump an elevated oxer jump backward so that the highest part of the jump is in front of the jump. Because of the horse's limited depth perception, it sometimes misjudges the height of the jump and strikes the highest part of the jump as it crosses the fence. Thus, the next time the horse jumps in competition, it will jump higher than normal to keep from hitting the jump.

12.4 Addressing of These Issues by Breed Associations and Show Organizations

Many of the practices discussed above have been, or are being, addressed by the leaders of the industry. For example, in the summer of 2008 the American Association of Equine Practitioners developed a White Paper calling for the total elimination of soring in the Tennessee Walking Horse. The following suggestions were recommended (AAEP, 2008):

White Paper

Putting the Horse First:

Veterinary Recommendations for Ending

the Soring of Tennessee Walking Horses

As the world's largest professional organization dedicated to equine veterinary medicine, with a membership of nearly 10 000 veterinarians and veterinary students who dedicate their life's work to caring for the horse, the American Association of Equine Practitioners (AAEP) takes very seriously its responsibility when offering a position statement regarding the treatment of horses. The AAEP condemns the abusive practice of 'soring' and formed the Tennessee Walking Horse Task Force in 2007 with the goal of contributing the expertise of the veterinary community to efforts that will permanently eliminate one of the most significant welfare issues affecting any equine breed or discipline. The Task Force recognizes that any effective change in the current culture of the industry must come from within, but we genuinely hope that, with this white paper, we can provide support to those within the Tennessee Walking Horse (TWH) industry who endeavor to end the continuing abusive practices specifically prohibited by the Horse Protection Act (HPA) enacted by Congress in 1970.

A Culture of Abuse

Soring is the practice of inflicting pain to create an extravagant and exaggerated show gait for both padded and flat-shod horses and includes but is not limited to the use of irritants; the treatment of the pastern region to remove the visible effects of irritants or scar/callus remnants resulting from previous irritants and/or action devices; pressure shoeing and excessive paring of the sole and/or frog; and any method utilized to induce pain or laminitis. Its continued practice is documented by the US Department of Agriculture's (USDA) citation of 103 violations of HPA regulations during the 2007 Tennessee Walking Horse Celebration, the industry's championship event.[1] The failure of the HPA to eliminate the practice of soring can be traced to the woefully inadequate annual budget of $500 000 allocated to the USDA to enforce these rules and regulations. In the absence of adequate governmental funding, it is incumbent upon industry participants themselves – owners, trainers, and all support personnel – to take full responsibility for developing a program which succeeds in eliminating the recognized abuses that are at the core of the problem. Continued reliance on the use of traditional techniques dependant upon the subjective response of the horse would appear a wasted effort and funding for the development of objective methodology for use by qualified veterinary inspectors must be provided.

Improved Methods of Evaluation

Because the HPA has been in effect since 1970, no scarring, calluses or other skin conditions indicative of treatments directed at increasing sensitivity should be present in horses currently in competition and none should be tolerated. Likewise, no efforts to mask such treatments should be tolerated.

The Task Force recommended the following specific objective methods for evaluation of the horses both before and after each competition (class, not event) to ensure the health and welfare of the equine participants (AAEP, 2008):

1. Immediate institution of drug testing (plasma, serum and cutaneous swabs) based on the methodology and regulations established by the United States Equestrian Federation (USEF).
2. Prohibition of any medical treatments or syringes, therapeutic or otherwise, by any personnel in the make-up ring prior to each class, an area which should be supervised by trained stewards known to be otherwise uninvolved in the Walking Horse industry.
   a. Limitations on the number of individuals and equipment which may accompany the horse into the make-up ring.
      i. Forbid the use of any devices utilized to tighten the bands which secure the 'packages.' (Packages are defined as the pads and shoe.)

---

[1] USDA Veterinary Medical Officer Horse Protection Show Report for 2007.

3. In recognition of the fact that many acts associated with soring occur in the stabling areas of the show grounds, it is recommended that security personnel and supervising inspectors be present in these areas 24 hours each day of the competition to ensure that no violations of the HPA occur.

4. Physical inspection, by a veterinarian, of the horses prior to entering the ring to include:
    a. Visual inspection of the limbs and shoes.
    b. Removal of saddles/girths to check for pain-inducing objects.
    c. Thermographic screening of the limbs to assist in defining specific anatomical areas requiring additional clinical examination and/or surface swabbing to detect forbidden substances.
    d. Palpation of the limbs including:
        i.   Routine evaluation of the limbs.
        ii. Assessment of digital pulses.
        iii. Critical assessment of specific areas suggested to be abnormal on thermographic examination.
    e. Swabbing of the limbs for foreign substance testing.
        i.   Areas determined to exhibit an abnormal thermographic pattern should be included in the testing.
    f. Examination of the horses in a standard pattern at a walk and extended walk, on a loose rein, in hand and under tack.

5. Observation by qualified veterinarians of the horses during competition for lameness while at work.

6. Re-examination of selected horses as they exit the ring (with horses held in the make-up ring while examinations are completed) to include:
    a. Thermographic re-examination.
    b. Removal of both front shoes of randomly selected horses or horses with abnormal thermographic patterns:
        i.   Visual and hoof tester examination of unshod feet for evidence of methods directed at inducing pain, such as pressure devices and excessive paring of the sole and frog.
        ii. Weighing of shoes (flat-shod horses) or shoes and package (padded horses).
    c. Digital radiographs of the feet, in randomly selected horses or horses found to have any physical or thermographic abnormalities, to detect:
        i.   Laminitis, acute or chronic, as manifested by either rotation of the third phalanx or sinking of the bony column within the hoof capsule.
        ii. Sole thickness.
    d. Drug testing including *both* plasma and urine for the presence of prohibited substances.
    e. Swabbing of the limbs for foreign substance testing utilizing current standard methodology.
        i.   Areas determined to exhibit an abnormal thermographic pattern should be included in the testing.

12.5 Putting the Horse First

In comparison to other equine breed and discipline associations with which the AAEP is familiar, the TWH industry has several glaring differences that contribute to the difficulty of achieving the goal of eliminating soring. In conclusion, the AAEP recognizes that it has no regulatory authority over the TWH industry but offers on behalf of the horse these recommendations regarding governance structure, uniform regulations, and judging standards (AAEP, 2008):

1. Establishment of a single organization that has governance responsibilities for the industry is critical for the effective resolution of conflict and the establishment and enforcement of uniform standards and regulations. The current arrangement of multiple Horse Industry Organizations (HIOs) fails to accomplish this vital need and has resulted in competing interests. The USEF could serve as a model for such an organization, with fees collected from members and competitors to fund the organization, the regulatory personnel (veterinarians and stewards) and the drugs and medication testing program (systemic and topical).
2. The adoption and strict enforcement of meaningful uniform standards and regulations, combined with more stringent penalties, are the cornerstones of establishing fair and humane competitions. Penalties should be much more severe and consequential to owners, trainers and other support personnel than in the past. Lifetime disqualification of horses found not to be in compliance would penalize trainers and owners to a degree likely to mitigate against a second infraction. We believe that owners are the only individuals who can bring adequate pressure to bear on each other and their trainers to eliminate these intolerable abuses.
3. Establishing standards of judging which value the innate grace and beauty of this breed instead of rewarding the currently manufactured extravagant and exaggerated gaits will facilitate a rapid return to horsemanship and training devoid of the intolerable abuses of soring in all its manifestations. The AAEP, in its mission to act in the best interest of the horse, remains willing to assist the TWH industry in prohibiting these cruel and inhumane practices. However, the decision to develop realistic and effective means of eliminating individuals who perpetuate this culture belongs to the TWH industry alone.

This paper resulted in considerable discussion within the breed, and that discussion continues today.

The industry is stepping forward and recognizing that it needs to make changes. Recently, the following changes were announced from a press release (HIO, 2009):

In an unprecedented move yesterday, the National Horse Show Commission voted to accept the proposal from Sound Horses, Honest Judging, Objective Inspections, Winning Fairly (SHOW), The Celebration® Horse Industry Organization (HIO), to assume all responsibilities currently conducted by the National Horse Show Commission (NHSC). The actual transfer will take place Wednesday, April 1, 2009. The NHSC Board of Directors voted unanimously to make the transfer after a lengthy discussion about assets and the ultimate dissolution of the Commission. The Tennessee Walking Horse National Celebration® (TWHNC®) Board of Directors voted last Thursday, to proceed with the proposed action and began immediately to initiate the revival of the horse show season. The United States Department of Agriculture (USDA) agreed to accept the transfer of Designated Qualified Persons (DQPs), all horse shows and sale affiliations previously contracted with NHSC, and all shows to begin operating under the SHOW HIO immediately. Pat Marsh, Chairman of the SHOW HIO Planning Committee and Dr. Doyle Meadows, CEO represented The Celebration® at the meeting. The biggest single factor in the entire transfer is the trainers and owners have removed themselves from the inspection process as well as the judges department.

When asked about what will be different effective April 1, 2009 when SHOW takes over? 'I can't assure you that anything will be different effective immediately,' said Meadows. 'What I can tell you is the single biggest difference will be the trainers and owners out of the inspection process,' concluded Meadows.

At the same time, the United States Department of Agriculture released the following announcement concerning the use of thermography as a detection tool (USDA, 2009):

Thermography to be Used in Detecting Soring

The following is a stakeholder update on the use of thermographic technology by Animal Care, a program within the US Department of Agriculture's Animal and Plant Health Inspection Service (APHIS). As many of you know, APHIS announced its intentions to consider the use of thermography during Horse Protection Act (HPA) inspections in 2007. Since then, APHIS has piloted the use of thermography and trained its Veterinary Medical Officers on the technology.

Thermography is a technology that can assist in identifying abnormalities indicative of soring. Through the use of infrared cameras, thermography measures the surface temperatures of an object. This technology has been incorporated into diagnostic equipment used by medical professionals, devices that enable firefighters to see through smoke, and some night-vision equipment. In thermographic images, cooler areas appear blue, black, green, or purple, while warmer areas appear yellow, orange, red or white.

Beginning with this show season, thermography will be integrated into the normal inspection process and used as an additional diagnostic tool for the detection of soring, the cruel and inhumane practice used to enhance the height and reach of a horse's gait. Horses can be sored in a number of ways including burning the animal's legs with caustic chemicals, using illegal shoes, or chains that are too heavy, among other methods.

During inspections, inspectors evaluate a horse's appearance and locomotion and physically examine the animal for any signs of pain, scars, blisters, or odors associated with soring practices. USDA also randomly swabs horses' legs to test for foreign substances.

The use of thermography will not replace these other methods of inspection nor will its use or associated protocols conflict with the operating plans in place for HPA enforcement. The technology will be used as a screening tool. Horse exhibitors, whose horses are deemed not normal based on thermographic results, will be given the option to either excuse themselves from the class without a penalty or undergo a more detailed inspection by an inspector. Flowcharts showing the inspection procedure are available on our website at www.aphis.usda.gov/animal_welfare/hp.

We remain committed to making continuous improvements to HPA enforcement and will do so both through the pursuit and use of technology as well as other methods. Our intention has always been to work with our industry partners and other interested parties to ensure that horses are protected from the cruel and inhumane practice of soring.

Certainly, all associations are trying to address actual inhumane practices or the appearance of any inhumane practices. However, the association that appears to be at the front of this effort is the world's largest breed association, the American Quarter Horse Association. In the fall of 2008, a blue-ribbon task force (the Horseman's Animal Welfare Task Force) was asked not only to identify inhumane practices taking place within the breed's shows but also to develop guidelines to eliminate these practices. The task force identified several practices to eliminate as well as procedures for eliminating them. The work of this task force and its effect on the entire show horse industry has the chance to be one of the most influential efforts to eliminate and begin to control the level of inhumane treatment that takes place in the show ring of all breeds. The AQHA Executive Committee approved the following recommendations from their task force, and listed them in the 2010 American Quarter Horse Association rulebook:

1. AQHA membership renewal forms should include a signature requirement stating the applicant has acknowledged and accepts to abide by Rule 401(b) which states: 'The standard by which conduct or treatment will be measured is that which a reasonable person, informed and experienced in generally accepted equine *care*, training, and exhibitor procedures and veterinary standards, would determine to be cruel, abusive or inhumane.'
2. Enforce the rules and Code of Ethics. Suspensions and fines should have more impact. Suspensions should include non-participation and denial of access to the show grounds for a given number of shows and/or days. Suspensions can be retroactive which would result in disqualification from previous show(s).
3. Professional Horsemen need to report to AQHA all conversations concerning abusive actions.
4. Change the equipment rule for Team Penning and Ranch Sorting to follow the Western equipment rules. A snaffle bit or hackamore must be used if the exhibitor is riding two handed. Use of a curb bit would require the rider to use only one hand.
5. Implement the following in the 2010 Rule Book under each of the designated disciplines:

Reining and Working Cow Horse

The practice of excessive fencing will not be allowed in the warm up and practice arenas.

No excessive spinning – excessive spinning is defined as no more than eight (8) consecutive turns and two (2) repetitions.

Working Cow Horse

It is the judge's responsibility to control the pen and the treatment of all cattle in cattle classes.

Dally Team Roping, Heading and Heeling

Prohibit excessive stretching of the steers. Definition of excessive stretching is intentional and continuous stretching of the steer after the horses have faced.

All Classes Over Fences

Disallow poling or schooling ramped oxers approaching backwards. No rail shall be higher than four feet in schooling areas. The definition of poling is when the obstacle is altered as the horse is negotiating said obstacle.

Any Time

There will be no excessive spurring, jerking of the reins or whipping with intent to cause discomfort, fear, distress, injury or intimidation. Excessive and continuous actions will result in disqualification and/or elimination from the show grounds.

Barrel Racing, Pole Bending, Team Penning, Ranch Sorting, Stakes Racing and Jumping

Revise rule 458(g) to read 'The judge must disqualify any contestant for excessive use of a whip, rope, crop, bat or reins anywhere on the horse.'

References

AAEP (2008) *Putting the Horse First: Veterinary Recommendations for Ending the Soring of Tennessee Walking Horses.* AAEP White Paper, August 2008. American Association of Equine Practitioners, 4075 Iron Works Parkway, Lexington, KY 40511, USA (www.aaep.org).

American Quarter Horse Association Rulebook (2010) Available at: http://siteexec.aqha.com/association/registration/handbook.html.

HIO (2009) *It's a Done Deal.* The Celebration Horse Industry Organization, Press release, April 15, 2009.

Reeves, M. (2006) After 7 of 10 horses ousted, remaining entries withdraw. *The Tennessean,* September 3, 2006. Available at: http://www.tennessean.com/article/20060903/NEWS01/101110016/Walking-Horse-finale-canceled.

Schrade, B. (2006) For months, USDA warned trainers about signs of soring. *The Tennessean,* September 3, 2006. Available at: http://www.tennessean.com/article/20060903/NEWS01/101290001/For-months-USDA-warned-trainers-about-signs-of-soring.

USDA (2009) *Thermography to be Used in Detecting Soring.* US Department of Agriculture, Press release, April 14, 2009.

The Horse as a Companion Animal

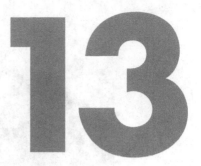

Nancy S. Loving

13.1 Introduction

While a horse does not occupy a place next to the hearth like a cat or a dog, the partnership that develops between horse and owner can be deep and satisfying. For those with a passion for horses, it is not difficult to understand how horses are viewed as 'companion animals' – the bond between horse and owner strengthens as these large animals wend their way into an owner's heart. The whicker of welcome, the soft blow of a horse's sweet breath on one's face, and the velvet touch of a warm muzzle add to the special emotional attachment an owner feels for a horse (Figure 13.1).

A horse, as a companion animal, often becomes the center of a rider's attention. A horse entering a person's life provides not only recreation and learning of skill sets, but also a platform for character development. Young riders learn to be responsible to another living being that flourishes from care and attention. Self-esteem may improve through accomplishments achieved with an equine partner. Training and competition provide outlets for demonstrating a rider's expertise, and also serve as practical excuses to spend more time in the companionship of a beloved horse at home and on the road. The horse provides the framework to meet and to network with others with a shared passion. A horse provides freedom and autonomy for those who feel constrained by busy life obligations or by a disability. Horse owners exclaim that being around horses is stress relief from the rat-race of busy lives. Riding, grooming, feeding, and cleaning chores are viewed as desirable activities that lend quietude to cherished hours of 'time-out.'

The backyard horse is often purchased with the intent that it will become part of the family, living out its days in this secure position. The barn is prepared, tack

Equine Welfare, First Edition. Edited by C. Wayne McIlwraith and Bernard E. Rollin.
© 2011 by UFAW. Published 2011 by Blackwell Publishing Ltd.

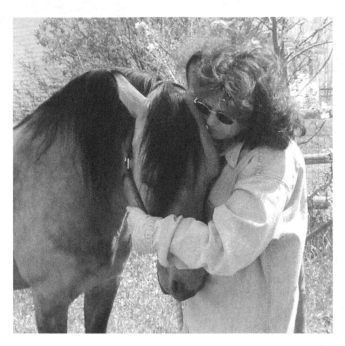

Figure 13.1 The emotional connection between horse and owner establishes the horse as a companion animal that is cherished and included as part of the family. (Reproduced with permission from Bill Cripe.)

cleaned and oiled, hay put up, and veterinary advice consulted. Horses stabled at training barns or turned out to pasture are no less part of a sentimental attachment despite being housed apart from a person's residence.

13.2 Use of the Horse for Athletic Pursuits

A horse, as a companionable animal, comes with bonus ability besides the bonding relationship that develops: it can be ridden. In a riding partnership, an owner takes pride in a horse's athletic talent along with personal accomplishments. Meticulous care is taken to ensure the horse looks its best – from the luster of a shiny coat to the dressings of tack. Together, horse and rider form a team during training and in competition. Bernie Rollin eloquently states the transforming effect of such a human–animal bond: 'We should keep as our root metaphor what must surely have informed the ancient vision of the centaur, the symbiotic unity of man and animal, mutually interdependent, rising to heights neither could scale alone' (Rollin, 2000) (Figure 13.2).

This sentiment of pairing horse and rider is embodied in art and literature, indelibly romanticizing the unique and co-dependent position of the horse in its integral

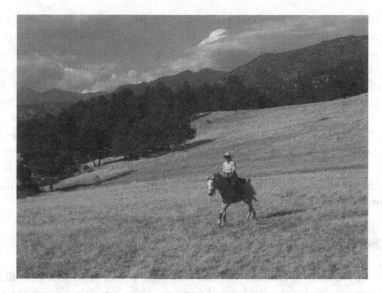

Figure 13.2 Horse and rider becomes a complete unit, experiencing the world in a unique way. (Reproduced with permission from Pat Jarvis.)

role in the forging of the civilized world. In today's modernized society, the horse no longer serves as beast of burden, transportation, or warhorse. Its interrelationship with humans has been transformed – as a companion animal and as recreation.

The horse, in its many roles as companion, riding partner, teacher, and traveling and adventuring partner fulfills many of an owner's equestrian dreams. In return, a fortunate horse is treated as a self-aware individual, provided with quality preventive medical care, nutrition, shelter, exercise, and opportunities for herd socialization; the horse flourishes within the nurturing atmosphere of an owner's companionable attention.

Yet, there are times when the anticipated outcome does not go quite as planned. Because a horse is a considerable investment not only in purchase price but also in persistent monthly costs imposed on its owner, practical logistics enter into decisions of how a horse is used. A horse may continue to be ridden regardless of failing soundness or vigor because that is the only riding horse in a person's stable. In other instances, the significance of a forged partnership and the comfort and security a rider feels on that horse's back become more important than the horse's lessened abilities. Medical therapies may be administered to alleviate pain from musculoskeletal concerns; this strategy may work to a point, but may not be able to ameliorate discomfort altogether or for the anticipated useful life of the horse. Training and competition persist despite the horse experiencing a slowly debilitating injury, degenerative condition, or advancing age. Such a horse may be ridden beyond its time; instead of being retired or ridden in a less-demanding athletic pursuit, there is an expectation for the horse to perform at a previous level, which may be more rigorous than his diminished capabilities can provide.

This kind of situation is not always abusive, but does have welfare implications. A horse may experience varying degrees of discomfort or anxiety when asked to work harder than he is able. Behavior may change, cooperation with a rider may falter, or the horse may simply tune out to the demands of the rider and refuse to perform. A veterinarian has the occasion during farm visits to observe the attitude and general health of a horse; this presents an opportunity to counsel an owner if it seems the horse is despondent, too thin, or more lame than usual. A dialog with an owner and/or trainer might encourage strategies to better prepare the horse for desired athletic demands or to explore optional careers for the horse, including retirement.

13.3 Breeding Ambitions

An owner with a mare or stallion that can no longer perform athletic pursuits due to injury or lameness is faced with limited options. They can either retire the horse to pasture with expenses accruing monthly, or find a way to achieve a valuable return on their investment by breeding the horse. An owner with an emotional attachment to the breeding prospect gains pleasure in perpetuating the genetic line of a favorite horse. To breed a horse that can no longer work as a riding partner makes sense, but an owner should be counseled in the practicality of this approach.

When considering a retired mare or stallion as a breeding prospect, it is relevant to factor in the cause of a career-limiting or career-ending lameness. A horse with lameness attributable to traumatic injury is likely to be a more desirable breeding candidate than a horse with a lameness issue related to a degenerative condition, especially if linked to conformation or structural characteristics. Continuing to propagate poor conformation or degenerative tendencies within the gene pool persists in creating an inevitable consequence of more lame horses in the future. This presents the potential for heartbreak for a future owner as well as putting a horse's welfare in jeopardy. Responsible ownership also carries with it the obligation of responsible selection of breeding stock.

13.4 The Overly Protected Foal

Foaling out a mare brings an owner full circle in the quest for excellence from the genetic line of a favorite horse. While all details are attended in preparation for welcoming a newborn foal to the family, sometimes the basic mental and physical needs of a foal are overlooked. A proud owner often has concerns that the foal might injure itself if given too much latitude to kick up its heels; a common tendency is to be overly protective of a young foal. The belief that it is 'safer' to confine mare and foal to a stall or small paddock rather than giving them freedom to

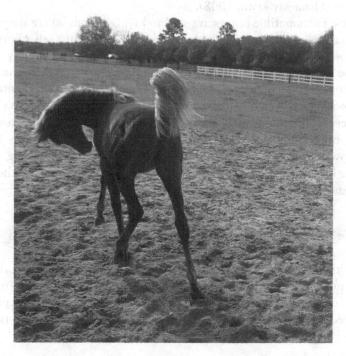

Figure 13.3 A young foal in turnout can kick up its heels in play and has the opportunity to socialize with others. (Photos Nancy Loving.)

run, play, and socialize in the pasture is not necessarily in the best interests of the horses. Current research indicates that confinement is counterproductive for optimal musculoskeletal development and structural strength for future riding pursuits (Smith and Goodship, 2008) (Figure 13.3). In addition, socialization of young horses within a herd of mares and foals is important to building confidence and behavioral compliance that carry over in cooperative relationships with people (Crowell-Davis, 1986).

An owner can gain from constructive education about the benefits of pasture turnout, exercise, and the lessons gleaned from interactive herd dynamics.

13.5 Incompatibility Issues

In the process of purchasing or raising a horse and accepting it into one's family, there is no way to know how well a new horse and new owner will mesh. Not all horses are suitable for all people. Sometimes, a person just doesn't like the horse, or vice versa, or the horse isn't able to do what the owner requires for an intended athletic pursuit. Unrealized expectations may result in wastage and potential welfare issues (Hennessy *et al.*, 2008).

Most times, incompatible horses are sold to loving homes where they transform into suitable companion horses; but sometimes, an owner must sell a horse as expediently as possible to recover an investment, and is willing to accept any reasonable offer. Or, the horse is sold at auction and there is little to guarantee that it will go to a good home rather than to one of neglect or abuse. Such a potential welfare scenario is not merely a fictionalized story, like a *Black Beauty* tale that follows a plot of misery until ending with a happy turn of events. Many horses sold to a prospective buyer may not receive a comparable quality of life as previously enjoyed. How a horse might fare in less-desirable living and working conditions depends to a large degree on the sensitivity of that horse's nature and the degree of difficulties encountered.

13.6 The Behavioral Challenge

If a horse with a dangerous vice, such as biting, rearing, striking, or rodeo-quality bucking, is put up for sale or sent to auction, an unsuspecting buyer (or innocent bystander) could be seriously injured (Figure 13.4). If all training options have been explored, with no improvement in the horse's temperament or in rider safety,

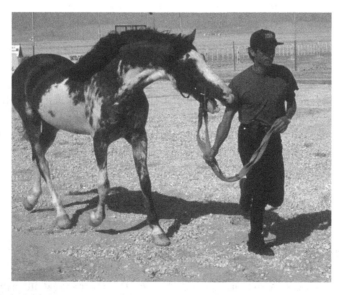

Figure 13.4 A horse that consistently displays menacing aggression may not fit in to the fabric of an owner's life as a good companion match. (Photos Nancy Loving.)

then other less ambiguous options include turning the horse out to pasture permanently or consideration of euthanasia if a true renegade. The concept of *caveat emptor* or 'buyer beware' is a common refrain, but responsibility ultimately rests with the horse owner and/or trainer who might be inclined to send a dangerous horse down the road for sale to the public. The Uniform Commercial Code has been adopted in many States in the USA as a guideline for private, commercial transactions, including sale of horses (Toby, 2007). This code covers express and implied warranties when a buyer and seller conduct a privately negotiated transaction. Besides ethical and welfare considerations related to placing a potentially dangerous animal as a companion horse in a new home, there are also legal ones related to intentional misrepresentation of a horse. At a public auction, however, there often isn't room for negotiating the terms of the sale, including warranties. In every case, private or public venue, a savvy buyer would be wise to ask many sensible questions in an attempt to uncover hazards and problems so the wrong horse doesn't end up in the wrong home.

13.7 Loss of Position in the Family

Even when the most perfect horse becomes part of a family, an owner may not realize at the time that taking on this ownership responsibility is a long-term commitment. The obligation may (and often does) extend as much as 20–30 years. The purchase price of the horse pales in comparison to accumulated costs of upkeep and care over years and decades. This lengthy time frame of obligated care can also lead to welfare issues, especially if the companion horse is later considered to be disposable.

As with any new acquisition, over time the excitement may fade and complacency sets in. Sometimes life gets in the way of a horse remaining an integral part of the family no matter how well it is loved – young riders grow up and move away from home, financial difficulties beset a family, or a busy job leaves little time to devote to the horse or may require a geographical move.

When a horse is no longer serviceable to the owner or family, attempts are made to donate the horse to a riding program, which can be at a university or privately, to a therapeutic center, or, in some instances, to non-painful research in universities. Such an offering provides a charitable tax deduction for the owner, and also may create a new opportunity for the horse, such as entering into a breeding or riding program that includes good care and attention. A horse's new-found position may assist in training future veterinarians or horse caretakers, or in the discovery of scientific information that might be used to relieve pain and suffering of a future equine patient.

Other efforts are made by conscientious owners to place a less than perfectly sound campaigner to a home with less grandiose expectations, where a skilled and experienced horse can train a budding equestrian to the particulars of competition.

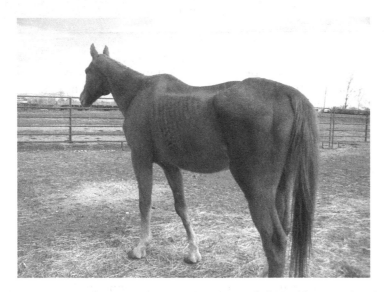

Figure 13.5 A neglected horse or one with underlying metabolic problems may lose body condition to the point of starvation, which may not be noticeable until after a winter coat has shed out. (Photos Nancy Loving.)

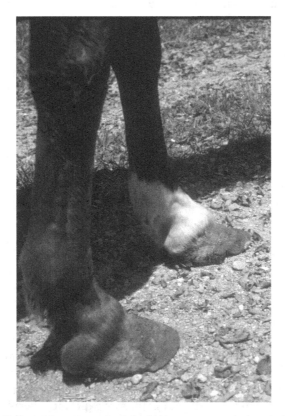

Figure 13.6 A neglected horse may be left with hooves untended and allowed to overgrow, which might create painful problems in the feet and/or joints. (Photos Nancy Loving.)

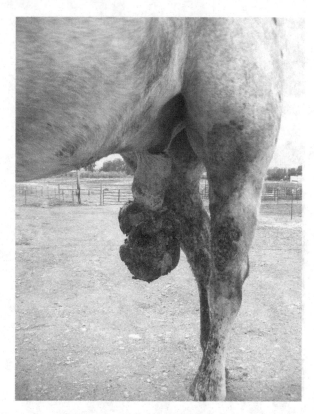

Figure 13.7 A neglected horse may be left to endure severe medical problems, as in this case, in which a severely invasive penile squamous cell carcinoma caused life-threatening blockage of urination accompanied by pain and distress. (Photos Nancy Loving.)

Or, a more crippling disability might prematurely retire a gentle horse to a new role as companion to an equine athlete living alone on a farm.

One of the biggest challenges faced today in equine welfare is that of abandonment, or the 'unwanted' horse. In some cases, a horse may be 'wanted' but an owner is unable to support the costs of horse keeping. At other times, a child owner grows up and pursues different interests or goes away to college, leaving the horse behind in the care of non-horse-savvy parents. These horses may be left in the field or paddock with below-par care given by well-meaning yet unknowledgeable people, or the horse may be offered free to a new home or to a rescue organization. Horse rescue sanctuaries are one adoption haven for unwanted horses, while therapeutic riding centers accept cooperative horses that can no longer perform rigorous athletics but can still be ridden. The number of unwanted horses far exceeds the available number of spots for them.

Another welfare challenge that the horse, as a companion animal, faces is neglect. In spite of the best intentions, a busy owner or an under-informed caretaker may

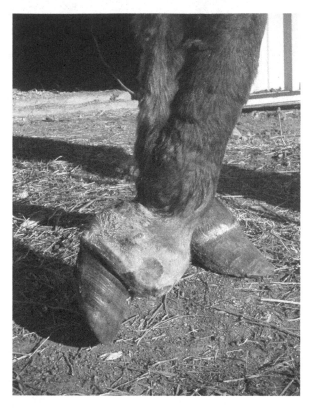

Figure 13.8 This horse experienced severe pain from a suppurative wound of the coffin joint and surrounding tissues that went untended due to owner neglect. His rescue came too late to be of any help, and euthanasia was the humane option. (Photos Nancy Loving.)

not realize the needs of a horse lingering in the backyard. Thick winter fur often hides a gaunt frame with a caretaker unaware of a steady process of starvation (Figure 13.5). Parasite control is ignored or forgotten, hooves are left untended to overgrow (Figure 13.6), and the horse must fend for itself, regardless of the size of acreage or the quality (or lack thereof) of pasture available. Economic considerations often affect whether or not a horse receives adequate feed or preventive, let alone more intensive, medical care (Figures 13.7 and 13.8). Not all owners can afford to treat or have the time to manage a horse with ongoing medical needs.

With increasing economic pressures in recent times, more horses are being considered as 'throw-away' commodities, with little regard for the fact that these are living, sentient creatures with not just basic needs of food, water, and shelter, but emotional needs as well. While many horses are purchased with the intent to use them for athletic activities, an owner should venture into horse ownership with full awareness of the full extent of responsibility – a horse cannot be put away like

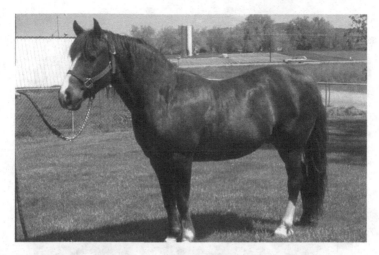

Figure 13.9 Overfeeding of the companion horse causes obesity, which can create numerous medical problems that cause pain and suffering, and ill-health. This horse is very fat (body condition score of 8 on a scale of 1 to 9), with a cresty neck and noticeable fat pads over the ribs, and along the shoulders and rump. (Photos Nancy Loving.)

a mountain bike or set of skis when interest lapses; its care entails basic needs that persist for the lifetime of the horse. An owner is obligated to fulfill that commitment or find the horse an appropriate home where all needs can be met. Or an alternative option, like leasing or joint ownership, might help in sharing the financial burden of maintaining a horse in the best of health. It could save everyone, and affected horses, the anguish of welfare conflicts if professional guidance and education precede the purchase of a horse, particularly for those families unfamiliar with the long-term consequences of horse ownership.

13.8 Killing Them with Kindness

In contrast, another welfare issue that is all too often encountered is the beloved companion horse that is lavished with too much care, and in particular too much food or rich pasturage. The horse becomes obese, which is a form of malnourishment. Excess body condition (Figure 13.9) adds to the burden of a horse with a musculoskeletal problem, and too much body fat makes it harder for a horse to dissipate heat in the summer months. Obesity leads to metabolic and hormonal imbalances, with debilitating laminitis as an ultimate consequence (Johnson, 2002) (Figure 13.10).

Similarly, active riding horses that seem well cared for are sometimes the recipients of overly ambitious attentions and micromanagement: they receive little to no turnout or exercise, are housed in barns with airways affected adversely by dust, ammonia fumes, and pathogens that flourish in warm places (Couteil *et al.*, 2007),

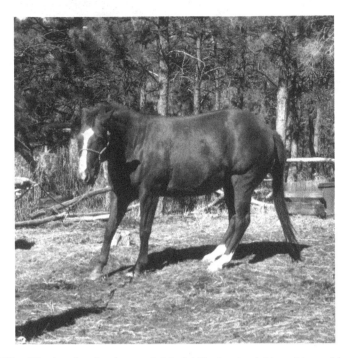

Figure 13.10 Obesity often leads to painful, debilitating laminitis, evidenced by the grimace and reluctance of this horse to walk and turn when asked. (Photos Nancy Loving.)

and confinement restricts their social interaction and stimulation. Carefully explained veterinary advice is important to help an owner maintain a horse's nutritional needs for optimal body condition, to prevent medical and behavioral problems that arise from too little exercise, and to facilitate a horse's emotional stability by encouraging living arrangements that include herd interaction and the chance to stretch its legs and run (Figure 13.11).

13.9 The Slow Demise

There are cases where a horse lives in a steady state of decline, such as the old horse with few teeth and an inability to maintain enough flesh on its frame despite being offered a high-calorie, gruel diet. There may be underlying malabsorption or metabolic problems, and no amount of feed provides sufficient nourishment. For some, flesh seems to evaporate from bones as chronic pain deadens the appetite along with pain-induced muscle catabolism (Figure 13.12). A crippled mare salvaged for breeding may be unable to conceive as her reproductive system shuts down in response to pain and weight loss.

An owner may hold on to false hope and be blinded to the reality of what their companion horse must endure. Because an owner sees their horse each day, there

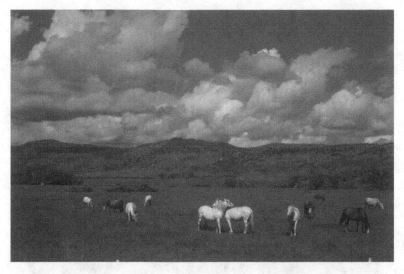

Figure 13.11 Pasture turnout is good for a horse's mental health, allows opportunities for herd socialization, and maximizes muscle tone and joint health. (Photos Nancy Loving.)

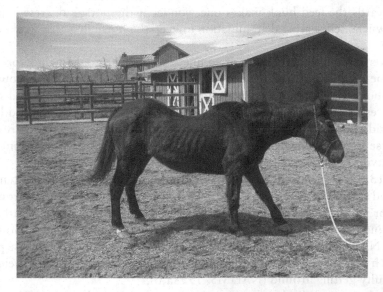

Figure 13.12 An old mare such as this is in constant pain from debilitating arthritis as well as suffering from continued weight loss related to pain and age-associated metabolic changes. (Photos Nancy Loving.)

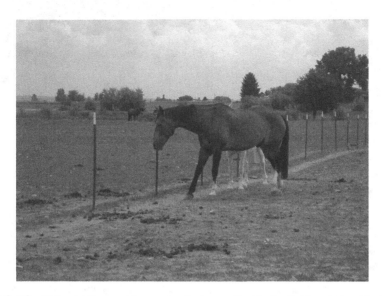

Figure 13.13　This middle-aged horse stands despondent in the field, pointing his chronically painful foot, unable to do much other than try to find a point of comfort. Quality of life is an important element to factor into a horse's care. (Photos Nancy Loving.)

isn't always the advantage of a time interval that marks notable changes in a horse's condition or demeanor. Watching a despondent horse shuffling its way across the field towards the feed bunk makes one wonder if the horse's distress is justified by an owner's self-serving determination to keep the horse in active work, or even just alive.

As veterinarians or advocates of equine welfare, our goals include preserving life to the best of our abilities. In so doing, it is important also to counsel an owner about their horse's quality of life. If pain-relieving medicines and surgical procedures fail to keep a horse alert and attentive to the world around him, he may spend a large part of his day trying to find a position of comfort (Figure 13.13). The horse may lie down more frequently than normal, speaking volumes with this behavior (Figure 13.14). A horse with advanced tarsal or carpal osteoarthritis (Figure 13.15) may have difficulty rising from the ground; being cast often causes panic and anxiety for both horse and owner. A horse in unrelenting, chronic pain is one for whom it is easier to make a decision to alleviate suffering, rather than postponing the inevitable. In reports by the National Animal Health Monitoring System (NAHMS), death was attributable to old age in 30% of the horse population, with nearly 65% of these old horses euthanized due to chronic weight loss or difficulty getting around (NAHMS, 1998a,b).

In a non-acute medical situation, it is sometimes difficult to recognize when a horse is experiencing pain or distress. A caring horse owner appeals to their veterinarian for an analytical assessment of the horse's condition. Tolerance to pain is a

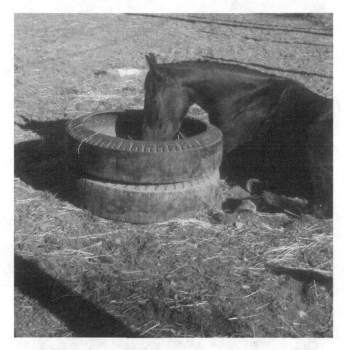

Figure 13.14 A horse that is in constant discomfort may lie down more than usual, even to the point of preferring to eat while lying on the ground. (Photos Nancy Loving.)

subjective process, and while humans verbalize their pain, it can be argued that behavioral changes in a horse also depict levels of discomfort. Horses respond to external and internal stimuli in similar ways as do people, with individual differences dependent upon the degree of stoicism inherent to that individual.

Expression of a horse's discomfort or stress takes many forms – some individuals display aggressive tendencies, with the horse lashing out at people or other horses for no apparent reason. Some chew on fences or inflict self-trauma. Others withdraw from the bombardment of stimuli around them. A listless or apathetic attitude in an otherwise alert individual, depressed appetite, a tendency to stand apart from the herd – these behaviors indicate an ailing equine body and mind (Taylor *et al.*, 2002).

On a less drastic note, when a horse is no longer serviceably sound for athletic pursuits due to a chronic but relatively 'mild' arthritic condition, navicular syndrome, old muscle or tendon injury, or chronic obstructive respiratory disease, one assumes responsibility for this horse's remaining life. No matter the age of the horse, when its quality of life begins to pale and an owner is sensitive to helping that horse, veterinarians search their scientific armamentarium and alternative therapies looking for solutions to alleviate the discomfort. Multiple medical procedures may be offered through the horse's lifetime to alleviate degenerative processes and forestall chronic

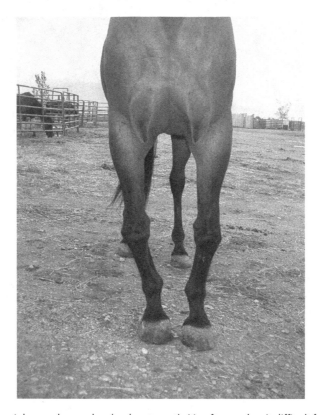

Figure 13.15 Advanced carpal or hock osteoarthritis often makes it difficult for a horse to get up off the ground in addition to affecting a horse's overall quality of life. (Photos Nancy Loving.)

pain. These procedures may not work for all individuals or for all time to keep the horse in riding condition; retirement to pasture may be an appropriate course.

Not everyone is endowed with acres of retirement pasturage, or the finances to keep a retired horse on the property, so other solutions are looked to, such as donation to horse rescue operations, therapeutic riding centers, or as a companion to another horse or to a person desiring a horse to look after but not necessarily to ride. Compassionate options and placement in a welcoming home are not always readily available. Sometimes a decision for euthanasia is considered.

There is the possibility that such a request may be abused as 'convenience euthanasia,' when an owner means to 'sacrifice' a healthy animal due to circumstances such as geographical relocation, or monetary constraints in attending to a non-life-threatening medical problem. In cases where a horse is truly suffering, euthanasia may be viewed as an act of kindness and compassion. An owner looks for guidance by seeking personal and professional opinions. In the final analysis, and with the horse's best welfare in mind, a decision of what next steps to take for a cherished equine companion must come from an owner's heart, coupled with sage medical advice.

13.10 Acute Medical Crisis

Inevitably, the years roll by and in most cases horses rarely outlive their owners. It is unusual for a horse to lie down quietly one night and not reawaken. For most, the door closes on life in a dramatic way, through the agony of colic (Figure 13.16), some irreparable trauma, or the wasting away of flesh and vigor.

The adage 'they shoot horses, don't they?' used to be more fact than fiction. Yet, with the advent of sophisticated medical and surgical measures to repair fractures, surgically correct intestinal displacements, or treat arthritic joints with injection of anti-inflammatory medications, previously unimagined options are now readily available through veterinary expertise and technology. In many cases, the decision to send a horse for emergency surgical care or to consider euthanasia of a trusty equine friend needs to be made on the spur of the moment, under the duress of an owner witnessing an animal to be in pain or distress. At times, not even heroic measures may be able to save a horse's life. A veterinarian's important role is to be there as counsel to assist an owner in making appropriate decisions in the best interests of the horse. It is optimal for a veterinarian to have a medical plan and end-of-life discussion with an owner in advance, so thoughtful consideration can be deliberated when emotions are calm rather than in the face of a calamity. In this way, a timely decision can be reached without prolonging a horse's pain or suffering.

With a horse's best welfare in mind, it is helpful to have on file, both at the barn and with the horse's veterinarian, an owner's desired medical directives for their

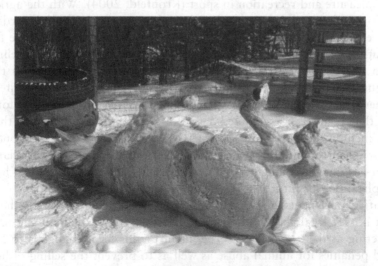

Figure 13.16 An acute medical crisis, like colic, may necessitate rapid decision-making by the owner to pursue aggressive medical treatment, surgery, or euthanasia. Haste is critical to minimize pain and suffering. (Photos Nancy Loving.)

horse and an agent listed who will act in their stead if the owner cannot be contacted during an emergency. Specifics should be delineated as to how much money may be invested in medical care and at what point the owner authorizes surgery or euthanasia if that is the most humane option.

Not everyone can afford or justify the financial burden of advanced medical procedures, no matter how well-loved a horse may be. Or, it may be necessary to provide a horse with a calm ending to its life rather than being subjected to the difficulties of complicated surgery or lasting pain.

The hardest part of this decision-making process is to decide when it is time to ease a horse's distress state. Today, the debate rages over the legality and societal ethics of a person requesting human euthanasia to relieve suffering and pain from terminal illness. Because horses in our society are still considered as personal property, owners are entitled to make such requests of their animal care doctors, and a veterinarian is able to act on these requests, in the best interest of each horse. (See Chapter 8 for a detailed discussion on euthanasia.)

13.11 Legislative Considerations

As an example of how welfare concerns can quickly change based on legislative policy, it is relevant to look at a current trend in the USA. At this time, horses in the USA are still legally considered 'livestock' and thus are viewed as personal property. Livestock implies that a domestic animal may be used for production and profit; intrinsic value is added to the horse as a companion animal in that it also provides pleasure and recreation in sport (Kronfeld, 2004). With the agricultural designation as 'livestock,' an owner has the right to make decisions regarding sale, lease, breeding, showing, and racing, as well as proffering medical care for their horse. Euthanasia is permissible; this decision is based on practical guidelines concerning a horse's welfare (AAEP, 2008). A 'livestock' classification in the USA places equine care and regulation under the governing umbrella of the United States Department of Agriculture (USDA) and similar State agricultural enforcement agencies that regulate horse-related activities and provide funding for the entire industry, including research projects (such as equine infectious disease outbreaks) and enforcement of the Horse Protection Act and the Safe Commercial Transportation of Equine to Slaughter Act (AHC/AAEP, 1999). Such funding has favorable implications for future equine welfare issues.

Legislative movements are being pursued by animal rights activists in the USA to change a horse's legal classification from 'livestock' to 'companion animal,' with people acting as their 'guardians.' The intent of this legal change is to facilitate increased penalties for animal abuse as well as to prevent the selling of horses to slaughter or to overseas sales for human consumption. Ironically, if this wording change occurs not just in terminology but also in legal intent, there may be limitations to the usefulness of a horse as a working animal, with more restrictions placed on equestrian sports, such as, for example, jumping, dressage, distance riding, gymkhana, or rodeo events. If the horse becomes a legal 'ward' and an owner is considered a 'guardian,' then a guardian is mandated to protect the rights of a less competent individual, much as they would a child, even at the expense of the guardian's rights (Toby, 2007). Fewer options may then exist for an owner, now considered 'guardian,' to elect to sell, give away, or breed their horse, or even to euthanize it in the face of suffering. In the end, the horse, as a legally considered companion animal/ward, would have fewer welfare protections than currently exist.

13.12 The Unique Joys of the Horse as a Companion

The designation of a horse as livestock does not preclude an owner from exploring a relationship and partnership with a horse and enjoying that animal in every way as a companion. To those entrusted with its care, the horse gives back intangible riches and pleasure. With its beautiful eye, sweet smell, strong stature, and tractable nature, the horse is a most unique companion animal, deserving of an owner's lifelong commitment to its well-being. It is not unusual to see the face of a horse owner light up in animated delight in speaking of their close bond with a horse, or of accomplishments in equestrian pursuits. It is these people who promote the best welfare conditions for the horse, and who sing the praises of the horse in its role as companion.

References

AAEP (2008) *Euthanasia Guidelines*. American Association of Equine Practitioners, Resource Guide and Membership Directory, Ethical and Professional Guidelines, pp. 43–44.

AHC/AAEP (1999) *Legal Status of Horses as Livestock*. White Paper, Committees of the American Horse Council, and the American Association of Equine Practitioners.

Crowell-Davis, S. (1986) Developmental behavior. *Veterinary Clinics of North America: Equine Practice* 2(3), 573–590.

Couteil, L., Hoffman, A., Hodgson, J. *et al*. (2007) Inflammatory airway disease in horses. *Journal of Veterinary Internal Medicine* 21, 356–361.

Hennessy, K., Quinn, K. and Murphy, J. (2008) Producer or purchaser: different expectations may lead to equine wastage and welfare concerns. *Journal of Applied Animal Welfare Science*, 11(3), 232–235.

Johnson, P. (2002) The equine metabolic syndrome peripheral Cushing's syndrome. *Veterinary Clinics of North America: Equine Practice* 18(2), 271–293.

Kronfeld, D. (2004) The horse – livestock or companion? *Virginia Horse Journal*, April.

NAHMS (1998a) *Equine Morbidity and Mortality*. Info Sheet, National Animal Health Monitoring System. US Department of Agriculture, Animal and Plant Health Inspection Service (APHIS), Washington, DC.

NAHMS (1998b) *Deaths in US Horses, 1997 and Spring 1998–Spring 1999*. Info Sheet, National Animal Health Monitoring System. US Department of Agriculture, Animal and Plant Health Inspection Service (APHIS), Washington, DC.

Rollin, B. (2000) Equine welfare and emerging social ethics. *Journal of the American Veterinary Medical Association* **216**(8), 1237.

Smith, R. and Goodship, A. (2008) The effect of early training and the adaptation and conditioning of skeletal tissues. *Veterinary Clinics of North America: Equine Practice* **24**(1), 37–51.

Taylor, P., Pascoe, P. and Mama, R. (2002) Diagnosing and treating pain in the horse: where are we today? *Veterinary Clinics of North America: Equine Practice* **18**(1), 8–10.

Toby, M.C. (2007) *The Complete Equine Legal & Business Handbook*, pp. 14 and 164–165. Eclipse Press, Lexington, KY.

Welfare Issues in the Rodeo Horse

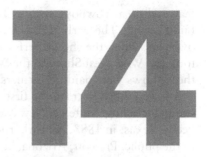

Doug Corey

14.1 Introduction

The unique appreciation of both the human and animal athlete is obvious in professional rodeo, and one that has prompted special attention to ensure that both are well cared for before, during, and after a performance. Like any other activity involving the use of animals, rodeo has been under scrutiny regarding the care and use of the livestock that are such an integral part of the sport. Rodeo organizations have been self-regulating, with rules to protect the livestock since the 1940s. Events sanctioned by the Professional Rodeo Cowboys Association (PRCA) have 60 rules that govern the equipment, competition, and handling of the livestock (see the Appendix to this chapter, section 14.13, where these rules are listed). Self-enforcement regarding livestock welfare has been a priority of the PRCA as a proactive stance to ensure all equine welfare concerns are addressed.

14.2 History

Rodeo as we know it did not exist until the late 1800s, but its roots in North America can be traced back to the Spanish settling California and becoming cattle ranchers. The word 'rodeo' originates from the Spanish word *rodear* meaning 'to surround' or 'to round up.' The skills of the early Spanish *vaqueros* were eventually passed along to the American cowboy after the Civil War, when the frontier territories were heavily expanding. The difference between Spanish rodeo and American rodeo is that the Spanish version focuses on style, while the American version focuses on speed and technique.

In the late 1800s, Wild West Shows began traveling the eastern States and did so for about 50 years. Today's rodeos are an offspring of these early shows, which

Equine Welfare, First Edition. Edited by C. Wayne McIlwraith and Bernard E. Rollin.
© 2011 by UFAW. Published 2011 by Blackwell Publishing Ltd.

featured great cowboys such as Buffalo Bill Cody and Bill Pickett, who invented bulldogging. The early 1900s marked the introduction of the Wild West Show overseas, when the shows performed in the UK, Europe, and Africa. Casey Tibbs took the Wild West Show to the World's Fair in Brussels, Belgium. The cowboys in these shows were paid performers and it wasn't a contest like modern rodeos.

It is very hard to trace the first rodeo in North America. Many places make this claim, including: Sante Fe, New Mexico, in 1847; Deer Trail, Colorado, in 1869; and Pecos, Texas, in 1883. All early rodeos varied greatly by events, and most were free to the public. Prescott, Arizona, held their first rodeo on July 4, 1888. Much of what we know today in the sport of rodeo grew from the Prescott Rodeo. The committee established the following, which still hold true today: prizes awarded, rules for competition, admission charged, cowboys invited to compete, and a committee to organize. The events included bronco riding, steer roping, and cow pony races. In 1889, the first steer riding competition was held, and later this event evolved into modern bull riding. By 1917, calf roping was added to the list of events at Prescott.

14.2.1 The Professional Rodeo Cowboys Association

In the 1920s, rodeo began to organize to combat problems of the rapid expansion of the sport. The Rodeo Association of America, made up of rodeo committees and producers, was formed in 1929. World Champions were to be selected in the following events: bronc riding, bull riding, bareback riding, calf roping, steer roping, bulldogging, team roping, and wild cow milking. The name was changed in 1946 to the International Rodeo Association. By 1936, the cowboys decided to form their own organization after going on strike at the Boston Garden Rodeo. The organization was named the Cowboys Turtle Association because they were slow to organize, but eventually 'stuck their neck out.' The organization wanted to ensure fair prize money, equality in judging, and honest advertising of the sport. In 1945, the name was changed to the Rodeo Cowboys Association. By 1955, the International Rodeo Association recognized the Rodeo Cowboys Association as superior and closed down. The inception of the Professional Rodeo Cowboys Association came in 1974 when the Rodeo Cowboys Association added 'Professional' to their name. Today, the PRCA is the largest sanctioning organization, with nearly 650 rodeos sanctioned yearly.

14.2.2 Rodeo organizations

Modern rodeos are held throughout the USA, and they are sanctioned by many different organizations catering to many different levels of competitors, ranging from youth and senior to amateur and professional. The PRCA, headquartered in Colorado Springs, Colorado, is the largest organization in the world representing the professional rodeo cowboy, as well as stock contractors, rodeo producers, rodeo committees, entertainers, and others associated with the pageantry of rodeo. It is estimated that there are a minimum of 10000 rodeos held annually in the USA, with an estimated one-half of them sanctioned by the PRCA, National High School Rodeo Association, National Intercollegiate Rodeo Association, National Little Britches Rodeo Association, Women's Professional Rodeo Association, International Gay

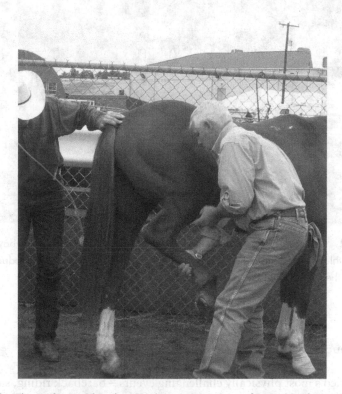

Figure 14.1 The Professional Rodeo Cowboys Association enforces 60 rules to provide for the proper care and handling of rodeo livestock. These rules require a veterinarian on-site for competition. Here, the author examines a roping horse at the Pendleton Round-up, in Pendleton, OR. (Reproduced with permission from the Professional Rodeo Cowboys Association.)

Rodeo Association, and others. This chapter will focus on American rodeos, which offer a variety of events, including tie-down roping, team roping, steer roping, steer wrestling, bareback riding, saddle bronc riding, barrel racing, and bull riding.

14.2.3 Rules
The PRCA has been the leader in creating animal welfare procedures, rules, and standards for American rodeo, and they network with other rodeo associations to ensure the welfare of the livestock participating. The PRCA first began implementing rules to ensure proper care and treatment of rodeo livestock in 1947. Since that time, the PRCA has successfully built the animal welfare program to serve as a model to all rodeo associations. All sanctioned rodeos have rules governing the care and handling of the livestock. All PRCA rodeos and many other rodeo associations listed above and others require a veterinarian to be on-site or on-call for the duration of the competition (Figure 14.1).

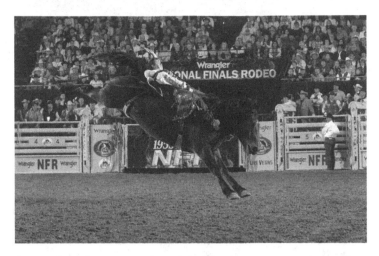

Figure 14.2 Bareback horses are talented athletes that team up with a cowboy to put on a spectacular athletic endeavor. (PRCA ProRodeo photo by Mike Copeman. Reproduced with permission from the Professional Rodeo Cowboys Association.)

14.3 Roughstock Events

Three of rodeo's most physically challenging events – bareback riding, saddle bronc riding, and bull riding – rely on horses and bulls that can kick high and buck powerfully. To understand the livestock involved as well as the care afforded to them, it should be helpful to have an explanation of these events. Livestock welfare issues in the roughstock events include the use of the cattle prod, spurs, and flank straps. All of this equipment is humane when used properly and regulated by the sanctioning rodeo organization.

14.3.1 Bareback riding

Bareback riding consistently produces some of the wildest action in the sport (Figure 14.2). A bareback rider begins his ride with his feet placed above the break of the horse's shoulder. If the cowboy's feet are not in the correct position when the horse hits the ground on its first jump out of the chute, the cowboy has failed to 'mark out' the horse properly and is disqualified. Throughout the eight-second ride, the cowboy must grasp the rigging (a handhold made of leather and rawhide) with only one hand. A rider is disqualified if he touches his equipment, himself or the animal with his free hand or bucks off. The rider is judged on his control during the ride and on his spurring technique (spurring will be addressed in a separate section). The score also is based on the rider's 'exposure' to the strength of the horse. In addition, the horse's performance accounts for half the potential score.

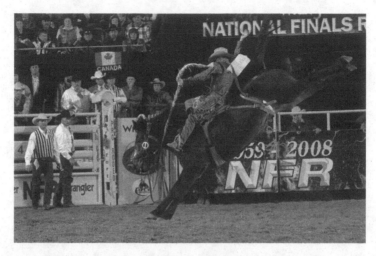

Figure 14.3 Saddle bronc riding horses are generally larger and have a more consistent bucking pattern than the bareback horses. (PRCA ProRodeo photo by Mike Copeman. Reproduced with permission from the Professional Rodeo Cowboys Association.)

14.3.2 Saddle bronc riding

Rodeo's 'classic' event, saddle bronc riding, has roots that run deep in the history of the Old West. Ranch hands would often gather and compete among themselves to see who could display the best style while riding untrained horses. It was from this early competition that today's event was born (Figure 14.3). Each rider must begin his ride with his feet over the bronc's shoulders to give the horse the advantage. A rider who synchronizes his spurring action with the animal's bucking efforts will receive a high score. Other factors considered in the scoring are the cowboy's control throughout the ride, the length of his spurring stroke, and how hard the horse bucks. Disqualification results if, prior to the buzzer, which sounds after eight seconds, the rider touches the animal, himself or his equipment with his free hand; either foot slips out of a stirrup; he drops the bronc rein; he fails to have his feet in the proper 'mark out' position at the beginning of the ride; or he bucks off.

14.3.3 Bull riding

Unlike the other roughstock contestants, bull riders are not required to spur. No wonder. It's usually impressive enough just to remain seated for eight seconds on an animal that may weigh more than a ton (about 900 kg) and is as quick as he is big (Figure 14.4). Upper body control and strong legs are essential to riding bulls. The rider tries to remain forward, or 'over his hand,' at all times. Leaning back could cause him to be whipped forward when the bull bucks. Judges watch for good body position and other factors, including use of the free arm and spurring action. Although not required, spurring will add points to a rider's score. As in all the

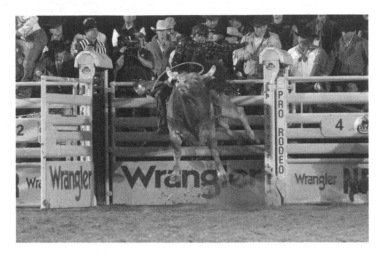

Figure 14.4 The bucking bulls used in modern rodeo are bred to be especially athletic. (PRCA photo by Mike Copeman. Reproduced with permission from the Professional Rodeo Cowboys Association.)

riding events, half of the score in bull riding is determined by the contestant's performance, and the other half is based on the animal's efforts. A bull rider will be disqualified for touching the animal, himself or his equipment with his free hand or bucking off.

Critics of these events have said that some of the equipment – the flank strap, prod, and spurs – compel the animals to perform. As a veterinarian, I am familiar with the behavior of large animals, and know otherwise. These are not animals that are forced to buck and perform in the arena. If a flank strap is pulled so tight as to be uncomfortable, the horses and bulls will likely cease to buck or not perform to the best of their ability. Rodeo livestock are those with a natural inclination to buck for the purpose of unseating a rider. In my opinion, many of these horses have found their niche in life as an athlete in the rodeo arena.

14.3.4 Born to buck
Rodeo stock contractors, who spend a lot of time and money to breed and buy top bucking animals, know better than anyone that only a small percentage of animals have the desire to buck. Today, a number of breeding programs are in place specifically to breed bucking animals (Figure 14.5). Rodeo contestants and stock contractors, who have a substantial investment in the animals, share a similar philosophy, which includes a sincere regard for the talent of the animals and the need for quality and humane care for them. And remember, most bulls weigh more than 1500 pounds (almost 700 kg), compared with the 150 pounds (about 70 kg) of the average bull rider. Additionally, bulls have a hide that is up to seven times thicker than human skin (Sisson and Grossman, 1953).

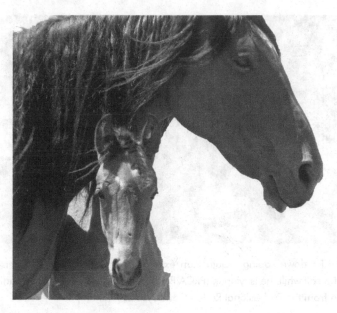

Figure 14.5 Today's bucking horses and bulls are produced in specialized breeding programs. Champion bucking horse Miss Congeniality is shown here with one of her 'born to buck' foals. They are owned by the Powder River Rodeo Company. (Reproduced with permission from the Professional Rodeo Cowboys Association.)

As with any discipline, bucking bulls and horses are introduced into rodeo competition in a number of different ways. The age of introduction depends on the stock contractor and the maturity of the livestock. The introduction to competition begins with familiarizing them with alleys and bucking chutes, and getting them accustomed to loading into and leaving the bucking chutes. Generally, when they are first bucked out, it is with remote control 'dummies' on their back. This introduction to competition has evolved into 'futurities,' especially in the bucking bull industry, where young bulls, not ready for competition with cowboys, will be judged only on their bucking ability with the 'dummies' on their backs.

14.4 Timed Events

Rodeo's roping events, tie-down roping, team roping, and steer roping, have origins in everyday ranch life. When cattle on a ranch need medical attention or other care, a rope is really the only way to catch them. In competition, the roping events showcase the talents of both the contestant and his horse. To successfully compete in any of the three, the contestant needs not only well-honed roping skills, but also a well-trained and intuitive horse. Roping in the competition arena closely resembles what the animals would undergo routinely on a ranch.

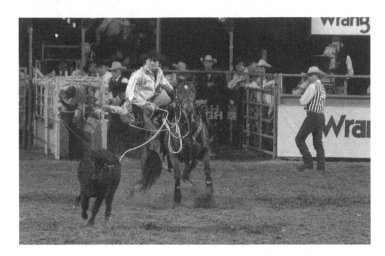

Figure 14.6 Tie-down roping requires an extremely athletic mount in order to assist the cowboy work the calf while he is tying it. (PRCA ProRodeo photo by Mike Copeman. Reproduced with permission from the Professional Rodeo Cowboys Association.)

14.4.1 Tie-down roping

Tie-down roping is an event born on the ranches of the Old West. Sick calves were roped and tied down for medical treatment. Today, success in tie-down roping depends largely on the teamwork between a cowboy and his horse. After the calf is given a head start, horse and rider give chase. The contestant ropes the calf, then dismounts and runs to the animal (Figure 14.6). After catching and flanking the calf (lifting calf from the standing position and laying on the ground), the cowboy ties any three of the animal's legs together using a 'pigging string' he carries in his teeth until needed. If the calf is not standing when the contestant reaches it, the cowboy must allow the animal to stand. When the cowboy completes his tie, he throws his hands in the air as a signal to the judge. He then remounts and allows the rope to become slack. The run is declared invalid if the calf kicks free within six seconds. As with any timed event, a 10-second penalty is added if the roper does not allow the calf the proper head start – this is known as 'breaking the barrier.'

An issue that rodeo is addressing is that of 'jerking' a calf down or over backwards. This occurs after the calf is roped, and, depending on how the rope is handled by the competitor or if the horse may move one way or the other, the calf may come over backwards. With this action, the calf may land on the side or on the back and head. The perception is that the 'jerking' of a calf is a welfare concern. However, the perception is much improved if the calf is pulled down on its side or actually just spun around without losing its footing. The roping of a calf can be perceived negatively, especially by a more urbanized society who do not

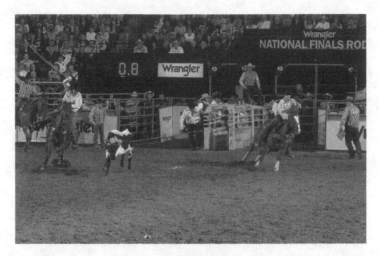

Figure 14.7 The team roping event requires excellent teamwork with both the riders and their mounts. (PRCA ProRodeo photo by Mike Copeman. Reproduced with permission from the Professional Rodeo Cowboys Association.)

have experience with ranch work. The sport of rodeo has made many reforms in an effort to provide for the safety of livestock and improve the perception of the event, including imposing weight limits that allow for the calves that are used to be of an optimum weight for this type of competition.

14.4.2 Team roping

Team roping is unique in that two cowboys (header and heeler) work together for a shared time. The first cowboy, known as the 'header,' ropes the steer either by the horns, around the neck, or 'half-head,' which is one horn and the neck. After this catch is made, the header wraps his rope around the saddle horn, commonly known as dallying, and turns the steer in a wide arc to the left (Figure 14.7). The second cowboy is known as the 'heeler.' He trails along beside the steer until the header turns the steer, then moves in behind the steer and attempts to rope the back feet. If he only manages one hind foot, the team receives a five-second penalty. Time is stopped when both cowboys' horses are facing each other. Welfare concerns in this event are minimal. Some steers may have rope burns on their hind legs, but generally the livestock is well suited for the event.

14.4.3 Steer wrestling

Steer wrestling is a one-on-one match between an animal weighing at least 450 pounds (about 200 kg) and a man who more than likely weighs less than half that amount. It's highly improbable that a man could injure a steer during the steer wrestling event. A cowboy who hopes to win at steer wrestling must employ finesse.

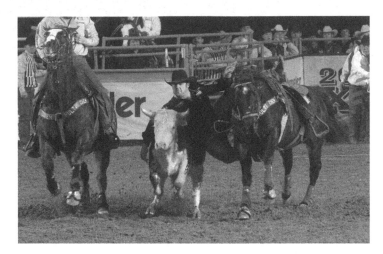

Figure 14.8 The steer wrestling event allows the cowboy to have a helper, called a hazer, and requires two horses – the steer wrestling horse that gets the cowboy right up to the steer, and the hazing horse that helps the hazer keep the steer in position. (PRCA ProRodeo photo by Mike Copeman. Reproduced with permission from the Professional Rodeo Cowboys Association.)

Steer wrestling involves careful positioning and leverage to enable the animal to be placed on its side.

Wrestling a steer requires more than brute strength. The successful steer wrestler, or bulldogger, is strong, to be sure, but he also understands the principles of leverage. The steer wrestler on horseback starts behind a barrier, and begins his chase after the steer has been given a head start. If the bulldogger leaves too soon and breaks the barrier, he receives a 10-second penalty. The steer wrestler is assisted by a hazer, another cowboy on horseback tasked with keeping the steer running in a straight line. When the bulldogger's horse pulls even with the steer, he eases down the right side of the horse and reaches for the steer's horns. After grasping the horns and sliding down off his horse (Figure 14.8), he digs his heels into the dirt. As the steer slows, the cowboy turns the animal, lifts up on its right horn, and pushes down with his left hand in an effort to tip the steer over. After the catch, the steer wrestler must either bring the steer to a stop or change the direction of the animal's body before the throw or he is disqualified. The clock stops when the steer is on his side with all four legs pointing the same direction. The welfare concerns in this event include the twisting of a steer's neck, the possibility of a broken horn, as well as a leg catching in the dirt. Perception is often much worse than reality, with the event utilizing tough Corriente steers and momentum being the way the contestants wrestle the steer rather than a twisting motion. The use of whips and bats on the bulldogging horses can also be a welfare concern and is discussed further in this chapter.

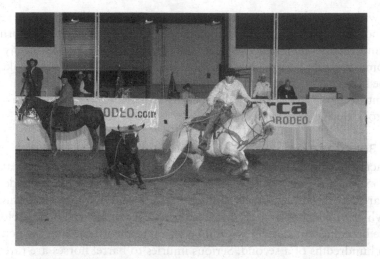

Figure 14.9 The steer roping horse must be strong and dependable to assist the contestant in laying down the steer and working the rope while the cowboy ties the legs. (PRCA ProRodeo photo by Dudley Barker. Reproduced with permission from the Professional Rodeo Cowboys Association.)

14.4.4 Steer roping

The steer roping event is started much like the other timed events with a steer in the chute and the contestant and horse behind a barrier in the roping box. The steer is released and given a head start, and the steer roping contestant throws a rope aiming to catch the steer around the horns, which are reinforced with plaster and reinforcement bar (rebar) and protected with horn wraps (Figure 14.9). If the contestant catches the steer by the horns or around the neck with a legal catch, he will proceed to moving his horse around the steer, positioning the rope around the back end of the steer to lay the steer down. As in tie-down roping, the contestant then ties the steer's legs with a smaller rope called a 'piggin string.' It differs from the tie-down roping in that the steer must remain laying down and the contestant will tie the steer facing the steer's legs. The horses are trained to keep the rope taught to assist in keeping the steer laying down. The steer must stay tied for six seconds, and then the judge will signal the tie is legal. The time begins when the contestant leaves the roping box and ends when the tie is complete. This event is sanctioned by the Professional Rodeo Cowboys Association, but it is not a mandatory event and is only held at about 10% of PRCA-sanctioned events, mostly those in rural and ranching communities, who can understand the skill needed to successfully compete in this event. Steer roping also requires a large arena, which does not allow it to be held at every rodeo arena.

The event has also been referred to as 'steer tripping.' As the event involved laying down or 'tripping' of the steer, the perception of the event to the public not familiar with livestock can be a problem. The steers used in this event are Corriente breed, known for their toughness, and the steers are protected with horn wraps, plaster, and rebar – therefore the steers handle the event well. As in any athletic event, some steers do become injured, most being minimal strains or broken horns and some broken legs. The practice of the event could be problematic, but since the contestants own the steers, they will generally work hard to minimize any harm to the livestock during practice sessions.

14.4.5 Barrel racing
Barrel racing is a timed event that involves a rider completing a cloverleaf pattern of three 55 gallon drums or barrels. The object is simply to complete the designated pattern around the three barrels with the fastest time without knocking over a barrel, which will incur a five-second penalty. Most horses are Quarter Horse type with race breeding. An electric eye will be set up to record the time, which is often down to hundredths of a second. Serious injuries to barrel horses are rare and the minor injuries that do occur are generally soft tissue injuries; rarely do catastrophic injuries such as fractures occur. The greatest concern in this event is the use of medications in a non-therapeutic manner to gain a competitive advantage. Excessive whipping can occur, and sanctioning organizations need to have rules and enforcement procedures to punish this activity.

14.5 Welfare of Rodeo Livestock During Transit

Transportation of any livestock can come with welfare concerns (Figure 14.10). The sport of rodeo involves a lot of travel, and therefore many precautions must be taken to insure that rodeo livestock arrive safe and ready to compete at rodeo events. Cowgirls and cowboys who compete in rodeos understand that a big part of the success of a timed event horse is its ability to adapt to traveling long distances, standing at a trailer for long periods of time, and adapting to different climates. No matter how talented a horse used for barrel racing, tie-down roping, steer wrestling or team roping is, if that horse does not do well being transported long distances and handling different situations, it will not be a successful rodeo horse. In order to assist rodeo's equine timed event athletes in handling the vast travel requirements, rodeo competitors purchase the highest-quality trailers and plan ahead as much as possible regarding feed, water, and stabling requirements.

Roughstock used in rodeos also must travel extensively but generally not nearly as much as timed event horses, due to the fact that a stock contractor will generally have one rodeo in a weekend, and the livestock will arrive at the rodeo grounds a few days before the rodeo and stay throughout the duration of the rodeo. In contrast, timed event competitors will compete in up to four rodeos in a weekend. Rodeo bucking horses and bulls are housed at ranches of various sizes in a herd

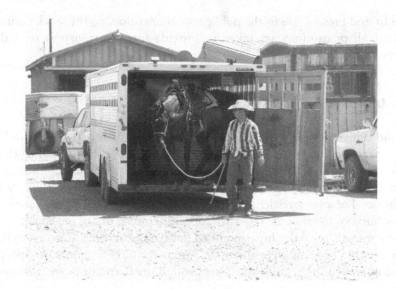

Figure 14.10 Horses involved in the sport of rodeo are accustomed to travel. In this photo, pickup horses unload after making a short trip from the livestock holding facilities to the arena. (PRCA ProRodeo photo by Susan Kanode. Reproduced with permission from the Professional Rodeo Cowboys Association.)

environment until such time as it is necessary to transport them to a rodeo. Stock contractors have various types of trailers to transport roughstock that include: standard gooseneck trailers pulled by pickups, straight deck trailers pulled by tractor trailers, and double deck trailers pulled by tractor trailers. The least understood and most utilized are the double deck trailers – these will be used to haul bucking horses, saddle horses, calves, steers, and bulls in different combinations. The use of double deck trailers has come under scrutiny recently when trailers designed for cattle have been used without being modified to haul horses to processing plants. The United States Department of Agriculture (USDA) has phased out the use of these trailers for this use in the guidelines for transporting slaughter horses. This is due in large part to the fact that the horses being hauled to processing plants for slaughter are not familiar with this mode of transport, the trailers do not have adequate headroom (mostly in doors), and the horses are not familiar with each other, causing a higher risk of injury to the slaughter horses. In contrast, the bucking horses that are being hauled in double deck trailers are generally bred specifically for the sport of rodeo, and have become accustomed to being hauled in these trailers from a young age along with herd mates they are very familiar with. Additionally, many rodeo stock contractors modify trailers to insure that there is adequate headroom for the horses and that the doors and ramps offer safe loading and unloading to bucking horses. As with any performance horse, bucking horses must be fit and presentable to the public for competition, so the stock contractors insure that all precautions are taken to provide for safe transport to and from rodeo events for all livestock.

14.6 Use of Whips and Similar Devices

Whips and similar devices to encourage horses to run faster are used in barrel racing and steer wrestling similarly to other horse racing events. In steer wrestling the hazer (the cowboy who assists the steer wrestler by keeping the steer running straight) often uses a modified flat whip to assist with encouraging speed as well as guidance for the hazing horse. The steer wrestler may also use a whip or similar device to encourage the quick burst of speed needed to catch the steer coming out of the chute.

In barrel racing, regular whips, modified flat bats, and ropes attached to the saddle horn referred to as an 'over and under' are used to try to gain more speed from the horse as well as often guide the horse around the barrel or move the horse into position.

Any time a whip is used in rodeo speed events or any other horse discipline, care must be taken for the whip or similar device not to be used in an abusive manner. The PRCA has general rules that prohibit 'abuse or mistreatment' that allow a rodeo judge to fine a contestant if it is determined that the contestant has gone beyond encouraging speed or guiding the horse.

14.7 Drug and Medication Policies

The sport of rodeo has not formulated extensive drug and medication policies. The PRCA has a rule prohibiting 'stimulants or hypnotics' in competition that would allow for rodeo judges to use their judgment if there is an issue at a rodeo involving harmful use of drugs on any of the livestock. The sport of rodeo needs to extensively study the types of medications that are being used for competition livestock. If such a study shows welfare issues involving inappropriate medication use, policies must be formulated to protect the livestock. Non-steroidal anti-inflammatory drugs (NSAIDs) are used commonly and in various combinations – this relates to the issue that the livestock travels long distances and many times will perform daily. Additionally, timed event horses will often be used more than once during a rodeo performance. Some rodeo horses may also receive multiple joint injections. This may sometimes be done for non-therapeutic reasons.

Barrel horses may be administered various medications before competition. Barrel racing is a speed event and many competitors may feel some of these medications allow for an edge. The perception can be that the barrel racing competitor that has the most successful combination of drugs may be the winner. Barrel racing associations need to formulate policies that protect the welfare of the competition horse.

14.8 Non-Sanctioned Rodeo Events

In addition to the standard sanctioned events decried in this chapter, many rodeos will have ancillary events that are not sanctioned by the rodeo organization and, in many cases, not sanctioned by *any* organization. These events include mutton busting (riding sheep), wild horse race, wild cow milking, calf dressing, horse races, chuck wagon races, and various others. It is up to the organizing rodeo committee to insure that the animals that take part in these events are provided proper care and handling, since they are not sanctioned and not covered by the rules of the sanctioning body of the rodeo. Some of the events such as the wild horse race (also referred to as team bronc riding) may be sanctioned by a separate organization with separate rules; again, it is up to the organizing committee of the rodeo to insure that the animals are covered by rules.

Historically, some of these events may have an 'anything goes' mentality, as the contestants are not required to be members of the sanctioning organization, and other rules may not be in place. This raises many concerns regarding how any rules are enforced and how the livestock are handled. As in any athletic endeavor, injuries may occur, and some of these events may have a higher rate or be perceived as having a higher rate of injury. The organizing committee should put into place safety measures, insure a veterinarian is on-site, and possibly conduct their own injury surveys to give them the needed data either to show the low rate of injury, or to improve the event, or consider not having that event at all. Some high-profile injuries and the nature of the wild horse race leave questions in the mind of some, and if rodeo committees choose to continue to have this event, they should definitely insure all procedures are in place to protect the horses involved.

Most rodeo committees are adapting to a greater concern shown by the public and either eliminating questionable unsanctioned events or creating their own guidelines and procedures to insure their fans, sponsors, and others that the livestock is handled properly. As a veterinarian, I applaud these steps.

14.9 Non-Competitive Rodeo Activity

As with any sporting activity, there are many practice sessions that take place before the actual competition. The same is true with the sport of rodeo, and the athletes that compete must practice their event before entering an actual rodeo competition. Many rodeo competitors own their own practice arenas and livestock. In other situations, rodeo athletes may practice at other arenas where many competitors practice for rodeo competition. These activities are not governed by rules of sanctioning organizations, and the competitors who are practicing are responsible for insuring the proper care and handling of the livestock involved. In my opinion, as attitudes towards the welfare of animals has changed over the years, I believe rodeo contestants are improving the care and handling of their own livestock. The PRCA and other rodeo associations are continually working to educate their membership regarding the health and welfare of livestock and the overall issue of animal welfare.

14.10 Welfare of Rodeo's Animal Athletes

Economics dictate that livestock owners ensure the health and welfare of their cattle. This applies not only to timed-event stock in the roping and steer wrestling events, but also to cattle on ranches that are handled with similar methods for sorting and branding.

PRCA rules, stock contractors, judges, and cowboys all play integral parts in assuring that roping stock are treated humanely. In tie-down roping, a calf must weigh between 220 and 280 pounds (about 100 to 130 kg). PRCA rules also stipulate the calf must be strong and healthy, and PRCA judges inspect the animals to ensure that no sick or injured livestock is used. Most calves don't participate in rodeos more than a few times in their lives because of weight and usage restrictions and the fact that calves grow so rapidly. Steers are used in the remaining two roping events, and the tough and robust Mexican Corrientes are the animals of choice for team roping and steer roping because of their endurance and strength. The steers used in team roping have a 650-pound limit (almost 300 kg). PRCA rules stipulate that the horns on the steers used in team roping and steer roping must be protected during performances. Also, steer roping cattle must be inspected two weeks before an event to make sure they're in good health.

14.10.1 Equipment and animal welfare

Veterinarians familiar with the sport of rodeo and the equipment used say that rodeo gear is safe to the animals involved, including the flank strap, spurs, and livestock prod. Each piece of equipment has a specific purpose and PRCA rules governing its use and placement. Veterinarians with on-site rodeo experience contacted for this report indicate the equipment used in rodeo is not dangerous, painful, or cruel. Some, in fact, have testified before legislative bodies that the equipment might provide some slight irritation but does not injure animals.

14.10.1.1 Flank strap

Bucking animals are born, not made, and the flank strap cannot magically turn a placid animal into a championship bucker, according to stock contractors and cowboys. When placed on an animal naturally inclined to buck, the flank strap simply augments the bucking action, encouraging a bucking bronc or bull to kick high with its back feet.

PRCA rules stipulate that flank straps must be lined with sheepskin or neoprene and must utilize a quick-release fastener (Figure 14.11). No sharp or cutting objects may be placed between the strap and the animal, and the sheepskin-covered portion must be placed over both flanks and the belly of the animal. The straps never cover

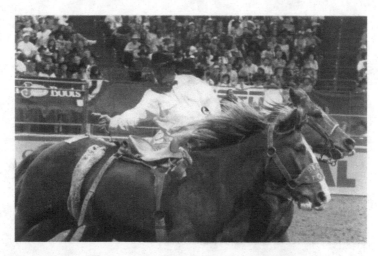

Figure 14.11 The flank strap used in the bucking horse events is fleece- or neoprene-lined and is equipped with a quick-release mechanism that is operated by the pickup man after the ride is complete. (PRCA ProRodeo photo. Reproduced with permission from the Professional Rodeo Cowboys Association.)

the genitalia or fasten so tightly as to cause pain. Equine experts, both with and without ties to rodeo, agree on use of the flank strap. In my opinion, having been involved with rodeo for 32 years as a veterinarian, the flank strap produces mild pressure on the flanks, but not so much as to hurt the animal. It might be compared to wearing a snug belt that may cause some mild irritation. Bucking is simply the horse's action to rid itself of a foreign object. The flank straps used in rodeo are never tight enough to immobilize or cause pain, and they don't injure an animal. A horse has 18 ribs, which protect its kidneys. The flank strap is placed behind the rib cage. In the author's opinion, properly used flank straps cause no harm to bucking horses and bulls.

14.10.1.2 Livestock prod
The livestock prod, powered by flashlight batteries, is used to move livestock humanely on ranches and, on occasion, at professional rodeos. PRCA rules only allow using the prod 'as little as possible.' The prod may only be used to move livestock if the animal is stalled in the chute or if it is at risk of injury. The rules also state that the prod can be used only on the animal's hip or shoulder areas. A horse's hide is almost three times as thick as human skin, and the hide of a bull is virtually seven times thicker. A horse's hide might be compared to the thickness of leather used in a woman's purse, and bull's hide is similar in thickness to the sole of a shoe.

The prod produces low voltage, but virtually no amperage (current). The prod causes a mild shock but does not cause burns because current (amperes), not voltage (volts), causes burns. Sometimes, it is necessary to touch an animal with an electric stock prod to get it to go where you want. The prod is not a damaging

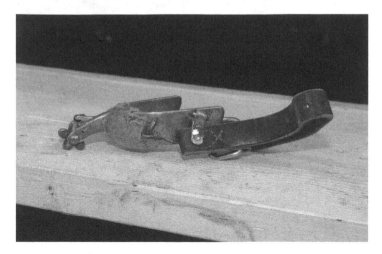

Figure 14.12 Spurs used in rodeo's roughstock events are governed by rules that require them to be dulled. (PRCA ProRodeo photo by Kirt Steinke. Reproduced with permission from the Professional Rodeo Cowboys Association.)

stimulant and presents no danger to the animal's health, but rather is an effective way to move the animals where they need to be in a timely fashion. In my opinion, there is a misconception that the livestock prod is similar to a taser stun gun – this is simply not true. The taser stun gun is many times (at least ten times) more powerful than a livestock prod. In my opinion, the electric livestock prod should be used minimally (for safety reasons) or not at all on a horse.

14.10.1.3 Spurs

A variety of spurs are used in rodeo, each with a different purpose, but all are dulled to avoid any harm to the livestock (Figure 14.12). Timed-event contestants often use spurs to cue the horse to speed up or turn. In saddle bronc and bareback riding, the spurs enhance the contestant's leg action while rolling over the horse's thick hide. Bull riders' spurs assist them in gripping the bulls, which have loose hides. In the saddle bronc riding and bareback riding events, PRCA rules prohibit the use of sharpened spurs, locked rowels (the star-shaped wheel on spurs) or rowels that lock. Specifically, acceptable spurs have rowels that are blunt and are about one-eighth of an inch thick so they will not cut the animals. The rowels must be loose so they will roll over the horse's hide, rather than dragging or cutting. Bull riding spurs have loosely locked rowels to aid in gripping the loose-hided animals, but the rowels are still dull. The thickness of the skin of rodeo livestock is important to take into consideration. The book *Sisson's Anatomy of Domestic Animals* states that the hide of a horse is up to 5 mm thick and bull hide is up to 7 mm thick (Sisson and Grossman, 1953).

14.10.2 Welfare issues

The sport of rodeo has continuously faced challenges in the development of the sport, many coming from animal rights extremists who don't believe that humans should be interacting with animals in entertainment, sport, industry, and recreation. Animal rights extremists provide barriers that the PRCA is constantly addressing. Programs to overcome these negative insinuations and to educate the public include contestant, stock contractor, and fan education and school programs. The PRCA believes that its animal welfare program is exceptional and works to educate the public concerning the care and treatment of livestock used in PRCA-sanctioned rodeos. The PRCA and the rodeo industry have for many years addressed negative legislation introduced by animal rights extremists who wish to ban or negatively affect rodeo. By maintaining an active presence in the political arena on the national, State, and local level, the PRCA is able to monitor legislation on all levels.

The rodeo industry has learned that the loss of our rural society means the loss of those who understand the practices surrounding livestock. This has created a barrier of misunderstanding surrounding the use of animals in the sport of rodeo. The PRCA hopes to keep the link to land and agriculture with city dwellers through the sport of rodeo. In addition, the PRCA sponsors youth rodeo organizations to encourage youth to become involved in horse activities and rodeo. PRCA involvement includes conducting seminars on animal welfare as well as event safety. Through these programs, young people are educated on sound horsemanship practices, animal welfare issues, and safety for both horse and rider in rodeo events. By educating youth, the PRCA hopes to encourage participation in rodeo and horse-related sports by assisting in building a foundation for safe, successful competition in youth rodeo and horse-related activities.

The PRCA has been very successful in its development of an animal welfare program. However, the PRCA only sanctions a small percentage of all rodeos. But, because the PRCA is a leader in the rodeo industry, they have held rodeo industry conferences, and developed minimal care guidelines for rodeo livestock and guidelines for veterinarians working rodeos. This has been done as a proactive step and to encourage other rodeo organizations to make changes as needed and create guidelines and rules similar to the PRCA. This has been done with the health and welfare of the animal at the forefront.

14.10.3 Livestock welfare surveys

In 1995, the PRCA amended its rule concerning veterinarians at PRCA rodeos to require a veterinarian on-site at all PRCA-sanctioned events. Before that, a rodeo committee was allowed to have a veterinarian on-site or on-call. The on-site veterinarian rule allowed the PRCA to add comments on rodeo reports from the veterinarian and the veterinarian's signature, plus any injury information and follow-up. This enables the PRCA to continuously monitor the success of the animal welfare program and update animal welfare concerns as needed. The 2008 injury survey, conducted by on-site veterinarians at PRCA rodeos, showed that the injury rate was extremely low.

All of the veterinarians are contracted by the rodeo committee, not the PRCA, and the forms must be signed by the veterinarian to be included in the statistics. The survey included 58 656 animal exposures at 148 rodeo performances and 55 sections of slack (extra competitors who do not compete in the rodeo performances). The rate of injury was calculated to 0.05%. These surveys have been conducted by veterinarians since 1995 and have shown similar rates throughout the years.

14.11 Maintaining Equine Welfare at Rodeos

Putting into place rules and enforcement procedures to safeguard the equine athletes that participate in rodeo is the first line of defense in advancing their welfare. The second line is the preparation of the facilities as well as preparing for any eventuality, including injury. Injuries to livestock in rodeo events are similar to those to livestock in other sports, and include strains, sprains, abrasions, and rarely broken bones. Most rodeos in the USA are produced by local rodeo committees who organize the events as community fundraisers. It is the sanctioning body's duty to assist in educating these committees to insure that the livestock at the event are afforded proper care and handling. Educational programs that assist committees in preparing their facilities and procedures, creating optimum ground conditions, and creating a procedure to deal with a livestock illness or injury, are paramount.

Rodeo committees should inspect their stock holding facilities and arena, preferably with their veterinarian, to insure that all areas are free from obstructions that may injure the livestock. All areas, including holding pens, bucking and roping chutes, arena fences, and gates and alleyways, should be a part of the inspection.

Creating a well-thought-out, practiced plan to effectively handle an injury to livestock involved in a rodeo is an essential part of planning for a rodeo (Figure 14.13). The rodeo committee should assemble all involved in handling a potential injury to discuss this plan, including the stock contractor, arena director, veterinarian, and livestock handling personnel. A written plan should be put into place that includes the following:

- Where the veterinarian will be stationed.
- Supplies the veterinarian will have with them.
- Where the veterinarian's vehicle with further supplies will be parked.
- Communication method with veterinarian.
- What conveyance will be used for small or large animals.
- Who will make the decision to transport an injured animal out of the arena.
- When will an animal be transported to a clinic rather than treated on-site.
- Where the animal will be taken for further treatment.
- How the veterinarian will communicate with the owner of the animal and for permission to treat.
- Other details necessary to insure that any injury is handled with the welfare of the livestock at the forefront and with the goal of immediate treatment.

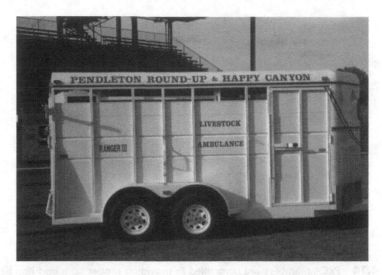

Figure 14.13 Even though veterinarian-conducted surveys show the rate of injury to ProRodeo livestock to be extremely low, as a precaution, PRCA rules require a conveyance to transport injured livestock – this is the Pendleton Round-up's animal ambulance. (PRCA ProRodeo photo. Reproduced with permission from the Professional Rodeo Cowboys Association.)

Those responsible for organizing a rodeo have the obligation to insure that proper procedures and planning are in place to elevate the welfare of the livestock involved to the highest level possible.

14.12 Summary and Conclusions

Equine welfare issues and initiatives are not new to the sport of rodeo, and members of the rodeo industry have had to be proactive, create positive programs to insure animal welfare, and put procedures in place to enforce rules protecting horses and other livestock involved in rodeos. While, like any program, it is not perfect and there are always improvements to be made, the sport of rodeo has made positive changes through the years as welfare issues have arisen.

The PRCA and its members are committed to promoting the proper care and treatment of the animals used in rodeo (Figure 14.14). As an association, the PRCA has been very proactive in establishing rules and regulations governing animal welfare and in creating a veterinary advisory group and an animal welfare committee to assist in the association's efforts in this important area. In addition, the PRCA employs a full-time Director of Livestock Welfare to further the positive efforts and assure the public that animal welfare is an extremely high priority. Recently, the

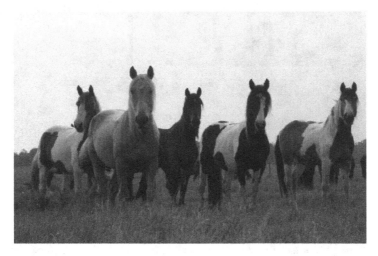

Figure 14.14 PRCA members are committed to providing proper care and handling for all rodeo livestock. In this photo, bucking horses at the J Bar J Ranch in Michigan enjoy time away from the rodeo in lush green pastures. (PRCA ProRodeo photo courtesy of J Bar J Rodeo. Reproduced with permission from the Professional Rodeo Cowboys Association.)

PRCA created the position of Livestock Welfare Superintendent, who travels to rodeos to serve as an on-site liaison to rodeo committees, stock contractors, and contestants on livestock welfare. The PRCA prides itself on implementing the highest standards for treatment of rodeo livestock in the business, as well as encouraging other rodeo associations to adopt similar standards. The animals involved in PRCA-sanctioned events are afforded proper care and treatment through a comprehensive, award-winning (American Association of Equine Practitioners, Lavin Cup Animal Welfare Award) animal welfare program and the enforcement of animal-related rules and regulations.

14.13 Appendix

PRCA rules governing the care and treatment of livestock at PRCA-sanctioned rodeos
Reproduced with permission from the Professional Rodeo Cowboys Association
The Professional Rodeo Cowboys Association (PRCA) has been enforcing rules to protect the livestock participating in their sanctioned events since 1947. Through the years, the PRCA has created the most comprehensive set of animal welfare rules in the sport of rodeo, creating a model for other rodeo associations to follow.

1. *Rule 9.0. General.* These rules are intended to ensure the humane treatment of rodeo animals and shall be in effect for all PRCA-sanctioned events. No animal shall be treated inhumanely by any Member.

2. *Rule 9.1. Sore, lame, sick or injured animal.* Animals for all events will be inspected before the draw, and no sore, lame, sick or injured animal or animal with impaired eyesight shall be permitted in the draw at any time. Should an animal become sick or incapacitated between the time it is drawn and the time it is scheduled to be used in competition, that animal shall not be used in competition and another animal shall be drawn for the contestant.

3. *Rule 9.1.1. Veterinarian.* A rodeo committee shall ensure that a veterinarian is present and on-site for every performance and/or section of slack. Any rodeo committee failing to do so shall be subject to a fine of $500 per performance and/ or section of slack per rodeo.

4. *Rule 9.2. Rowels.* No locked rowels, or rowels that will be locked on spurs, may be used on bareback or saddle bronc horses. Spurs must be dulled.

5. *Rule 9.2.1. Removal of an injured animal.* A conveyance must be available, supplied by the stock contractor, and shall be used, where practicable, to remove animals from the arena in case of injury. The conveyance must be large enough to remove a horse or bull. Injured calves shall be removed from the arena in a pickup truck, calf stretcher or by conveyance. Animals removed from the arena pursuant to this section shall be placed in a situation as isolated and comfortable as possible to reduce stress.

6. *Rule 9.2.2. Must be humane.* Any injured livestock shall be humanely removed from the arena before continuing the rodeo contest or performance.

7. *Rule 9.3. No sharp objects in cinch, saddle, girth or flank straps.* No sharp or cutting objects in cinch, saddle girth, or flank straps shall be permitted. Flank straps used for horses must either be sheepskin-lined or neoprene-lined and shall be of the quick release type. Sheepskin-lined or neoprene-lined flank straps shall be placed on the animal so the lined portion is over both flanks of the animals. In the bull riding, a soft cotton rope at least 5/8 inch in diameter is acceptable as a flank strap and does not require the sheepskin or neoprene lining.

8. *Rule 9.4. Prods and other artificial stimuli.* Standard electric prods shall be used only as specified in these Official Rodeo Rules and in the Bylaws. If a prod is used, the animal shall only be touched on the hip or shoulder area. No other artificial stimuli shall be used (with the exception of rodeo equipment and gear commonly used and accepted in connection with the respective events at PRCA-sanctioned rodeos.)

9. *Rule 10.1.5. Prods.* In the riding events, use of prods and similar devices is prohibited. The only exceptions shall be in the saddle bronc riding and bareback riding, and only in the case of a known chute stalling animals, and only if agreed upon by the contestant, the stock contractor and the judge before the contestant's competition begins. In this instance, the prod shall not exceed 12 inches in length. Use of a prod without the agreement of the contestant, stock contractor, and the judge before the

contestant's competition begins in the saddle bronc and the bareback riding, or use of a prod in the bull riding at any time shall result in a fine of $1000, doubling with each violation to the stock contractor and the contestant will receive the automatic option of a reride.

10. *Rule 3.2.2. No animal may be in the draw twice on the same day.* In all riding events, stock can not be placed in the draw twice in the same say, with the exception of rerides, unless approved by the Event Representative and the Director of Rodeo Administration.

11. *Rule 4.8.3. Unsafe arena conditions.* If the arena conditions are deemed at any time to be unsafe by the arena director, a majority of the Event Representatives present, any judge, or the primary stock contractor, competition may be stopped until which time the arena conditions are deemed satisfactory by the individual or individuals who initially determined that arena conditions were unsafe.

12. *Rule 8.4. No hold overs.* No cattle that have been used may be held over from one calendar year to the next.

13. *Rule 8.4.1. No switching of events.* No steers may be switched in events unless approved by the Event Representative or the Director of Rodeo Administration.

14. *Rule 8.5. Running of timed-event stock.* All timed-event stock shall be run though event chutes and through the arena prior to the start of contest where conditions permit.

15. *Rule 8.8. Unsatisfactory animals.* An Event Representative may declare a particular animal unsatisfactory. Upon notification, either written or verbal, the stock contractor or Rodeo Committee shall eliminate such animal(s) from competition draw.

16. *Rule 8.8.1. No change of events.* If an animal has been declared unsatisfactory for an event, that animal may not be used for another event without the approval of the Event Representative.

17. *Rule 8.9.1. Trimming the horns.* Stock contractors and the Rodeo Committee will be expected to cooperate in trimming the horns of steers that are not able to pass through the timed-event chute.

18. *Rule 8.9.2. Steer wrestling cattle.* The horns on steer wrestling cattle must be blunted to the size of a dime.

19. *Rule 8.9.3. Steer roping cattle.* Plaster and rebar must be placed around the horns of steer roping cattle prior to contesting, and all such steers should have horn wraps that extend 4 inches down the jaw from the base of the horns. The horns must be blunted to the size of a quarter.

20. *Rule 8.8.4. Team roping cattle.* All team roping cattle shall be protected by horn wraps. The horns on all team roping cattle must be blunted to the size of a dime.

21. *Rule 8.9.5.1. Blunting of bulls horns.* All horned animals used in the PRCA bull riding shall have their horns blunted to at least the diameter of a half-dollar.

22. *Rule 8.10.1. No use other than contest events.* An animal used in the contest events of a PRCA rodeo may not be used in any way, other than in the contest events of

that rodeo, until after the last time that animal has been used in the contest events at that rodeo, unless otherwise approved by the Event Representative.

23. *Rule 8.11.2. Injured animals at rodeo.* The stock contractor of record shall be responsible for notifying the Central Entry Office of riding event stock that becomes injured and is in the draw for later competition time.

24. *Rule 11.2.1. Ineligibility time.* If a riding event animal is replaced in the draw at a rodeo, that animal cannot be used for a period of 48 hours following the first performance that the animal was replaced.

25. *Rule 8.12.1. Roping calves.* All roping calves must be either native, brahma, or of a similar cross. Weight for the calves shall be a minimum of 220 pounds and a maximum of 280 pounds with fresh calves not to exceed a maximum of 260 pounds.

26. *Rule 8.12.2. Steer wrestling cattle.* All steer wrestling cattle must be Mexican Corriente steers. All steer wrestling cattle must weigh a minimum of 450 pounds and a maximum of 600 pounds.

27. *Rule 8.12.3. Team roping.* The maximum weight for animals that are to be used in team roping is 650 per head and the minimum is 450 per head. All team roping steers must be Corriente steers.

28. *Rule 8.12.4. Steer roping.* All steer roping steers must be Mexican Corriente steers. All steers used in the steer roping event must weigh a minimum of 450 pounds and a maximum of 600 pounds.

29. *Rule 9.5.1. Construction of chutes.* Chutes must be constructed to prevent injury to an animal. Maintenance men and equipment shall be available at chutes to assist in removal of any animal should it become necessary.

30. *Rule 9.5.2. Conditions of arena.* The arena shall be as free as possible of rocks, holes and unnecessary obstacles.

31. *Rule 9.5.3. No small animals.* No small animals or pets allowed in the arena, unless part of a contract act.

32. *Rule 9.5.4. Removal of livestock after competition.* Livestock must be removed from the arena after each competition is completed.

33. *Rule 9.6. Neckrope must be used in tie-down roping.* In tie-down roping, a neckrope must be used. Calves may not be intentionally flipped backward. Contestant must adjust rope and reins in such a manner that will prevent horse from dragging calf. Rope to be removed from calf's body as soon as possible after 'tie' is approved. Roping claves shall be strong and healthy.

34. *Rule 9.7. No stimulants or hypnotics.* No stimulants or hypnotics may be given to any animal used for contest purposes.

35. *Rule 9.8. Animals excessively excited in chute.* Any animal that becomes excessively excited and lays down in the chute repeatedly, or tries repeatedly to jump out of the chute, or in any way appears to be in danger of injuring himself, may be released immediately.

36. *Rule 9.9. Confinement and transportation.* No stock shall be confined or transported in vehicles beyond a period of 24 hours without being unloaded, properly fed and watered.

37. *Rule 9.10. Abuse of animal.* If a member abuses an animal by any unnecessary non-competitive or competitive action, he may be disqualified for the remainder of the rodeo and fined $250 for the first offense, with that fine progressively doubling with each offense therafter.

38. *Rule 9.11. Mistreatment of animal.* Any member guilty of mistreatment of livestock anywhere on the rodeo grounds shall be fined $250 for the first offense, with that fine progressively doubling with any offense thereafter.

39. *Rule 9.12. Tie downs covered.* All chain, metal and wire tie-downs and bosals must be covered.

Riding event rules

40. *Rule 9.13. Apparent injury during competition.* Should a riding event animal show evidence of injury inflicted by a contestant during competition, that contestant will be fined $250 for the first offense and $500 for the second offense, and $1000 for the third and subsequent offenses.

41. *Rule 9.13.1. Delay further use of animal injured.* Should a riding event animal be apparently injured by a contestant during competition, thus resulting in the contestant being reported for such a violation, that animal cannot be used until such time the injury has completely healed.

42. *Rule 9.1. Drawn animal becomes sick or crippled.* If an animal that is drawn in a riding event becomes sick or crippled before it is competed on, a judge must pass on the animal's inability to be used before it can be shipped or replaced in the draw.

43. *Rule 10.4.2. Bareback riding. Cinches and latigos.* Cinches on the bareback riggings shall be made of mohair or neoprene and shall be at least 8 inches in width at the center, but must be tapered to accommodate cinch 'D' rings. Latigos must be of leather only.

44. *Rule 10.4.2.1. Bareback pads.* Required bareback pads are to completely cover the underside of the ridding, and are to extend a full 2 inches behind the rigging.

45. *Rule 10.4.2.2. Pads must cover underside of rigging.* Pads used under riggings must be leather-covered on both sides. No hair pads will be allowed. Only a high density foam pad, at least 3/4 inch thick will be allowed. In addition, the pad must have leather over the bars 3/19 inch thick extending at least 1/2 inch on either side of the handle bars.

46. *Disqualification.* A rider shall be disqualified if riding with rowels too sharp or locked.

47. *Rule 10.4.6.1. Spur rowels.* Spur rowels must have five or more points.

48. *Rule 10.5.5. Saddle bronc rider disqualification.* A saddle bronc rider shall be disqualified for riding with locked rowels, or rowels that will lock on spurs, and/or rowels not dulled.

49. *Rule 10.6.3.1. Bull riding. No bull tails under flank straps.* No bull tails will be allowed under flank straps.

50. *Rule 10.6.4. No sharp spurs.* Rider shall not use sharp spurs.

51. *Disqualification of a bull rider.* A bull rider shall be disqualified for using sharp spurs.

Timed event rules

52. *Rule 11.1.4.1. Lining for timed event boxes.* In order to protect the contestant's horse, the back and the side opposite the timed event chute of the timed event boxes shall either have a lower rail which is no less than 3 inches above ground level and have no obstruction in the area from the ground level up to the lower rail or be lined from the ground level up to a minimum of 3 inches high with a solid panel. Box pads are likewise required for each timed event box.

53. *Rule 11.3.8. Drawn animal becomes sick or crippled.* If an animal that is drawn in a pen in a timed event becomes sick or crippled before it is competed on, a judge must pass on the animal's inability to be used before it can be shipped or replaced in the draw.

54. *Rule 11.3.13.2. No consecutive runs on same horse.* In timed events, provided there are other qualified horses on the rodeo grounds, no consecutive runs shall be allowed on the same horse, or horses, unless approval is granted by the arena director, arena boss and/or stock contractor.

55. *Rule 11.6.3. Tie-down roping time limit.* There will be a 25-second elapsed time limit in the tie-down roping. A whistle indicating 'no time' shall be blown by the timer at the end of a 25-second span. Roping a calf after the 25 second whistle has sounded shall be a Class III Offense for mistreatment of animals.

56. *Rule 11.6.4. No dragging of calf.* A neck rope must be used on the horse, and contestant must prevent horse from dragging calf.

57. *Rule 11.6.5. No jerk down.* Rodeo Committees have the option to request a special ground rule for 'no jerk down' in the tie-down roping.

58. *Rule 11.7.8. Steer wrestling time limit.* There will be a 60-second elapsed time limit in the steer wrestling. A whistle indicating 'no time' shall be blown by the timer at the end of he 60-second span.

59. *Rule 11.8.10. Team roping time limit.* There will be a 30-second elapsed time limit in the team roping. A whistle indicating 'no time' shall be blown by the timer at the end of the 30-second span.

60. *Rule 11.9.10. Excessive dragging of steer.* Steer roping contestant, who in the opinion of the judge, excessively drags a steer may be disqualified and/or fined.

Acknowledgement

The author wishes to acknowledge the help of Cindy Schonholtz in preparation of this chapter.

Reference

Sisson, S. and Grossman, J.D. (1953) *Sisson's Anatomy of Domestic Animals*, 4th edn, pp. 909 (horse), and 920 (bovine). W.B. Saunders, Philadelphia, PA.

Welfare Concerns in the Training and Competition of the Cutting, Reining, and Reined Cow Horse

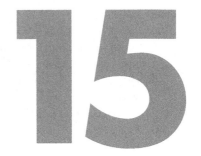

Jerry B. Black
and David Frisbie

Western performance horse events have become some of the most popular and successful equine disciplines competing in the world today. The popularity of the events is in part due to the USA's love of Western history and culture. Most of us have at one time or another been intrigued by the 'cowboy way of life.' Over time, the international equestrian community recognized the athletic appeal of the Western horse, allowing international competitions to grow significantly. Reining is now an event at the World Equestrian Games and is being considered as an Olympic event.

In order to discuss welfare issues that affect the Western performance stock horse, it is important to understand the history of the sport as well as the concept of training. Although each type of horse is trained differently to some extent, the cutting horse fairly represents the group as a whole in both history and training methodology.

Equine Welfare, First Edition. Edited by C. Wayne McIlwraith and Bernard E. Rollin.
© 2011 by UFAW. Published 2011 by Blackwell Publishing Ltd.

15.1 Description and History of Western Stock Horse Sports

15.1.1 Cutting horse

According to publications produced by the National Cutting Horse Association, the cutting horse was born of necessity long ago on the open grass plains of west Texas. This was the era of Western history that included big cattle drives from the open ranges of ranches – such as the Burnett 6666 Ranch, the Waggoner Ranch, the Pitchfork Ranch, and the Matador Ranch – to Dodge City, Kansas. On these big country ranches, where no barbed wire fences existed, cutting horses were the only means of working vast herds of cattle. In those days the task of the horse was quite simple, at least by definition. Guided by his rider, the cutting horse would enter a herd of cattle quietly and deliberately. A single cow was cut, or separated, from the herd. The natural instinct of the cow is to return to the safety of the rest of the herd. The cutting horse, through breeding and training, controlled the cow with a series of moves and counter-moves. The speed, agility, balance, and quickness of the cutting horse kept the cow from the herd, where other cowboys would hold the cut. The horse and rider would re-enter the herd again and again, repeatedly cutting cattle out until the work was done. Only the top hands earned the right to ride the best horses of the *remuda* (the herd of horses from which the hands selected their mounts), the cutting horses (Steenberge, 1990).

The unique skills of the cutting horse were a great source of pride to the frontier cowboy. This often led to impromptu or jackpot cuttings on the open range or in later years, around the turn of the century, in outdoor pens of the large ranches. From this love of the cutting horse and the subsequent competition to determine who had the best horse came the roots of cutting as we know it today. The first cutting horse contest for money was held at the 1898 Cowboy Reunion in Haskell, Texas. Twelve cutting horses competed for a purse of $150. From this start, regular events occurred on ranches of the southwest and at the Fort Worth Stockyards. Rules and prizes varied greatly, but the ability of the cutting horse to separate single calves from the herd always was and continues to be the goal of the competition. From these roots, the National Cutting Horse Association (NCHA) was formed in 1946 during the Fort Worth Exposition and Fat Stock Show. The stated purpose of the organization was to standardize the rules and judging of competition, and to preserve the tradition and history of the cutting horse with the ranching and livestock industry.

15.1.2 Reining horse

The origins of the reining horse are similar to those of the cutting horse and date back to the earliest Spanish settlers in what today is Mexico and the southwestern USA. Large ranches managed their cattle herds from horseback. Cattle were moved, branded, doctored, sorted, and herded on open range with no holding equipment. Cowboys needed good horses that could change directions quickly, stop 'on a dime,' and sprint after a wayward cow. The cowboy's horse needed to be controlled mostly by legs and weight shifts, ridden with only one hand and a light touch on the reins, so the cowboy could handle a lariat (to rope cattle), open a gate, or countless other tasks to move a cattle herd. As in cutting, friendly competitions to show off these ideal characteristics of good horses amongst cowboys and vaqueros evolved into the sport of reining.

Reining as a sport was first recognized by the American Quarter Horse Association (AQHA) in 1949 and by the United States Equestrian Federation (USEF) in its western division shortly thereafter. The National Reining Horse Association (NRHA) was formed in the USA in 1966 and quickly developed worldwide. Standardized rules and patterns were gradually adopted in whole or part by all organizations that sanction reining horse events. The sport of reining became an International Equestrian Federation (FEI) recognized discipline in 2000, and international competitions such as the World Equestrian Games are now governed by the FEI in cooperation with the NRHA. Reining is growing in popularity around the world and is considered one of the world's fastest-growing equestrian sports.

Today, competitions approved by the NCHA, NRHA, and NRCHA (National Reined Cow Horse Association) occur throughout the USA and Canada. In addition, many members of these organizations from other continents including Europe, Australia, and South America are conducting competitions outside North America. It is the format of these competitions and other Western performance horse disciplines that present a unique challenge to the equine veterinarian.

15.2 Introduction to Training the Western Stock Horse

Training of the cutting horse begins early in their two-year-old year. Usually 60 to 90 days are spent in basic training before the horse is introduced to cattle. This is generally accomplished by turning one cow into a round pen that is approximately 125 feet (38 m) to 175 feet (53 m) in diameter. The horse is taught to mirror the movements of the cow as it moves around the perimeter of the large circular arena. This is a repetitive process done time and time again, several days a week for months.

The object of training is for the horse to develop an ability to perform identical movements to the cow. Simply put, when the cow stops, or stops and turns, the horse does the same maneuver. This type of training is accomplished by asking the horse to stop with the aid of the bridle and turning the horse to move with the cow. The key to training is the complete and balanced stop. With time, the stop will ultimately be followed by the ability of the horse to 'read' the movement of the cow and turn in the direction the cow is going. Because this ability to watch the cow and respond to its movement is instinctive to the working stock horse, breeding is of the utmost importance. Without this genetic instinct, the horse will simply not respond to the movement of the cow and will not initiate the stop or turn necessary to continue to track the animal. Like training the well-bred hunting dog, a good cutting horse trainer will know in a relatively short period of time if the young horse has the instinctive and athletic ability to be a successful cutting horse (Black, 2003).

The finished cutting horse must perform the necessary moves to keep the cow in proper position away from the herd without any hand cues from the rider, relying on the instinct to read the movement of the cow alone. Using the reins to guide the horse is permitted only to make the cut of a single cow out of the herd. After the cut is successfully made, the reins are placed in a relaxed position on the horse's neck and only leg cues are permitted from the rider during the actual working time. The ability of working cutting horses to contain the individual cow provides the excitement of competition in cutting.

Training of the cutting horse prospect that has shown good potential will continue as a three-year-old, preparing it for the first major competitions, the futurities. The futurity is the first of the horse's 'aged event' competitions that will continue for four years. No horse can compete in aged events beyond six years of age. Aged events typically will consist of two elimination go-rounds followed by semi-finals and, ultimately, the final competition. Significant musculoskeletal stress is placed on these athletic performance horses with multi-day competitions over a short period of time. In addition, the horses are usually 'practiced' on cattle daily, including the day of competition, to sharpen their performance skills.

Competition in these aged events is heavy, with the major shows having well over 500 entries in a single age division. Purses in this type of event can exceed a total of $1000000. The nature of this 'aged event' competition, with large purses in numerous events over a four-year period of time, has caused the cutting horse economy to grow rapidly over the last several years. Select yearling and training sales are conducted annually that are beginning to parallel the racing industry in financial return on sales. This has contributed to the current popularity and resurgence of breeding of the cutting and Western stock horse, which in turn will ensure the preservation of the tradition and heritage that this horse played in the history of the great Old West.

Reining horses are trained to perform a precise pattern of circles, spins, and stops. All work is done at a lope or gallop (the fastest of the horse gaits). The lope is a slow relaxed version of the horse gait most commonly known as the canter. Reining is often described as a Western form of dressage riding, as it requires the horse to be responsive and in tune with its rider. The horse should be willingly guided or controlled with minimal aids that are not easily seen. Judging is based upon the horse's ability to perform a set pattern of movements.

The reining pattern includes an average of eight to twelve movements that must be executed by the horse. Patterns require the following movements:

(1) *Circles*. The horse must perform large, fast circles at a near-gallop, and smaller, slow circles at a lope. The circles should be perfectly round, with the rider dictating the speed of the horse. Most circles incorporate changes of direction that require a flying change of lead.

(2) *Flying lead change*. The horse changes its leading front and hind legs at a lope mid-stride. The horse should not break gait nor change speed. The precision of the flying lead change is the most important factor in judging.

(3) *Rundown*. The horse gallops or 'runs' along the long side of the arena, at least 20 feet (6 m) from the fence or rail. The rundown is a required movement prior to a sliding stop or rollback.

(4) *Sliding stop*. The horse goes from a gallop to a complete halt, planting its hind feet in the arena footing and allowing its hind feet to slide several feet, while continuing to let its front feet 'walk' forward. The back should be rounded, raised upward to the withers and the hindquarters come well underneath the horse. The movement should finish in a straight line.

(5) *Back or backup*. The horse backs up quickly for at least 10 feet (3 m). The backup must be in a perfectly straight line, completely stopped when asked, and hesitate for a moment before the next movement.

(6) *Rollback*. The horse immediately, without hesitation, performs a 180-degree turn after halting from a sliding stop, and immediately goes forward again into a lope. The horse must turn on its hindquarters, bringing its hocks well under the back and the motion should be continuous with no hesitation.

(7) *Spins or turnarounds*. Beginning from a standstill, the horse spins 360 degrees or more (up to four and one-quarter full turns) in place around its stationary inside hind leg. The hind pivot foot remains in essentially the same location throughout the spin, though the horse will pick it up and put it down as it turns. Spins are judged on correctness, smoothness, and cadence. Speed adds to the degree of difficulty and will improve the score of a correctly done spin.

(8) *Pause or hesitate*. The horse is asked to stand still for a few seconds to 'settle' between movements in the reining pattern, particularly after the spin. Horses that are ill-mannered or behave with impatience during the pause will be penalized.

Training the reining horse requires time and patience to master the combinations of maneuvers required in a competition pattern. Repetitive training as in the cutting horse occurs throughout the horse's career and is the key factor in training the young reining or reined cow horse prospect. Reining may be performed by any horse but the stock horse breeds, particularly the American Quarter Horse, dominate the industry. The reining horse must be agile, quick, and very responsive to the rider's commands. Powerful hindquarters typical of the Quarter Horse are necessary to hold the correct position in a sliding stop or rollback. Good conformation is essential to withstand the stresses of training and competition. In addition, the horse must have an excellent temperament to perform with both the speed and the precision to be a successful show horse.

The increasing popularity of the cutting and reining horse as a show and performance individual is occurring both nationwide and on an international level. Sales of this type of horse have increased to Europe, South America, and other countries. In North America, the revival of interest stems primarily from excellent programs instituted by associations such as the National Cutting Horse Association (NCHA), National Reining Horse Association (NRHA) and the National Reined Cow Horse Association (NRCHA). Collectively, theses three associations approve the vast majority of the competitions in the Western stock horse disciplines. All of these associations encourage owner participation at the amateur or non-professional level in their major events, increasing the popularity of cutting, reining, and reined cow horse competitions as the premier Western performance horse sports. This owner/rider participation in turn attracts significant sponsorships from major corporations, increasing the overall purse amounts distributed within the industry.

It is the intensity of repetitive training over many years, the significant stresses placed on the individual athlete during multi-day competitions, and the inevitable pressure placed upon trainers and competitors when large purses are at stake that create many of the welfare challenges that are present in the working stock horse industry today.

15.3 Industry Welfare Concerns

15.3.1 Early training of the young Western stock horse

Training of the young Western stock horse begins early in their two-year-old year, with the first futurity competitions for many horses beginning in the late summer of their three-year-old year. Many people involved in the industry have expressed concern regarding the early training and competition of these young equine athletes. There has been no research completed to date that evaluates the incidence of athletic injuries in cutting horses relative to the age they are started. Studies conducted on Thoroughbred racehorses indicate that a key factor in injury prevention of the athletic horse is not necessarily delayed training of the two-year-old but rather the proper conditioning of the musculoskeletal system to achieve the necessary remodeling of the bones, cartilage, ligaments, and tendons to increase overall strength. Investigations as part of an international study involving the Equine Orthopaedic Research Center at Colorado State University indicate that exercise of the very young Thoroughbred horse is not harmful and can provide benefit to the articular cartilage (Rogers et al., 2008a, b).

Experience from the racing industry further indicates that factors such as increased competition demanding increased levels of training and more stress on the musculoskeletal system must be considered when evaluating the incidence of injury. It is reasonable to believe that these same factors are the principal cause of increased injury rates in the cutting horse at this time. Future research is needed in the improvement of the understanding of the pathogenesis of exercise-induced traumatic disease, early diagnosis of bone and joint disease, as well as conditioning and training methods to strengthen the musculoskeletal system in the young athletic cutting and reining horse (McIlwraith and Black, 2008).

Based on current knowledge, it is unlikely that starting young cutting horses a year later as three-year-olds would decrease the incidence of athletic injury in the industry. Further research is needed to help determine the cause of athletic injuries in this group of performance horses. Future research will likely focus on multiple possible causes of musculoskeletal trauma, including genetics, medication use during competition and training, surfaces of show arenas, training and warm-up facilities, as well as general conditioning and training methods. Other areas of concern include fatigue related to show schedules as well as fatigue associated with excessive training practices. The cutting, reining, and reined cow horse industries must be responsible for the health and safety of their horses and be responsible for funding adequate research to protect these trusted equine athletes.

15.3.2 Other training considerations

Training the young working stock horse requires considerable time and patience. Good trainers recognize that individual variations in maturity, physical strength, desire, and genetic ability require different approaches to training methods and often different work schedules. Many young horses are naturally talented and progress in their training at a very rapid pace. Care must be taken not to move forward too quickly, thus not allowing the musculoskeletal system to adapt to the stresses being placed on the individual. Common areas of trauma include synovitis and/or capsulitis of the hocks and stifles, as well as tendonitis or desmitis of the suspensory apparatus that occurs in either the fore or hind limbs. The tendency to medicate and continue training is common and re-injury often occurs. It is the responsibility of the veterinarian, trainer, and owner to make good decisions based upon the welfare of the horse, and often reduced training or rest should be considered. It has been the authors' personal experience that young horses in particular need short periods of time out of training to rest and rejuvenate themselves. Ideally, individual pasture or grass paddock turnout should be available to the horse, allowing it to enjoy a natural environment and some instinctive behavior. Good horses tend to return to work with a better attitude and willingness to accept training. This is particularly true if the individual had low-grade musculoskeletal pain prior to the rest period.

Excessive use of training aids continues to be a welfare concern in the industry today. Many are considered part of the training and showing equipment but always should be used in an appropriate manner that does not inflict undue pain to the horse. Young horses are typically started in a snaffle bit attached to a headstall and split reins. This type of bit allows control with minimum force placed on the tongue, bars, and commissars of the lips. The mouthpiece should be a minimum of 5/16 inch (8 mm) in diameter measured 1 inch (25 mm) from the inside of the ring of the snaffle bit, with a gradual decrease to the center of the snaffle. The mouthpiece should be round, oval or egg-shaped, and made of smooth and unwrapped metal. The chin strap should be made of leather or other woven material, avoiding those made of iron, chain or other similar materials. These bits must be designed and used in such a way that, when the reins are pulled, no undue leverage is applied that causes pain to the horse (NRCHA, 2009a). Young horses are commonly trained in the snaffle bit for one to two years and slowly graduated into the hackamore and more traditional bits over time. As training progresses, bits with unbroken mouthpieces and longer cheekpieces are commonly used to allow more control using significantly less leverage. The Western bit normally has a curb configuration to the mouthpiece, allowing pressure to be placed on the bars as well as the lower jaw through the curb strap. The finished bridle horse often wears a vaquero-styled spade bit that requires very minimal leverage to achieve full control and a complete stop from a gallop (Martin and Martin, 1999). Achieving this level of ability takes years of slow progressive training putting the horse 'in the bridle.' It requires the patience of an excellent horseman or horsewoman and the unyielding trust of the finished bridle horse. Unfortunately, there are no real shortcuts in training the Western stock horse and abuse of the bridle can occur. Any bridle equipment that causes bleeding of the mouth or face, damage to the bars of the mouth, lacerations of the tongue, or unnecessary pain to the horse should be considered abusive and is a welfare concern.

Spurs are used on the vast majority of Western stock horses for both training and competition. The use of spurs dates back to the Romans, when they were used to aid positioning of the horse during warfare. The Western spur used today is a modern version of the Spanish spur worn by the *vaqueros* and *charros* from Mexico who were sent to the West to manage the large number of cattle raised on the vast ranchlands of the Spanish Colonial days. The first known spurs made in the West were at the Spanish Missions in the early 1800s. From this beginning the 'California spur' evolved that is very similar to the spurs worn today (Martin and Martin, 1999). The contact point of the spur to the horse is the points of the rowel. Rowels come in myriad sizes and styles as well as number of points. Used correctly, the spur provides a cue to the horse either to accelerate, initiate lateral movement or maintain a position while in motion. Well-trained horses need very little spur action to initiate a response, although the presence of the spur is an aid much like a bit. Often, no more than a touch or holding a spur against the side of the horse achieves the desired response. Training may begin with rowels that have five blunt points and progress to higher numbers or shape of rowels depending on the sensitivity of the individual horse. Excessive use of the spur to punish a horse can inflict significant pain and trauma to the horse and is a serious welfare concern. Horses that have been spurred to the point of lacerated skin lesions or soft tissue blunt force trauma to the point of muscle atrophy are considered, by today's standards of welfare, to have been treated inhumanely.

15.4 Other Humane Considerations

15.4.1 Inhumane treatments

The American Quarter Horse Association (AQHA) approves many events each year that include cutting, reining, and stock horse competitions. The AQHA rules clearly define additional practices that constitute inhumane treatment and are worthy of consideration for all Western stock horse disciplines (AQHA, 2009a). Inhumane treatment includes, but is not limited to, the following:

(1) Exhibiting any horse that appears to be sullen, dull, lethargic, emaciated, drawn or overly tired.
(2) Placing an object in a horse's mouth so as to cause undue discomfort or distress.
(3) Tying a horse up or around in a stall or when lounging or riding in a manner as to cause undue discomfort or distress.
(4) Use of inhumane training techniques or methods including excessive spurring and/or excessive jerking of reins.
(5) Use of inhumane equipment, such as saw tooth bits, tack collars, tack hackamores or other equipment used specifically to inflict pain, excessive discomfort or bleeding.
(6) Use of any item or appliance that restricts movement or circulation of the tail. Specifically, tail blocking is prohibited and will be discussed in more detail below.

Tail blocking – using substances, usually ethyl alcohol (ethanol), injected around the nerves that supply the muscle that elevate the tail, to block the movement of the tail – is commonplace in Western performance horses. The legality of this practice is beyond the scope of this chapter and will vary from State to State depending on the credentials of the person performing the procedure. However, the AQHA has taken a stance that this is not an acceptable procedure at events they sanction. They have instituted guidelines as well as testing policies to attempt to control this procedure. The American Association of Equine Practitioners (AAEP) has also condemned this practice as unethical by their membership through their support for AQHA policies. Because associations such as the AQHA have stated that veterinarians signing medication forms and participating as official show veterinarians must be members in good standing of the AAEP, such stances by the AAEP have impact with the veterinary community. It does however come with a price. Specifically, it drives such procedures into 'back alleys,' and the mainstay of people providing such a service are veterinarians or lay people with inadequate medical training to perform the procedures, which is the unethical practice of veterinary medicine. The horse typically suffers in either case. The AQHA (2009b) has made significant inroads on addressing this issue but more still needs to be done. Horses with marginal use of their tail (enough use to pass the tail test but not normal use) are still being used (placing well) in AQHA classes, which is a factor that drives the continuation of this practice. The NCHA, NRCHA or NRHA have no restrictions on the practice of tail blocks. Because tail-blocked horses are perceived as more desirable in the show ring, the associations by their judging promote the practice of blocking tails. It will take some specific rules and enforcement policies to change this conduct globally in Western performance horses.

15.4.2 Welfare concerns at shows and events

The three major Western stock horse associations have rules in place that strictly prohibits the inhumane treatment of horses of any kind in the show arena, warm-up areas, and practice pens, or on the show grounds in general. In 2003 the NCHA enacted a zero-tolerance policy under standing rule 35 prohibiting inhumane treatment or abuse at any time during approved competitions. The zero-tolerance policy requires that any of the following acts should be reported to show management. The reportable offenses are summarized as follows:

(1) Slapping or hitting a horse on the head, or any other part of the body either with the rider's hand, reins or any other object.
(2) Using a bit in such a way that a horse is caused to bleed from its mouth or face.
(3) Any act that the general public would perceive to be a violation of rule 35b dealing with inhumane treatment.
(4) The exhibition of a crippled or injured horse, or a horse with any other health abnormality, which could thereby result in the horse's undue discomfort or distress is considered inhumane treatment.

Abuse is defined under the zero-tolerance policy as inhumane and includes excessive jerking, spurring, whipping, slapping, use of lip wire or similar device, or any other act intended to cause trauma or injury to the horse. In addition, any act of abuse on the show grounds which could also potentially endanger the safety of other persons or animals is strictly prohibited NCHA (2009a).

The NRHA has less terminology describing abuse or inhumane treatment but clearly defines abuse as a major cause for disciplinary action. The rule book under Section E defines abuse as an action, or failure to act, which a reasonably prudent person, informed and experienced in the customs, accepted training techniques and exhibition procedures, would determine to be cruel, abusive, inhumane or detrimental to the horse's health (NRHA, 2009a). International Equestrian Federation (Fédération Equestre Internationale, FEI) rules and guidelines apply to reining horses competing in international competitions that are approved by the FEI.

The National Reined Cow Horse Association clearly defines inhumane treatment in rules 14.1.7–14.1.9 stating that the NRCHA takes very seriously the welfare of these great horses to which we are devoted (NRCHA, 2009b). The content of the rules are very similar to those of the NCHA.

It is important that all performance horse associations have clear-cut rules in place to prohibit inhumane or abusive treatment of horses with mechanisms in place to actively enforce violations in an appropriate and timely manner. It is equally important that show management, competition officials, judges, contestants, and association members protect the welfare of the horses participating in events by reporting inhumane or abusive actions of contestants or trainers to appropriate authorities immediately.

As previously mentioned, the NCHA has convened a subcommittee to assess and address concerns with use and husbandry of cattle. The NCHA feels that there are appropriate guidelines in place for both NCHA events and NCHA-sanctioned events. Further, the NCHA feels that good compliance at NCHA events is being realized, and further inquiry into compliance at NCHA-sanctioned events is underway.

15.5 Medications

15.5.1 General use of medications

It is interesting that little to no regulation of medications is present in nationally sanctioned events for the Western performance horse, at least by the parent organizations (i.e., NCHA, NRHA, and NRCHA). It is likely that this stems from early days when these events were local competitions between cowboys. Subsequently, with the gradual increase in popularity over the years, the topic of medication policies is just recently being addressed by these organizations. Today, the individual earnings of horses and riders in these disciplines go well into the millions of dollars. This clearly has an effect on the landscape of competitiveness, which is one factor that translates into reasons for medication usage. Certainly, the use of medication is not unique to the reining or the cutting horse industry. As alluded to above, what is unique is the way these three organizations (NCHA, NRHA, and NRCHA) regulate themselves at sanctioned events compared to other organizations.

Specifically, most other large organizations have adopted medication policies. One commonly used policy is that of the United States Equestrian Federation (USEF, 2009). The USEF policy allows the use of medication for a therapeutic purpose. More specifically, certain medications, such as most non-steroidal anti-inflammatory drugs (NSAIDs), cannot be administered within 12 hours of competition and have a certain daily limit as well as number of consecutive days the medication can be administered. Certain NSAIDs can be administered without turning in a medication form. Most other therapeutic substances require the horse not to compete for 24 hours post-administration and a medication form to be filed with the organization. The ability to give therapeutic substances, which in some instances may be sedation for a medical procedure or local anesthesia for diagnostic blocks, in the authors' opinion is very germane to the welfare of the horse. The way in which the USEF medication policy is written does not significantly encumber the use of medications and hence medical treatment of horses for therapeutic purposes, which is a very important issue. It does require the horse not to compete for 24 hours allowing for a negligible physiologic effect of the medication. One important consideration is that the USEF also has an extensive method for testing for medications so their guidelines can be enforced.

This is in contrast to the NCHA rulebook (NCHA, 2009b), which has a single paragraph on the use of medications at competitions:

> Administration of drugs while on the show grounds, including show arena, and practice
> arena is strictly prohibited unless administered in a lifesaving situation. Such an instance
> must be reported to show management. The decision of show management as to lifesaving
> treatment should be based on consultation with a veterinarian. Show management shall
> disqualify and/or refuse entry to any contestant and/or owner for violation of this rule.

As written, this rule would exclude the administration of many medications that could be beneficial to cutting horses at competitions, such as NSAIDs, which certainly have been recognized as having a place in equine competitions. The use of NSAIDs is permitted at most US competitions and is allowed with certain restrictions by the USEF medication rules. Furthermore, the authors would suggest that the judicious uses of some medications, as outlined by organizations like USEF, are in fact relevant to the humane and ethical treatment of horses at such competitions.

The NCHA has formed a subcommittee on horse and cattle welfare that is currently addressing this rule. In speaking with Lindy Burch, the Chairperson of the committee, the organization in the short term is trying to restrict the use of medication in the show and practice arena. These areas can be visually monitored by the organization, but because no testing policy is in place, there is no mechanism whereby the NCHA can enforce medication rules past this point. The reality of medication use currently at NCHA events is that they are effectively uninhibited. This is an issue the subcommittee is actively working on but they will be faced with some challenges. The issue most likely will not be with the therapeutic use of medications as defined by USEF; it will be with the use of tranquilizers, sedatives, and other psychotropic medications for performance alteration during the competition. Currently a subset of cutting trainers that might be considered 'propsychotropic' would suggest that it is more humane to give a horse some sedation and lope it for 2 hours versus 8 hours of loping without medication prior to the event. There are obviously a multitude of issues with this example, but it does embody a position that will need to be addressed as the NCHA proceeds forward with their medication policy.

The NRHA rulebook (NRHA, 2009b) has no reference to medications or drugs outside of the section pertaining to combined events with USEF. At these events, exhibitors must comply with USEF rules. Thus excluding these combined events or events sanctioned by other organizations (FEI), the NRHA does not have medication rule. Like the NCHA, the NRHA has been working toward a medication policy. They have proposed some novel ideas but have yet to implement a policy. In 2006, Steve Harris chaired an NRHA subcommittee that was charged with addressing the medication issue. This committee took a few actions, one of which was education of their membership on the use and issues surrounding medication in the NRHA. They also drafted a medication policy that would be funded by a $1 entry fee. This policy was mainly aimed at surveillance but did propose restriction of local anesthetics for desensitizing structures above the pastern region or 'high blocks'. In this proposal, exhibitors would be allowed to use any medication but need to declare what was in the horse's system. Using the collected fees, random testing was to be used to ensure accurate reporting by the exhibitors. If inconsistencies were documented between the test results and the declaration, a penalty system was to be in place. This proposed policy was to expire two years after implementation. All of the data was to be kept confidential but used to formulate a drug policy based on documented usage. This policy suffered a landslide defeat in 2007 by the general membership of the NRHA. This same year the NRHA endorsed an affiliate reining group of the USEF, which would allow the rules of the USEF to be utilized at events but would not be an official part of the NRHA. In 2008 the NRHA formed a new committee to address animal welfare issues. The current president of the NRHA, Rick Weaver, is committed to development and implementation of a medication policy that is beneficial to the horse. The use of psychotropic medication in reining is similar to those in the NCHA and will need to be addressed as medication policies are considered in the organization.

There are benefits to the lack of medication policies. For example, exhibitors at either NCHA or NRHA events, with the noted exceptions, are typically effectively able to use medications as they see fit or as directed by their veterinarian. An advantage of the system is that it allows horses in these events to be treated as necessary. For example, the treatment of horses suffering from 'gas colic' at NCHA and NRHA events is unimpeded compared to horses competing at USEF events. Horses at NCHA and NRHA events could be treated with a dose of flunixin meglumine 10 hours prior to a class. In USEF jurisdiction, the horse would not be able to receive a full dose of flunixin meglumine without having time off and in many cases be hand walked to see what response is achieved. Specifically, in the USEF situation the horse would be unable to compete in less than 12 hours post-treatment assuming a standard 1 mg/kg dose. An extreme example might be the unknowing desensitization of a stress fracture prior to competition risking a potential catastrophic outcome.

In a 'grayer' ethical area would be the example of psychotropic medication use during competitions, which is common place in practice. Specifically, the use of non-therapeutic medication has been justified by trainers and veterinarians. For example, in the case of a young horse, the use of psychotropic medication to take the edge off will be beneficial and humane for the horse compared to overwork of the horse, and will yield similar results. The authors have not personally witnessed ill-effects of either example. But the risk seems inevitable and this is an issue that needs to be addressed. In addition to the concern for horse and rider, the perception by the public regarding the above described practice will also have to be factored into decisions made by the association. Rules, such as exist for all events in the State of California, have shown that sometimes politicians will provide governances on the horse industry. If a uniform set of rules is a goal, a proactive stance is warranted by the industry.

15.5.2 Maintenance injections

Similar to other equine disciplines, the cutting, reining, and cow horse industries are plagued with controversy over the issue of 'maintenance injections.' This would be the routine injecting of joints such as hocks and stifles because a certain time has lapsed or the horse is going to a major competition but has no perceptible lameness issues. Much debate occurs with both trainers and owners as well in the veterinary community on the correct use of intra-articular medications and the issues that potentially arise from it. Owners and trainers often have one of three perceptions regarding this issue:

(1) waiting until the horse exhibits signs of soreness is too late;
(2) starting to inject joints will lead to a slippery slope where the horse will need it all the time; and
(3) using cues from the horse to dictate when joint injections are necessary.

Veterinarians often report feeling pressured to inject joints on a routine basis or the customer will get someone else to do it. The authors believe that this issue on the surface is straightforward.

The medical treatment of joints should be undertaken when there is a perceptible issue and not as part of a scheduled maintenance program. The level of certainty that a particular practitioner uses to make this determination will vary greatly and will need to be based on their level of comfort and experience. In practice, the implementation of this approach will take cooperation from trainers, owners, and veterinarians. There are certainly times that full diagnostic workups are indicated. This would include diagnostic blocks as well as radiographic imaging. In some cases this degree of workup is not necessary and other methods of formulating therapeutic plans are justifiable. For example, in the authors' opinion, there are times when clinical presentation provides sufficient evidence for subsequent joint therapy. One such example might be a horse that had been previously worked up and responded to intra-articular treatment of the lower hock joints and it re-presents a year later with the same clinical signs. While most clinical signs are not definitive for locations, when multiple findings are used in conjunction with each other, a reasonable level of certainty can be reached. Examples would be the character of the gait under saddle, a positive response to hock flexion, as well as focal muscle pain. In such cases a discussion with the agent outlining the various options for further diagnostics and or treatment obviates questionable ethical issues. An example that would be considered at the other end of the spectrum would be the injection of a horse where no previous examination or experience is provided along with the lack of a clinical exam because it is 'time.' The responsibility for the treatment of a patient will always rest with the veterinarian. Thus through cooperation with the owner and/or agent, a comprehensive plan for each patient should be undertaken and the treating veterinarians should be able to defend the plan in front of their peers.

15.6 Genetics

It is clear genetics plays a large role in both the cutting and reining industries. While breeding horses of certain genetic characteristics can result in more talented horses with better performance, there are also questionable traits that can be passed on. Questionable traits range from minor conformational faults to serious medical conditions. For example, hyperkalemic periodic paralysis (HYPP) is an inherited disease of the muscle that occurs through a genetic point mutation. Through observation of the medical presentation, research into the cause, and final action of the breed registry, this disease is being controlled. A more recent example is hereditary equine regional dermal asthenia (HERDA). This is also a genetic skin disease predominantly found in the American Quarter Horse. Within the breed, the disease is prevalent in particular lines of cutting horses. HERDA is characterized by hyperextensible skin, scarring, and severe lesions along the back of affected horses. Affected foals rarely show symptoms at birth. The condition typically occurs by the age of two, most notably when the horse is first being broke to saddle. There is no cure, and the majority of diagnosed horses are euthanized because they are unable to be ridden and are inappropriate for future breeding.

More subtle genetic associations have been noticed through repository radiographs, such as osteochondrosis desiccans or other radiographic abnormalities in certain breeding lines. It is important to stress the open sharing of such information and the need for all factions of the industry to work together to try and better the breed based on sound scientific and ethical platforms. In some cases, it might be the eradication of HYPP or HERDA or the discovery that a perceived issue may not affect performance or health. An example of the latter would be interpretation of flattening on the medial femoral condyle, which was first assumed to be associated with subchondral bone cysts. This flattening is often seen in certain blood lines. More investigation into the occurrence and subsequent outcomes are needed to see if a relationship between performance-limiting issues and diagnosis exists. It is important to realize that the open discussion and sharing of information as it relates to genetic traits is important in the longevity and improvement of any breed.

15.7 Conclusion

As the cutting, reining, and reined cow horse events become more popular spectator sports, it is critical that the industry protects the welfare of these equine athletes in both competition and training environments. Professional horseman must take the responsibility of applying appropriate sanctions to those who abuse or treat a horse in an inhumane manner. These organizations along with groups such as the AAEP are currently actively addressing issues outlined in this chapter.

References

AQHA (2009a) *American Quarter Horse Association Rule Book*, Rule 441(h,k), Show Rules and Regulations. American Quarter Horse Association, Amarillo, TX.

AQHA (2009b) *American Quarter Horse Association Rule Book*, Rule 441, Prohibited Conduct. American Quarter Horse Association, Amarillo, TX.

Black, J. (2003) Lameness in the cutting horse. In *Diagnosis and Management of Lameness in the Horse*, pp. 1017–1020. Saunders, St. Louis, MO.

Martin, N. and Martin, J. (1999) *Bit and Spur Makers in the Vaquero Tradition*, pp. 19–25, and 47–48. Hawk Hill Press, Nicasio, CA.

McIlwraith, C.W. and Black, J. (2008) Training age and soundness in the cutting horse. In *The Horse*, October, Article No. 12831.

NCHA (2009a) *National Cutting Horse Association, Official Handbook of Rules and Regulations*, Section IV, Standing Rule 35, pp. 57–58. National Cutting Horse Association, Fort Worth, TX.

NCHA (2009b) *National Cutting Horse Association, Official Handbook of Rules and Regulations*, Section IV, Contestants, p. 58. Available at: http://www.nchacutting.com/ag/judges/pdf/rule_book.pdf.

NRCHA (2009a) *National Reined Cow Horse Association Official Handbook*, Section 5.6, p. 22. National Reined Cow Horse Association, Byars, OK.

NRCHA (2009b) *National Reined Cow Horse Association Official Handbook*, Sections 14.1.7–14.1.9, p. 39. National Reined Cow Horse Association, Byars, OK.

NRHA (2009a) *National Reining Horse Association Rule Book*, Rule E, Section 1, 2, p. 40. National Reining Horse Association, Oklahoma City, OK.

NRHA (2009b) *National Reining Horse Association Handbook*. National Reining Horse Association, Oklahoma City, OK. Available at: http://www.nrha.com/handbook/09handbook.pdf.

Rogers, C.W., Firth, E.C., McIlwraith, C.W., Barneveld, A., Goodship, A.E., Kawcak, C.E., Smith, R.K.W. and van Weeren, P.R. (2008a) Evaluation of a new strategy to modulate skeletal development in Thoroughbred performance horses by imposing track-based exercise during growth. *Equine Veterinary Journal*, 40, 111–118.

Rogers, C.W., Firth, E.C., McIlwraith, C.W., Barneveld, A., Goodship, A.E., Kawcak, C.E., Smith, R.K.W. and van Weeren, P.R. (2008b) Evaluation of a new strategy to modulate skeletal development in racehorses by improving track-based exercise during growth: the effects on 2-year-old and 3-year-old racing careers. *Equine Veterinary Journal*, 40, 119–127.

Steenberge, P. (1990) *The Cutting Horse*, p. 7. National Cutting Horse Association, Fort Worth, TX.

USEF (2009) *The United States Equestrian Federation Rulebook*, Chapter 4, Drugs and Medications Rule, GR408–413, and GR51–54. United States Equestrian Federation, Lexington, KY. Available at: http://www.usef.org/documents/ruleBook/2009/GeneralRules/Chapter%204.pdf.

PMU Ranching and Equine Welfare

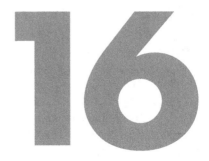

Nat T. Messer

16.1 Historical Perspectives

The discovery in the mid-1930s that pregnant mares' urine (PMU) contained estrogens that occurred naturally in a water-soluble, orally active form was the impetus for the beginning of PMU ranching (Zondek, 1934). Ayerst, McKenna & Harrison, Ltd., in cooperation with the Department of Biochemistry at McGill University, Montreal, Canada, under the direction of Dr. J.B. Collip, undertook extensive research to develop a process whereby the conjugated water-soluble, orally active estrogens of PMU could be produced for clinical use at a price that would enable their widespread use. By 1941, sufficient progress had been made to commence commercial production of the potent, orally active, conjugated estrogens of PMU in Canada. The following year it was approved for use in the USA (Stevenson, 1945). In 1943, the American Home Products Corp. purchased Ayerst, McKenna & Harrison, Ltd., later shortening the name to Ayerst Laboratories, and then merging it with Philadelphia-based Wyeth Laboratories in 1987. The company that now processes the urine to obtain the raw product is a subsidiary of Wyeth called Wyeth Organics.

Initially, the company either purchased pregnant mares to collect urine from or contracted with owners of pregnant mares in rural Quebec to allow the company to collect urine from their mares at several designated 'collection depots' ranging in size from only five or six mares to units with as many as 1000 mares. The actual collection of urine from the mares began by collecting the urine off the floor of the barns, grossly contaminated with bedding and feces. As this had detrimental effects on the water-soluble conjugated estrogens, the urine was then collected by several workers moving around the barns collecting the urine as the mares voided (Stevenson, 1945). Eventually, a harness apparatus was designed to automatically collect the urine and exclude the feces, and this is still in use on the PMU ranches

Equine Welfare, First Edition. Edited by C. Wayne McIlwraith and Bernard E. Rollin.
© 2011 by UFAW. Published 2011 by Blackwell Publishing Ltd.

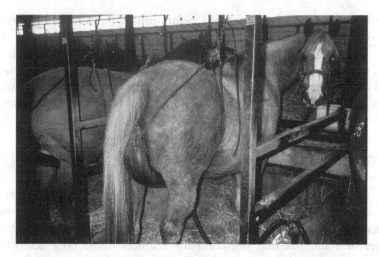

Figure 16.1 PMU mare with typical urine collection harness in place during the collection season.

today (Figure 16.1). In the larger units, prevention of disease was a major problem and concern; however, serious outbreaks of 'strangles,' influenza, and other infectious diseases were reportedly minimized due to measures adopted for early recognition of disease, isolation of infected animals, coupled with the liberal use of the then relatively new antimicrobial drug sulfanilamide (Stevenson, 1945).

As the use of estrogen replacement therapy by women increased, the company realized that it would not be able to contract with enough ranchers to meet the growing demand for PMU, so they expanded their network of mare owners to the Canadian prairies, where horses and pasture land were plentiful. In the mid-1960s a new processing plant was built in Brandon, Manitoba, where it has remained since. Consequently, PMU ranching became a significant agricultural enterprise in the midwestern Provinces of Alberta, Manitoba, and Saskatchewan in Canada and in the State of North Dakota in the USA. Ranchers constructed their own facilities to house their own pregnant mares rather than transporting their mares to collecting depots. Most of the ranchers were horse breeders before they became involved in the PMU industry.

Between 1960 and 1990, the number of PMU ranches reached nearly 500 ranches housing as many as 60 000–70 000 mares during the collection season, which typically ran from mid-October through mid-March. It was during this period of substantial growth and increased visibility that issues regarding the welfare of the mares and their offspring were raised because of the way in which the mares were maintained with limited access to outside corrals or pastures for approximately six months during their pregnancy and because of the disposition of the mares' offspring after weaning. This led to the first version of the Recommended Code of Practice for the

Care and Handling of Horses in PMU Operations (COP) published in 1990 by the Province of Manitoba that established guidelines for welfare and housing standards to be followed by the PMU ranchers (Manitoba Department of Agriculture, 1990). Since that time there have been four updated and revised versions, each version being approved by the Commissioner of the North Dakota Department of Agriculture, the Manitoba Minister of Agriculture, Food and Rural Initiatives, and the Saskatchewan Minister of Agriculture and Food (NAERIC, 2007).

16.2 General Information

Pregnant mare urine ranches are privately owned facilities. The owners of the ranches have applied for and have been granted contracts with Wyeth (now Pfizer) to produce a designated quantity of urine from pregnant mares annually based on a rigid set of standards that the company requires of its contracted ranchers. Ranchers are paid by the company based on grams of estrogen, independent of urine volume delivered, and the company pays for all urine transportation costs. Each ranch is required to conform to the COP, which was developed by a committee initiated by the Manitoba Department of Agriculture and the company and instituted in 1990 (Manitoba Department of Agriculture, 1990).

The ranches range in size from approximately 75 to 350 mares 'on-line,' i.e., mares confined to tie stalls with a collection apparatus (harness) in place (Figure 16.2). Mares go 'on-line' beginning approximately October 15th and are taken off-line on approximately March 23rd each year. This means most mares are stabled for approximately 5–6 months during their pregnancy. The rest of the year,

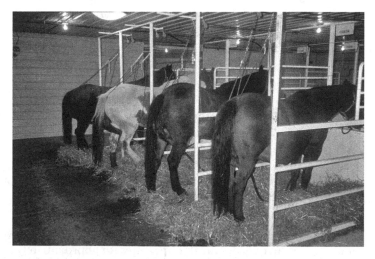

Figure 16.2 Inside a PMU barn during the collection season; mares have access to good-quality forage and water delivered by one of several watering systems.

the mares are turned out in either improved or native pastures to deliver their foals, for re-breeding, and for rearing their foals. Most ranches have other horses on the premises being kept either on pasture or in corrals. Other horses include younger replacement stock, pregnant mares not 'on-line,' barren mares, stallions, and riding horses used by the owners. Some ranches have pasture contiguous to the property where the barn is located, while others are more fragmented, with land scattered in different locations in the general vicinity of the main facility.

A variety of horse breeds are represented in the population of mares on these ranches, including Belgian, Shire, Percheron, Clydesdale, Quarter Horse, Appaloosa, Arabian, Curly Coats, Paints, as well as a variety of crossbred (Thoroughbred–draft horse cross also known as a Canadian sport horse) and grade types. Initially, the heavy breeds were overrepresented in the population of mares on PMU ranches, but currently there are more light breeds represented than heavy breeds. Likewise, there were initially more grade horses utilized for collection of PMU, but now the majority of mares are purebred mares due to the incentives available to ranchers for maintaining purebred mares and producing more marketable foals. The ranches with purebred horses have their own private production sales of foals in the fall after weaning; those farms with crossbred and grade horses sell their foals through public auction after weaning.

16.3 Welfare Issues with PMU Ranching

In 1995, the Canadian Farm Animal Care Trust (CANFACT) arranged and carried out an industry-wide inspection of randomly selected PMU farms in Manitoba Province (11 farms), Saskatchewan Province (11 farms), Alberta Province (10 farms), and the State of North Dakota (five farms) by a team of 12 inspectors consisting of equine veterinarians and equine welfare advocates. This inspection occurred during the collection season during the months of February and March, 1995. The purpose of the inspections was to determine if the management practices employed on these farms ensured that the care and welfare of the mares was satisfactory and if this industry represented a responsible and humane use of horses. Accompanying the inspection team during all farm visits were two representatives of the company. These representatives were in charge of their own team of inspectors who were employed by the company that monitors compliance by the ranchers with the COP. The inspectors employed by the company at that time were assigned to a specific number of farms in a geographic area. There were six inspectors and two supervisors, one of whom served as a seventh inspector. Each farm was inspected every 4–6 weeks to determine if the owner was in compliance with all aspects of the COP, and a report was filed with the company. These inspection reports were one of the determinants used to justify renewal of the annual contracts that ranchers enter into with the company. The inspectors also serve as consultants to the rancher in regards to equipment, feed, or other management issues.

During this inspection, approximately 5000 mares were observed housed in tie stalls with a collection harness suspended around them for the purpose of collecting PMU. The CANFACT inspectors were allowed full access to the facilities, barns, the mares, and any available records, and were able to talk with the ranchers, ask questions about PMU ranching, and take photographs. The ranchers were aware that the inspection team was in their vicinity, but they did not know which ranches were slated for inspection until the morning of the inspection, as the team randomly selected which ranches to inspect between 7 and 8 a.m. each day. Overall, the inspection revealed that the mares used for collection of PMU were in good to excellent physical condition; were housed in clean, well-ventilated barns; were fed good-quality hay and concentrate; and were free from signs of infectious diseases commonly encountered in groups of horses held in close confinement (Figure 16.3). Despite allegations by animal activists, the mares are able to lie down in their tie stalls. It appeared that the ranchers were in compliance with the current COP in the majority of cases and, where they may not have been exactly in compliance, there were no particular adverse consequences for the mares.

The inspection team did identify a few areas of concern and made the following recommendations that would hopefully improve the health and welfare of the mares used for the collection of PMU:

(1) Develop a more comprehensive inspection process and report form, which addresses all aspects of PMU ranches; no inspector be allowed to inspect a farm more than four times per year; all farms be inspected by all inspectors each year; each farm have unannounced veterinary inspections at least annually during the production season; annual inspection reports summary be reviewed by an independent review board and be provided to the producer; enforce the COP wherever the rancher fails to comply.

(2) Ensure that lead rope and/or chain ties are of sufficient length to allow the horse to lie down comfortably; a quick-release mechanism should be provided for each tie in case of fire or entanglement; establish guidelines to be added to the COP for fire prevention and evacuation of horses in case of fire; fund studies to determine the merits of exercise in pregnant mares confined to stalls for 5–6 months of their pregnancy, concentrating on defining the underlying causes of problems currently blamed on lack of exercise; construct exercise yards so they are more convenient and safe, so that exercise yards mentioned be located adjacent or connected to the barn by alleys which make turnout of all (including 'unbroken') mares convenient and possible.

(3) The company should fund research from monies collected from ranchers via the research check-off system which will determine what dietary factors including water, if any, affect urine quality, by what mechanisms, and are these dietary adjustments safe for the mares; these results should be distributed to the rancher in understandable format to be applied on each farm. Production of the highest-quality urine from the smallest number of mares to meet industry

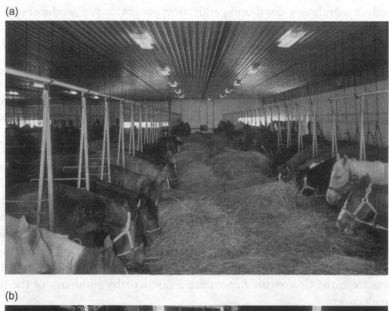

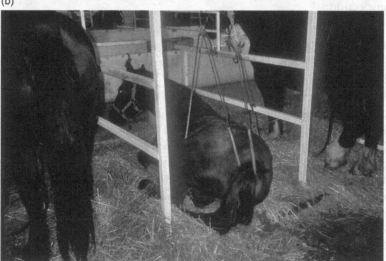

Figure 16.3 (a) PMU mares in their tie stalls during the collection season. (b) PMU mare lying down in a tie stall with collection harness in place.

demands should be everyone's goal; no more mares should be kept on-line than is necessary to meet demands of the industry.

(4) Use enough bedding and/or replace existing bedding frequently enough that the floors of the stall and the area just behind the stall is covered with enough bedding to provide a cushion between the floor and hoof /horse for the majority of the day.

(5) Conduct mandatory continuing education programs for producers on equine health care relevant to the PMU industry. Make regular visits by a licensed veterinarian a necessary part of the health-care program for each farm.

In 1997, a smaller team of inspectors made up of individuals from the 1995 CANFACT inspection team and representing the Canadian Veterinary Medical Association, the American Association of Equine Practitioners, and the International League for the Protection of Horses made a follow-up inspection of a number of PMU ranches during the collection season. The purpose of the follow-up visits was to evaluate the progress made in responding to recommendations from the CANFACT inspections, as well as to evaluate the Continuous Improvement Process (CIP) initiated by Wyeth to address more proactively the health and welfare of mares used for the collection of PMU. The results of that inspection were summarized in a document called the *Equine Veterinarians' Consensus Report on the Care of Horses on PMU Ranches*, which was submitted to Wyeth and to the respective organizations of the inspection team members (NAERIC, 1997). The following statements from the *Consensus Report* are a noteworthy summary of the findings of this inspection:

- The use of PMU horses to produce a commodity for the benefit of mankind is responsible and justified, as long as the horses receive the type of humane care observed on these ranches.
- There is evidence that Wyeth-Ayerst and the PMU ranchers are concerned with maintaining and improving the care, health, and welfare of horses on PMU ranches.
- The ranchers showed a pride in their animals and a concern for their well-being. The facilities and management are good. Horses observed were bright, alert, and apparently free of significant vices or stereotypic behaviors.
- There has been progress as a result of the 1995 inspection by 12 inspectors with the Canadian Farm Animal Care Trust. Their recommendations have either been implemented, such as enhanced field inspections and veterinary care, or are being investigated in well-designed studies.
- Notwithstanding the progress that has been made since the 1995 inspection, two areas of management, water and exercise, should continue to be given priority to evaluate to what extent modifications to existing practices may be appropriate.
- PMU mares receive quality feed and water, and in many respects the care is comparable to that given horses, or for that matter any livestock, used for other purposes in North America.
- Compliance with the recommended COP, a self-imposed, self-regulated set of guidelines established several years ago and recently updated, was generally good. Where minor differences from the COP were noted by the inspection team on a few farms, at no time did they appear to adversely affect the health and welfare of the mares. The quality of management compensated for these differences.

- Wyeth-Ayerst's CIP addresses the unique management needs concerning urine collection. The field inspection, trailer inspection, veterinary health review and reporting procedures, barn improvement program, and the appointment of two advisory groups are all evidence of the company's dedication and commitment.
- The Linwood Equine Ranch, established by the company, provides the opportunity for research that would benefit the horse world in general as well as PMU mares in particular.

The 1997 inspection team made the following conclusions: the ranchers took pride in their animals, and Wyeth-Ayerst showed a commitment to continuing to improve the standards of equine welfare on the farms; the allegations of inhumane treatment of horses involved in PMU ranching are unfounded; the horses are very well cared for; the ranchers and the company have responded in a progressive and proactive manner to both professional and public interest; observations and recommendations for improvement have been taken seriously and continue to be acted upon by Wyeth-Ayerst and the PMU ranchers; and the public should be assured that the care and welfare of the horses involved in the production of an estrogen replacement medication is good, and is closely monitored.

16.4 Continuous Improvement Process

As a response both to recommendations put forth by the CANFACT inspectors and to continued outside criticism of PMU ranching from animal advocacy activists, Wyeth initiated a comprehensive program to demonstrate their ongoing commitment to the health and welfare of the horses within the PMU industry. The Continuous Improvement Program (CIP), which involves several components, was developed by equine veterinarians, quality assurance specialists, and ranchers to ensure the health and well-being of the horses involved, identifying issues within the industry, and developing strategies to improve mare and ranch management. These management strategies include such steps as monthly ranch inspections by field inspectors employed by Wyeth, a veterinary herd health review program conducted three times per year by independent veterinarians, and barn improvement programs, to name a few (Freeman, 2000). As part of the CIP, they also purchased and converted an existing PMU ranch into a model operating PMU ranch for research and educational purposes. Under the direction of the managing veterinarian at this research facility, they conduct ongoing research on issues that potentially improve the health and welfare of mares used for collection of PMU, such as watering methods, exercise and confinement of pregnant mares, and the effects of confinement on health and behavior. The CIP included the appointment and formation of two outside advisory boards that provide expertise on both the overall management of ranches (the Equine Management Group) and research efforts and needs within the industry (the Equine Research Advisory Board). As a consequence of all this, PMU ranching has in place more checks and balances to ensure animal care and welfare than virtually any other livestock industry, making it one of the most regulated and scrutinized equine activities in North America.

16.5 Research Initiatives

The most significant welfare concerns identified by outside inspectors and animal welfare advocates have been watering systems and protocols utilized on PMU ranches; behavioral and health consequences of continuous confinement of pregnant mares for six months; and the disposition of the foals after weaning. To address these concerns, both the company and independent outside investigators have conducted a number of studies that have been published as peer-reviewed articles.

The methods utilized to provide water for PMU mares while stabled during the collection season vary among the ranchers all the way from providing water in buckets to an automated, timed, intermittent delivery system. In one study, 22 light breed and 18 draft breed stabled mares were provided water continuously or by one of three intermittent water delivery systems (Freeman *et al.*, 1998, 1999). Various physical and laboratory parameters were measured on mares being provided water from each watering system and compared with one another. Such things as body temperature, attitude, appetite, water intake, urine output, and horse and stable hygiene were measured daily. Clinical measures of hydration (skin turgor, gum moisture, capillary refill time, and fecal consistency) and biochemical measures of hydration (packed-cell volume (PCV), plasma total protein concentration, serum osmolality, urine specific gravity, and urine osmolality) were measured three separate times during each phase of the study. The results of this study showed that all mares remained healthy for the duration of the study, clinical and biochemical measures of hydration did not differ among water delivery systems, and both horse and stable hygiene were worse when horses had continuous access to water. The study concluded that all of the water systems evaluated provided adequate amounts of water to stabled horses to maintain health and hydration status.

In another study looking at restricted water intake below *ad libitum* water intake in six pregnant mares, it was found that, as water intake decreased from an *ad libitum* water intake of 6.9 liters per 100 kg body weight (bwt) in stages down to 3 liters per 100 kg bwt, there was a corresponding proportional decrease in feed intake and decrease in body weight over the three-week study period (Houpt *et al.*, 2000). There was also an increase in serum osmolality as water intake decreased, but PCV and plasma total protein did not change significantly. Cortisol levels decreased as water intake decreased. The only change in behavior that occurred was a decrease in the time spent eating. The study concluded that water restriction below *ad libitum* intake (4 liters per 100 kg bwt or less) does cause dehydration in pregnant mares and may diminish their welfare, but is not life- or pregnancy-threatening.

Based on the guidelines for provision of water included in the COP, it appears that PMU mares receive adequate amounts of water and that, regardless of the watering system used, the mares remain healthy and reasonably well-hydrated if they consume at least 4 liters per 100 kg bwt of water per day.

The behavioral and health consequences of continuous stabling of pregnant mares being provided water by a variety of watering systems has been studied as well. One study compared quantitative measures and clinical assessments of behavior as an indication of psychologic well-being in stabled pregnant mares over a two-year period of time (McDonnell et al., 1998, 1999). In this study continuous 24-hour videotaped samples were used to compare quantitative measures and clinical assessments of behavior among groups of stabled mares provided water by various water delivery systems. A computer-based event recorder was used to record frequency and duration of each of the following behaviors: eating hay, drinking water, standing rest, recumbent rest, interacting with adjacent horse (on the basis of type of interaction, i.e., affiliative or aggressive, and role of interaction, i.e., initiator or target), stereotypy (e.g., cribbing and head bobbing), and object chewing. In addition, an experienced equine behavior clinician who was blinded as to the type of watering system reviewed the summary quantitative data of each horse to make an overall clinical assessment of behavior. This study concluded that all horses had clinically normal behavior regardless of the type of watering system used and despite being confined to a tie stall for extended periods of time.

In another behavioral study, the amount of time confined pregnant mares engaged in behavioral activities, also known as time budgets, was compared between light and draft mares under similar housing, feed, and water management, and also compared to time budgets of feral free-range horses (Flannigan and Stookey, 2002). Similar behaviors as described in previous studies were recorded from 55 light and 55 draft late pregnant mares housed in tie stalls using continuous video recording. Light mares spent significantly more time feeding and significantly less time standing active and standing resting. Time spent resting in a recumbent position, total time spent resting, and the amount of time spent drinking was not significantly different between light and draft mares. Likewise, the number of activity changes and interactions with neighboring mares were not significantly different between the two breed types. The time budget of both groups fell within the range of activity budgets of free-range feral horses. There was also no significant difference in the number of horses performing stereotypies between light and draft mares. When the time budgets of both light and draft mares that performed stereotypies were pooled, the activities did not differ significantly from their counterparts that did not perform stereotypies. This study concluded that, because of the low prevalence of stereotypies and because the time budgets were similar to those of free-range horses, the management practice of keeping large numbers of pregnant mares in tie stalls is rational and the welfare of mares is sound (Flannigan and Stookey, 2002).

In addition to the studies described previously regarding the effects of various methods of providing water for the mares on their health and welfare and the behavior of mares involved in the PMU industry, other studies have been performed to evaluate the effects of confinement of pregnant mares on their overall health. One study was designed to determine the effects of an extended period of restricted movement during the collection of PMU on aerobic fitness and well-being of pregnant mares (Sparks *et al.*, 1999). One group of mares in their seventh month of gestation were housed continuously for a 90-day period in tie stalls that were constructed according to guidelines in the COP. Another group of mares in their seventh month of gestation were maintained in pasture. One week before the trial began both groups of mares were subjected to an exercise test on a high-speed treadmill where heart rate was recorded during and following the exercise test. Blood samples were collected for determination of lactate levels before, during, and after exercise. On the last day of the study a second exercise test was administered, with each mare performing the exact work as she performed in the first exercise test, with heart rates and blood samples taken as during the first test. Of the parameters studied, there were no differences between the confined mares and the mares kept on pasture. Such things as length of gestation, viability of foals, heart rates, blood lactate concentrations, and tolerance for exercise did not differ between groups or between the beginning and end of the study. The study concluded that restriction of movement by housing in a tie stall for a 90-day period had no effect on aerobic fitness or on the ability to carry and deliver a healthy foal (Sparks *et al.*, 1999).

Another study looking at foal mortality rates between 466 PMU mares and 167 mares from extensively managed ranches found no significant difference in foal mortalities between the two types of ranches (Burwash *et al.*, 1999).

The disposition of the offspring of the pregnant mares used for the collection of PMU has been one of the most contentious welfare issues confronting the industry. In the earliest days of PMU ranching, when many of the mares were unregistered or grade mares, many of the foals were probably purchased after weaning at 4–5 months of age and taken to feedlots to be prepared for processing for human consumption. Some of the female offspring were retained by the ranchers as replacement mares for urine collection when they were old enough to be bred, and some of the male offspring were kept to be used for riding and ranch work. Contrary to popular belief, the foals were not slaughtered right after weaning at a very young age, but they were maintained in the feedlots and fed a nutritious diet until they were 2–3 years of age, at which time they were processed for food. Animal activists and the public in the USA have always opposed this practice and continue to do so today. But equine veterinarians, animal welfare advocates, the agricultural community, and PMU ranchers view processing of horses for human consumption as a legitimate and humane method of euthanasia (AAEP, 2008).

Because of the increasing concern and outside scrutiny directed at PMU ranching by animal activists, the ranchers themselves became more proactive in their own defense of the industry and became organized under the direction of the North

American Equine Ranching Information Council (NAERIC). Under this organization's guidance and direction, PMU ranchers have made significant improvements to the quality and marketability of their horses, so that the majority of offspring from PMU mares are now being raised and purchased for a variety of equine performance activities and events in North America rather than being purchased for consignment to the feedlot. Through NAERIC, several programs have been instituted to ensure that PMU ranching is able to realize its full potential. Such programs include, just to name a few: a breeding enhancement program to increase the use of Thoroughbred stallions in crossbreeding with mares to produce valuable sport horses; the NAERIC Advantage Program®, a value-added program for horses bred on NAERIC member ranches and registered with NAERIC, with more than 40 000 horses registered with NAERIC and eligible to earn NAERIC Advantage rewards; and the Mounted Police Horse Program. These various NAERIC incentive programs offered to PMU ranchers have significantly increased the number of registered horses raised and maintained by ranchers thereby, ensuring that the welfare of offspring from PMU mares is now greatly improved as compared to the early days of PMU ranching.

16.6 PMU Ranching Today

Beginning in 2003, Wyeth initiated significant downsizing of the PMU industry in response to reduced market demands for their product Prempro™ brought about by results from the Women's Health Initiative Studies (WHI, 2003) that indicated there were significant health risks for women taking the currently recommended doses of conjugated estrogens in combination with progestin. In order to impose this mandatory downsizing effort on the ranchers in a fair and equitable manner, Wyeth established a multi-million-dollar trust fund to help ranchers not getting their contracts renewed by the company to disperse their horses to markets other than feedlots and processing, and to help the ranchers themselves transition into other job opportunities. This meant that the displaced ranchers, with guidance and assistance from NAERIC and the Equine Placement Trust Fund (EPTF) Advisory Board, had to find suitable homes for nearly 25 000 mares in a period of 18–24 months. The financial assistance from the EPTF helped to pay for the upkeep of the mares in transition, in marketing the mares for sale, and with the costs of transportation and veterinary export expenses to the new homes for the mares, and included a reasonable severance package for the ranchers themselves. The downsizing brought the number of ranches down to approximately 80 ranches, and concentrated the ranches in Saskatchewan Province, Manitoba Province, and the State of North Dakota to reduce the costs of transportation of the bulk urine to the manufacturing plant in Brandon, Manitoba. This significantly reduced the number of mares used for collection of PMU, which was one of the recommendations and goals of the outside inspection teams, i.e., production of the highest-quality urine from the smallest number of mares to meet industry demands. The downsizing effort was carried out efficiently and from all accounts accomplished its goals with few exceptions.

Despite significant external and internal challenges, the PMU industry has survived and flourished. As PMU ranchers continue to work to demonstrate to the public that their practices are sound and the levels of care and welfare on PMU ranches are high, Wyeth, NAERIC, and the ranchers themselves have developed an unprecedented system of self-regulation not seen elsewhere in the equine industry. In recognition of these efforts, in 2009 the American Association of Equine Practitioners awarded NAERIC with the Lavin Cup, which is given out annually to a non-veterinary organization or individual that has demonstrated exceptional compassion or developed and enforced rules and guidelines for the welfare of horses.

References

AAEP (2008) Position on the transportation and processing of horses. *American Association of Equine Practitioners Resource Guide*. American Association of Equine Practitioners, Lexington, KY.

Burwash, L.D., Pritchard, J. and Coleman, R.J. (1999) Foal mortality on extensively managed farms. In *Proceedings of the 16th Equine Nutrition and Physiology Society Symposium*, Raleigh, NC, pp. 247–248. Equine Science Society, Champaign, IL.

Flannigan, G. and Stookey, J.M. (2002) Day-time budgets of pregnant mares housed in tie stalls: a comparison of draft versus light mares. *Applied Animal Behavior Science* 78, 125–143.

Freeman, D.A. (2000) The pregnant mares' urine industry – management and research. *Journal of the American Veterinary Medical Association* 216, 1239–1242.

Freeman, D.A., Cymbaluk, N.F., Kyle, B., Schott, H.C., Hinchcliff, K.W. and McDonnell, S.M. (1998) Health and welfare of stabled PMU mares under varied water and turnout schedules: 1. Physiology. In *Proceedings of the 44th Annual Convention of the AAEP*, pp. 19–20.

Freeman, D.A., Cymbaluk, N.F., Schott, H.C., Schott, H.C., Hinchcliff, K., McDonnell, S.M. and Kyle, B. (1999) Clinical, biochemical, and hygiene assessment of stabled horses provided continuous or intermittent access to drinking water. *American Journal of Veterinary Research* 60, 1445–1450.

Houpt, K.A., Eggleston, A., Kunkle, K. and Houpt, T.R. (2000) Effect of water restriction on equine behavior and physiology. *Equine Veterinary Journal* 32, 341–344.

Manitoba Department of Agriculture (1990) *Recommended Code of Practice for the Care and Handling of Horses in PMU Operations*. Canadian Agri-Food Research Council, Ottawa.

McDonnell, S.M., Freeman, D.A., Cymbaluk, N.F. *et al.* (1998) Health and welfare of stabled PMU mares under various watering methods and turnout schedules: behavior. In *Proceedings of the 44th Annual Convention of the AAEP*, pp. 21–22.

McDonnell, S.M., Freeman, D.A., Cymbaluk, N.F., Schott, H.C., Hinchcliff, K. and Kyle, B. (1999) Behavior of stabled horses provided continuous or intermittent access to drinking water. *American Journal of Veterinary Research* 60, 1451–1456.

NAERIC (1997) *Equine Veterinarians' Consensus Report on the Care of Horses on PMU Ranches*. North American Equine Ranching Council, Louisville, KY.

NAERIC (2007) *Recommended Code of Practice for the Care and Handling of Horses in PMU Operations*. North American Equine Ranching Council, Louisville, KY. See: http://www.naeric.org/.

Sparks, C.R., Topliff, D.R., Collie, M.E., Freeman, D.W. and Breazile, J.E. (1999) The influence of restricted movement on the physical fitness and well-being of pregnant mares. In *Proceedings of the 16th Equine Nutrition and Physiology Society Symposium*, Raleigh, NC, pp. 251–252. Equine Science Society, Champaign, IL.

Stevenson, W.G. (1945) Pregnant mares' urine as a source of estrogens. *Canadian Journal of Comparative Medicine* 9, 293–301.

WHI (2003) *Women's Health Initiative Estrogen-Plus-Progestin Study*. Available at: http://www.nhlbi.nih.gov/whi/estro_pro.htm.

Zondek, B. (1934) Mass excretion of estrogenic hormone in the urine of the stallion. *Nature* 133, 209–210.

Welfare in the Discipline of Dressage

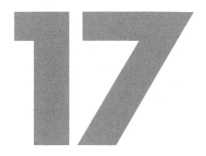

Midge Leitch

Possible problems with the welfare of horses in competition, while acknowledged to exist, have not traditionally been a concern of the general public or the veterinary profession involved in their care. Abusive training techniques, offensive in nature, are usually ignored by those dealing with their medical aftermath, while the audience engrossed in the spectacle gives little thought to the quality of the lives of the horses involved.

While dressage is not usually among those disciplines which initially come to mind when welfare is the topic under consideration, there are areas of concern that apply in general to horses in competition as well as specific issues that apply to these particular horses. As in many other areas of training, inexperience and incompetence can lead to misuse and abuse, which may or may not be intentional.

17.1 General Husbandry

The care and training of horses embarking on a career in dressage should be approached with a long-range plan. No other discipline requires the length of time in training to develop horses capable of the highest level of performance, the Grand Prix. The average dressage horse is expected to be prepared to perform at that level only after 5–7 years of training, at the age of 9–12. The most successful breeds tend to be slow to mature, larger in stature, and the result of the introduction of the hot-blooded strains into the more stolid carriage horse breeds. Such breeding efforts, initiated in Europe, decades ago, have resulted in the warmblood breeds that we recognize today as the most successful candidates for a career in dressage.

In the author's opinion, certain routine husbandry practices promote agitation and erratic behavior in horses, especially those involved in intensive training regimens. For instance, because of limited space in most European countries

Equine Welfare, First Edition. Edited by C. Wayne McIlwraith and Bernard E. Rollin.
© 2011 by UFAW. Published 2011 by Blackwell Publishing Ltd.

specializing in the breeding and training of warmblood horses intended for dressage, turnout exercise is not included in the daily routine of most horses past the age of two. Time spent on mechanical walking machines may promote an increase in the level of fitness but does not replace unsupervised exercise, which allows horses to unwind mentally as well as stretch and flex their musculoskeletal system without the restriction of either training aids or the weight of a rider.

Arguments against turnout exercise revolve primarily about admonitions concerning possible injury. In my experience, horses that have not had turnout exercise eliminated from their routines and horses to which turnout exercise is carefully introduced or reintroduced, which may involve the initial utilization of sedation, are unlikely to be at greater risk of injury than their stall-confined counterparts. More likely, the latter are often at greater risk from training injuries sustained as a result in inadequate opportunities to stretch and relax.

Mounting energy, which accompanies confinement, coupled with the anxiety associated with training demands, is, in my opinion, much more constructively dealt with by the freedom of turnout exercise than by additional training efforts or controlled exercise designed to produce fatigue or compliance. The latter frequently utilizes excessive longeing (lungeing) or exercise under tack, neither of which encourage relaxation and calm. In the adult horse, this uncontrolled energy results in a horse that is unable to relax during competitions and is often unable to participate in awards ceremonies without the likelihood of danger to itself and/or others.

17.2 Travel Preparations

Since most people who undertake serious dressage training have competition as an end-point, travel to events becomes an integral part of the horse's routine. Gradual introduction to shipping by restricting initial trailer or van trips to short excursions, while carefully training horses to load and unload without excitement, will diminish the anxiety that may be associated with these experiences. It should be readily apparent that a horse that arrives at a competition in a relaxed frame of mind, free of self-inflicted injury from kicking or pawing during transport, is more likely to perform at its best.

Long-distance transportation requires additional planning to ensure adequate hydration, protection from injury, and reasonable recovery time upon arrival. Transportation by air, in my experience, appears to be far less fatiguing for most horses than comparable time spent on the road. While airport quarantine, airplane loading and unloading, and takeoff and landing may be perceived as more stressful situations, the relaxation of the actual flight, without the stopping, starting and turning of vehicle transportation, usually lends itself to chewing hay, drinking, and napping. Horses arrive in remarkably rested condition, less leg-weary, though some may be a little stiff from confinement to a stall for the length of the trip. Providing time in the trip schedule to allow these horses a day or so to relax before they resume full work will usually restore them to their pre-trip status. Again, hand walking on the first day will provide the maximum benefit to muscles somewhat stiff from confinement and will lead to better comfort when work under saddle begins.

Withholding large carbohydrate loads during transportation is more likely to diminish the possibility of illness associated with incomplete digestion, which can result from less than optimal gastrointestinal function that often accompanies travel. Providing good-quality forage, to which the horse has already been accustomed at home, in conjunction with fresh water, again preferably brought from home, are the best preventive measures that one can take to avoid digestive upset.

17.3 Training Methods

As with any upper-level competition horse, the better the foundation, the more likely the success. Focus on this maxim during selection of a prospect may help to minimize the difficulties faced during training that result from conformational deficits. Innate talent, which of course may help to overcome physical imperfections, is an often indefinable characteristic in the very young horse, so building on the best foundation that can be discovered is the next best choice. The personal preference of the rider and/or trainer in type and attitude is naturally important and should be considered while assessing the strengths and weaknesses that accompany specific conformations. Flexibility must be accompanied by support and strength in these horses which are required to work in both collected and extended frames.

The dressage horse is generally described as the ballet dancer of the equine world when a more accurate description would be the weightlifter of the equine world. This discipline requires the development of impulsion without momentum, a considerably more difficult feat than producing speed (racehorses) or elevation (jumpers). Initial fitness should be addressed in the early stages of training in a similar fashion as it is in other non-racing performance disciplines. Work that continues in the face of fatigue is more likely to produce injury than effective fitness.

Overall fitness of dressage horses is often neglected. Many horses present at competitions, even at the upper level, overweight and unfit – conditions that may go unrecognized by their riders and trainers. Injuries directly related to fatigue are the result. These include suspensory desmitis, tendonitis (more often affecting the deep digital flexor tendons in the hind legs than the superficial digital flexor tendon), and muscular soreness. Many riders, trainers, and veterinarians involved with dressage horses are unfortunately unaware of the real danger of tendonitis and suspensory desmitis and often overlook these problems in the early stages when the possibility of complete resolution is possible. Too often, by the time such soft tissue lesions are recognized, permanent damage is the result and careers negatively impacted.

The epaxial musculature requires concentrated task-specific work in order to result in strength which will accommodate the amount and type of work that is the standard of training under saddle. More than in any other discipline, supporting the weight and movement as the rider engages the aids becomes a challenge for the dressage horse. The length of the daily training regimen is often considerably longer than in other disciplines, and riders may fail to recognize initial signs, requiring horses to continue to train while muscles fatigue.

Simultaneously, cardiovascular and respiratory fitness must not be overlooked, and this may remain unrecognized by inexperienced and poorly informed trainers and riders. The upper-level dressage horse is traditionally exposed to periods of intense exercise during the training regimen, the warm-up period prior to competition, as well as during the competition itself. The length of these periods may be deceptive, as the average test lasts about 12 minutes; however, the intensity of the work requires continuous maximal effort. Excessive length of the warm-up is a common training misunderstanding that results in many horses leaving their best efforts in the warm-up arena and producing disappointing efforts in the competition arena, which are then followed by additional corrective training efforts that are likely to be ineffective if not abusive.

Exhausted horses in the warm-up arena or following a performance, with sides heaving, nostrils flaring, and excessive lathering of the flanks and neck, are indications of work beyond a reasonable level of fitness, which should be addressed if the best interests of the horse are to be protected. Veterinarians and stewards need better guidelines and support if they are to monitor these aspects of competitions and enforce reasonable regulations.

17.4 Competition Regulations

The extent of required evaluations at the upper levels of competition are established by the Fédération Equestre Internationale (FEI, the International Equestrian Federation) (www.fei.org), which mandates pre-competition examinations. These consist of abbreviated physical examinations referred to as 'in-barn examinations' and the official jog or presentation of competing horses before the official FEI veterinarian and a member or members of the judging panel known as the Ground Jury in a check for soundness at the trot.

Stewarding at recognized competitions that fall under the auspices of the United States Equestrian Federation (USEF), the United States Dressage Federation (USDF) or the FEI endeavors to guard against excessive use of aids by the implementation of bit and spur checks as horses exit the ring. These examinations attempt to insure that the types of bit and spurs fall within the mandated guidelines and that there is no evidence of injury secondary to their use. The presence of blood in the commissures of the lips or on the tongue resulting from injury from bits or bleeding on the flanks secondary to inappropriate use of spurs is cause for elimination from competition. These examinations have virtually eliminated the practice of amputation of portions of the front of the tongue in an effort to prohibit protrusion of the tongue, which is a habit acquired by some horses during periods of tension. Considered an 'indication of resistance by the horse' during competition, unethical trainers utilized this barbaric method to camouflage the results of improper training techniques, which resulted in anxiety rather than comfort during the learning process.

The FEI website states that 'manufacturers of bits, saddlery and other horse equipment who wish to have their products approved under FEI Dressage Rules shall, as of fall 2008, submit samples for testing by the FEI/IDRC (International Dressage Riders Club) Panel.'

The Bitless Bridle™,[1] developed by Robert Cook, is proposed as a solution to the potential discomfort or abuse posed by a bit; however, its acceptance in the competition world has been slow.

Most competitions provide supervision during the hours of competition and precompetition warm-up. FEI-level competitions require horses to remain in their stalls, except during designated hours for which supervision is constant. Human traffic in the stabling area is closely monitored and even accompanied, when access after closure of the stables is necessary. Nonetheless, abusive training methods have not been completely eliminated. What constitutes abuse? 'When you see it, you will know it,' responds Elizabeth Williams, FEI Chief Steward General of Dressage for the USA. Besides excessive periods of exercise or abusive riding, these training abuses include, but are not limited to, the following:

(1) Nosebands tightened excessively and/or fitted too high on the face of the horse in an effort to eliminate any opening of the mouth which is considered a resistance, receiving negative marks.
(2) Improper bits and/or their improper use resulting in injury to the commissures of the lips or cuts in the dorsal surface of the tongue.
(3) Curb chains tightened excessively resulting in compression of the circulation to the tongue.
(4) Excessive use of the aids:
   • spurs
   • whips – the use of double whips has been outlawed
   • side reins extending from the bit to the girth – utilized without adequate length resulting in overflexion of the neck when horses are being longed or ridden
   • draw reins extending from the girth between the front legs, through the bit to the rider's hands – utilized to draw the horse's head to an excessively low position and/or to create overflexion of the neck when horses are being ridden.

The FEI addressed a specific method of training defined as 'over-bending or hyperflexion (ventroflexion),' commonly referred to as rollkur, in the report of

---

[1] See www.bitlessbridle.com.

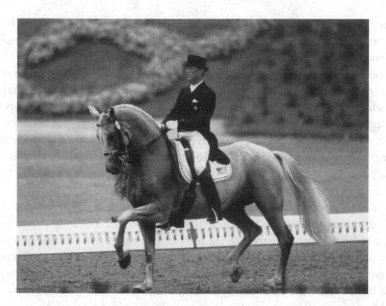

Figure 17.1 A horse being ridden in the rollkur position during training. (Courtesy of the FEI website.)

a combined meeting of the FEI Veterinary and Dressage Committees in May, 2006 (see Figure 17.1). Increasing public concern over this training method led to publications within the scientific literature (Van Breda, 2006) and the combined committee developed the following definition containing admonitions (FEI, 2006a):

> Hyperflexion of the neck is a technique of working/training to provide a degree of longitudinal flexion of the mid-region of the neck that cannot be self-maintained by the horse for a prolonged time without welfare implications. There must be an understanding that hyperflexion as a training aid must be used correctly, as the technique can be an abuse when attempted by an inexperienced/unskilled rider/trainer.

The FEI Veterinary Subcommittee on Welfare, founded as recently as 2004, agreed that the use of this training method by experienced and competent hands, for short periods of time during the training regimen, resulted in no apparent abuse or clinical side-effects. However, a strong assertion that 'hyperflexion is a welfare issue in the hands of the unskilled' (FEI, 2006b) was included in the report's conclusions. The Subcommittee was directed to identify research that would unequivocally determine the clinical effects on the horse of this training technique. Neither the specific nature of these research projects nor their findings have yet been made available.

Providing adequate means of relaxation at competitions is always a challenge, regardless of the discipline. Adequate space for quiet hand walking is almost never a primary concern of management. Thus, for most horses, any escape from stall confinement almost always necessitates their being ridden. An unfortunate result of this absence of hand walking in stress-filled environments is a horse that becomes nearly uncontrollable in hand in such circumstances and so is even more restricted to exercise under saddle. Such individuals are frequently seen at the official presentation before the Ground Jury presenting a danger to their handlers, spectators, and themselves. There are those unscrupulous trainers or riders who encourage such behavior in the belief that it may conceal lamenesses or discourage close examination for spur injuries, but these efforts are rarely met with success. The end-result is a horse that is deprived of the only remaining opportunity to stretch and relax at a competition.

Maintaining good nutrition and adequate hydration during competitions can prove challenging with some horses. Different grain and hay may prove unpalatable and, combined with the stress of the new and strange environment, may increase the tendency to drink and/or eat too little. Transporting grain, hay, and water from home may be optimal but may not be possible in many instances. Teaching horses to drink water that has been flavored with small amounts of electrolyte powder may help to camouflage an unfamiliar taste or smell. Salting hay to encourage water consumption can be effective as well.

Rules governing nutritional supplements must be considered, and assurances from manufacturers that their products are compliant will not serve as a successful defense if positive drug tests occur. It is especially difficult to have confidence in the reliability of herbal supplements to remain within the dictates of the regulations and to avoid resulting in positive tests. Both national and international governing bodies have forbidden the use of many herbs suggested to have calming effects, regardless of the proof of their effectiveness. Sprinkled liberally among examples of forbidden substances provided by the USEF in their *Drugs and Medications Guidelines* pamphlet (USEF, 2007) is a multitude of herbal compounds:

acepromazine, acetophenazine, acetylpromazine, albuterol, alfentanil, alprazolam, aminophylline, amitriptyline, amphetamines, antihistamines, apomorphine, arsenic, atropine azaperone, barbiturates, belladonna, benperidol, benzocaine, benzodiazepines, beta blockers, bethanechol chloride, bromperidol, bumetanide, bupivacaine, buprenorphine, buspirone, butorphanol, caffeine, camphor, capsaicin, carfentanil, carprofen, chamomile, chloral hydrate, chlorbutanol, chlorpheniramine, chlorpromazine, chlorprothixene, clenbuterol, clozapine, cocaine, codeine, comfrey, cyclobenzaprine, cyproheptadine, dantrolene, demethylpyrilamine, detomidine, devil's claw, dextromethorphan, dextromoramide, dezocine, diazepam, digoxin, diphenhydramine, dipremorphine, dipyrone, doxapram, doxepin, droperidol, dyphylline, ephedrine, epinephrine, epoetin alfa, erythropoietin, etamiphylline, ethacrynic acid, ethchlorvynol, ethyl alcohol, etidocaine, etodolac, etomidate, etorphine, eugenol, fenfluramine, fenspiride, fentanyl, fentiazac, fluanisone, fluoxetine, fluphenazine, furosemide, glycerol guaiacolate, glycopyrrolate, guaifenesin, guanabenz acetate, haloperidol, homatropine, hops, hydrochlorothiazide, hydrocodone, hydromorphone, hydroxyzine, imipramine, ipratropium, kava kava, ketamine, ketorolac, laurel, lavender, lemon balm, levallorphan, levorphanol, leopard's bane, lidocaine, lithium, lorazepam, LSD, mabuterol, mazindol, meclizine, medetomidine, meperidine, mepenzolate bromide, mephentermine, mepivacaine, meprylcaine, methadone, methamphetamine, methaqualone, methyldopa, methylphenidate, metomidate, milenperone, molindone, moperone, morphine, nalbuphine, nalmefene, naloxone, nefopam, night shade, nikethamide, nitrazepam, nitroglycerin, opiates, orphenadrine citrate, oxybutynin, oxymetazoline, oxymorphone, paroxetine, passion flower, pentazocine, pentoxifylline, pergolide mesylate, phencyclidine, Phenobarbital, phentermine, phenylephrine, phenylpropanolamine, phenytoin, piperacetazine, pirenperone, pramoxine, prazepam, prethcamide, prilocaine, procaine, procaine penicillin, procaterol, prochlorperazine, procyclidine, promazine, promethazine, propentofylline, propiomazine, propionylpromazine, propoxyphene, propranolol, pseudoephedrine, pyrilamine, rauwolfia, red poppy, reserpine, risperidone, romifidine, salmeterol, scopolamine, sertraline, skullcap, sodium cacodylate, spiperone, strychnine, sufentanil, sumatriptan, terbutaline sulfate, terfenadine, tetracaine, THC, theobromine, theophylline, tolmetin, tramadol, trazodone, trifluperidol, trihexyphenidyl, tripelennamine, tropicamide, valerian, vervain, xylazine, xylocaine, zolpidem.

Competitors are responsible for guarding against the presence of these and other substances, which are forbidden. The search for solutions to behavioral problems or simple excessive energy is unlikely to end, although the success of medications as the answer diminishes as the sophistication of drug testing advances. As in other disciplines, competitors occasionally turn to water and feed deprivation to produce an artificially quiet demeanor; however, the discipline of dressage is, for the most part, spared this abusive practice because of the sustained, high energy level required for performances.

In an effort to increase the height of the trot, passage, and piaffe, trainers have utilized weights in the form of pastern chains, similar to those used to elevate the gaits of the American Saddlebred. Applied while the horses are in the stall, as well as during training exercise by some, the intent is to increase the muscular effort required to lift the limbs as well as to exacerbate the effort because of the annoyance of the chain's action. In general, the effect is not a lasting one and the practice is not widespread.

17.5 Conclusion

Abuse in the discipline of dressage frequently occurs at the lower levels and involves incompetent training and riding techniques, which develop because the sport is perceived to be less dangerous than most equestrian activities. Individuals who are not mentally or physically equipped for more strenuous sports, such as eventing, hunting or jumping, select dressage as an outlet for their fondness for horses.

Subsequently they often expect their horses to learn to perform the movements without the proper training, which they are incapable of providing.

At the upper levels of the sport, abuse takes the form of training that forces the horse to attempt levels of collection, extension or complexity of movement for which it is not physically capable, or physically or mentally prepared.

Codes of behavior and regulations concerning equipment and medication are in place for competitors at both national and international level of competition. Further education of the stewards and veterinarians assigned to provide for the welfare of horses in competition is paramount if they are to recognize and prevent subtle forms of abusive riding and exercise beyond an individual horse's level of fitness and training.

References

FEI (2006a) *Report of the FEI Veterinary and Dressage Committees' Workshop: The Use of Over Bending ('Rollkur') in FEI Competition*, FEI Veterinary Committee Meeting at the Olympic Museum, Lausanne, January, p. 10. Fédération Equestre Internationale, Lausanne, Switzerland.

FEI (2006b) *Report of the FEI Veterinary and Dressage Committees' Workshop: The Use of Over Bending ('Rollkur') in FEI Competition*, FEI Veterinary Committee Meeting at the Olympic Museum, Lausanne, January, p. 11. Fédération Equestre Internationale, Lausanne, Switzerland.

USEF (2007) *Drugs and Medications Guidelines*, August. United States Equestrian Federation, Lexington, KY.

Van Breda, E. (2006) A non-natural head–neck position (rollkur) during training results in less acute stress in elite, trained, dressage horses. *Journal of Applied Animal Welfare Science* 9(1), 59–64.

Raising Welfare Standards for Endurance Riding

18

Nancy S. Loving

The horse has played a pivotal role in history, carrying humans into new frontiers as pioneers or warriors. Mounted man was more efficiently able to protect territorial borders, move livestock to verdant pastures, and reach other people for trade and communication. Whether serving as transportation or beast of burden, horses have secured their value in man's history for their ability to travel swiftly over long distances and difficult terrain.

The modern horse is now used mostly for recreational pursuits. The sport of endurance riding has capitalized on the equine capacity for stamina and fleetness of foot. In 1955, Californian Wendell Robie set out to prove that modern horses could accomplish long-distance travel comparable to that achieved by pioneers and the US Cavalry. Robie's vision was accurate: this first endurance ride emerged as the Western States Trail Ride (Tevis) – one rider, one horse ridden 100 miles in one day. (The Tevis still exists today; it is considered a distinct honor to complete.) The organization of the American Endurance Ride Conference (AERC) formed in 1972 to promote horse safety, rider education, and to standardize fair rules to prevent equine cruelty during these endurance tests (Frazier, 2000). In endurance pursuits, the welfare of the horse is the ultimate responsibility of the rider, but the organization of the ride by ride management and the quality of the veterinarian staff also affect the outcome.

18.1 What is Endurance Riding?

Distance riding takes many forms, each endurance discipline defined by its speed. Competitive trail horses move at a steady pace of 3.5–6 mph (about 5.6–9.6 km/h), where too fast or too slow accrues penalty points. Multi-day endurance rides cover 50 miles (80 km) each day for 3–5 days, with a steady pace of 6–10 mph (9.6–16 km/h)

Equine Welfare, First Edition. Edited by C. Wayne McIlwraith and Bernard E. Rollin.
© 2011 by UFAW. Published 2011 by Blackwell Publishing Ltd.

(a)

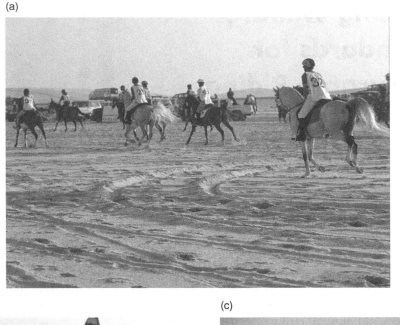

(b)   (c)

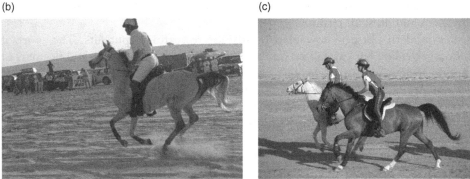

Figure 18.1 Desert competitions over 100 miles are often completed in less than 7 hours riding time.

giving the best chance of completing all days. These events are in contrast to higher-speed races against the clock as seen in endurance 'racing.' At the elite fulcrum of the sport, a well-prepared horse competing in Fédération Equestre Internationale (FEI, the International Equestrian Federation) competitions is able to transit 100 desert miles (160 km) in less than 7 hours riding time, maintaining an average speed of 14 mph (22.5 km/h) (Figure 18.1). In mountainous and wilderness terrain, front-running horses typically finish their 100-mile (160 km) journey in a riding time of 12–14 hours (Figure 18.2).

Most 100-mile competitions allow 24 hours for a horse to complete, while championship FEI endurance races require completion within 18 hours. Peppered within

(a)

(b)

(c)

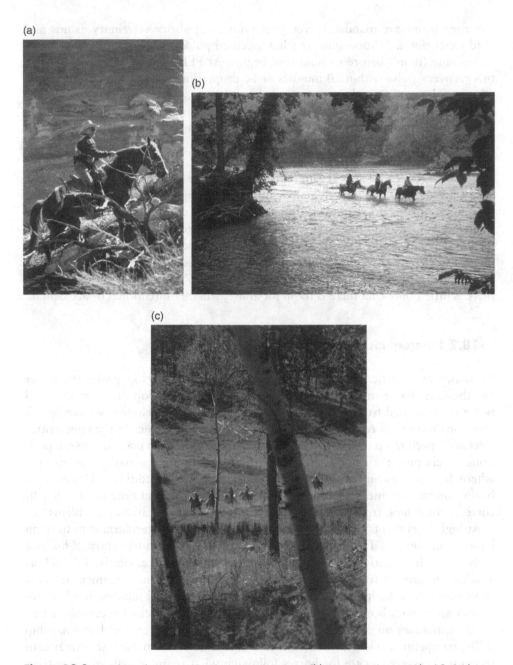

Figure 18.2 A 100-mile competition in mountainous or wilderness terrain may take 12–14 hours for the front runners to complete.

this time frame are mandatory vet gates with compulsory veterinary exams and hold (rest) times. A horse must reach a specified pulse criterion (usually 64 beats per minute (bpm)) before its hold time begins. At FEI events, a horse must reach this recovery pulse within 20 minutes or be disqualified. Mandatory holds generally provide up to three hours of rest and sustenance staggered in short periods of 20–60 minutes throughout a 100-mile course. Fifty-mile competitions are won in 3–6 hours of moving time along the trail, depending on terrain and weather conditions, yet horses are allowed 12 hours for completion, including up to 2 hours of hold time.

It is not very feasible to take an unfit, pasture horse and put him to these endurance tests – a rider must develop a horse's talent through training and conditioning spanning months and years. It is difficult to force an endurance horse to 'run' for hours on end – horses that excel in this sport are selected to perform based on their mental capacity to do the job, their innate and trained physiologic stamina, and musculoskeletal fortitude. When one considers the exacting physiological efficiency required for a horse to cover 100 miles in less than 7 hours or even in 24 hours, there is little doubt that there is room for abuse, whether intentional or accidental.

18.2 Inherent Risks of the Sport

As with any athletic discipline, endurance horses do develop problems, either metabolic issues or musculoskeletal injury. Ideally, a metabolically compromised horse is eliminated from continuing on the trail before developing serious health problems in time to recuperate through rest, food, and water. As the competitive level and speed ramp up with greater challenges for horses to place in top ten positions, riders push their horses closer to the edge, with more situations developing where horses are 'pulled' (disqualified) for metabolic conditions. Horses may border on the imminent need of treatment, but with rest and time most will self-correct. For others, treatment is necessary to resolve life-threatening problems.

At high-level events, it is not uncommon for attending veterinarians to have on hand a minimum of 15 liters of intravenous (IV) fluids per horse entry. While not all horses will be markedly compromised, many will receive restorative IV fluids as a safety precaution to avoid further metabolic deterioration. Treatment in most other equestrian disciplines largely concerns musculoskeletal injuries, but here we have a sport with horses ridden in such a way that necessitates metabolic treatment, sometimes on a large scale. With technology and improved horsemanship skills, competition has grown fiercer. It is cause for concern that field treatment triage is necessary to care for horses following what is supposedly an equestrian 'competition.' A lurking question persists: Is it really acceptable for consequences of these performance demands to require such intensive therapy?

Despite the physical and health challenges of long-distance events, endurance riders and organizations have worked hard to bring the sport of endurance to the mainstream of public acknowledgement, with a focusing prism of media attention on this fast-growing international sport. Welfare issues necessitate improvements in horse safety for practical purposes as well as public perception.

18.3 Drug-Free Policy

Those involved in distance sports pride themselves on being governed by 'drug-free' regulations, meaning a horse cannot receive any performance-enhancing or pain-relieving medications for 96 hours before the competition. This equalizes the playing field so that horses perform solely through talent, training, and rider skill, and without pharmaceutical masking of musculoskeletal issues. Drug testing is implemented at random national and at all high-level endurance competitions to assure compliance with the drug-free policy.

This drug-free policy is now in contention at the FEI level with a trend toward permitting non-steroidal anti-inflammatory drug (NSAID) use. Under the governing umbrella of FEI, this allowance includes endurance horses. The debate continues at the time of writing as it is not yet determined how this may impact horse welfare. It is too early to tell if this could provide beneficial relief for horses performing with mild problems or instead be tremendously dangerous for horses with significant structural problems. There is also concern for the increased risk of gastric or colonic ulcers or kidney damage when combining unavoidable dehydration with NSAIDs (Nieto et al., 2004).

18.4 The Challenge

The sport of endurance racing has evolved steadily over the past couple of decades, with horses accomplishing more over long distances than previously thought possible. This is in part due to the advent of newer technology to assist training and monitoring – heart rate monitors, thermistors to measure body temperature, and Global Positioning System (GPS) units to accurately calculate speed and distance. Light-weight saddles, heat-dissipating saddle pads, and hi-tech foot gear reduce weight or heat load for competitive advantage and horse comfort. Riders have a better understanding of equitation and improved nutritional and conditioning strategies. Competitors recognize and select for traits that characterize a talented equine athlete. Riders also understand how to better manage their horses during a competition in ways to cool, feed, and electrolyte, along with riding strategies that optimize performance from each horse. Coupling the information 'superhighway' with national and international relationships among riders and the wealth of published material on the subject of distance riding, competitors have improved their horsemanship knowledge to obtain the most from their horses' inbred potential.

Riders attend endurance rides for various reasons, with objectives dictated by time constraints, competitive intent, and financial ability. Goals include trail riding in beautiful wilderness and the joy of the camaraderie of like-minded riders. Some strive for personal satisfaction of accomplishment and development of a partnership with a horse while accruing high lifetime mileage. Others have a defined goal during a competition season such as a quest for points, year-end awards and honors, and/or to qualify for Championship and FEI competitions.

Many competitors ride with the intention of putting their horses' well-being first and foremost to the completion of a ride, riding under the laudable philosophy of 'to finish is to win.' Nonetheless, horses continue to be given IV fluids during and following competitions, particularly at high-caliber events. Weather conditions factor in to the number of necessary treatments, with heat and humidity inducing a higher incidence of metabolic compromise on otherwise reasonable trails. Endurance riding is an 'extreme' sport, with recognized physical demands exacted from the horses.

Whether a rider attends a local, 'backyard' ride with relatively casual goals, or competes in more prestigious FEI or championship races, riders and ride organizers should promote equal standards as a model for all involved in the sport, no matter the value of the prize or the degree of recognition. Distance riding organizations are instrumental in upholding this philosophy.

18.5 The Objectives of a Governing Body

Many governing bodies are national or international in scope, and oversee that the rules and regulations are implemented in the sport. Standards of care are expected to meet requirements of each governing body, with the horse's welfare foremost in importance. In the USA, for example, the oversight organization is the American Endurance Ride Conference (AERC). International competition falls under the auspices of the FEI. Governing bodies of endurance sports evolved to:

- protect the health and safety of the horses;
- equalize the playing field within a set guideline of rules and regulations;
- sanction rides that comply with a minimum standard of trail and ride logistics; and
- provide recognition and awards for accomplishments of horses and riders.

While rules and regulations within this sport are relatively limited so as not to overwhelm the spirit of competition, welfare issues arise when recommendations are not always followed or adhered to in the spirit in which they were intended, or when rides are sanctioned yet barely meet minimum requirements.

The FEI expects all those involved in international equestrian sports to adhere to the FEI's *Code of Conduct for the Welfare of the Horse* (FEI, 2009b) 'to acknowledge and accept that, at all times, the welfare of the horse must be paramount and must never be subordinated to competitive or commercial influences.' This Code also encourages all stages of preparation, training, and on-site competition to be guided by welfare concerns, including post-ride care and even once a horse's competition career has ended (FEI, 2009b).

The FEI also urges attainment of the highest levels of education by all involved in the sport. Throughout the world, research is steadily directed toward understanding the significance of clinical parameters as measured against completion rates and blood chemistries obtained before, during, and following competition stress. Data come from notable endurance events like the World Championships, World Cup Finals, the Pan American Championships, the Western States 100 (Tevis), the Old Dominion, and the previously popular Race of Champions, with a wealth of information continually forthcoming from future high-caliber events. In fact, veterinary accomplishments within endurance riding contributed to stimulating further studies that improved safety and welfare for eventing horses at the 1996 Atlanta Olympics. This success further improved the general public's view of equestrian events.

Keen competitors like to have as many rides scheduled as possible. Ride management and veterinarians desire high completion rates with few casualties. Ride management (in FEI this is the Organizing Committee) has a daunting task to negotiate all details required to organize an event that satisfies the sanctioning organization as well as competitors, veterinarians, and ride officials (AERC, 2008a). Among the many details, it is possible for ride management to overlook the importance of two crucial ingredients to a successful ride and horse safety: (a) necessary veterinary controls and vet check logistics; and (b) the hiring of competent and experienced veterinarians. Experience is paramount in being able to recognize impending problems in a competition horse.

18.6 Avoiding Metabolic Mishaps

To ensure that competition horses receive the best scrutiny and care and to avoid potential metabolic consequences, ride managers, veterinary staff, and riders all need to work together on behalf of the horses. Many issues for avoiding metabolic problems depend on the judgment and responsibility of each rider to his or her horse. Dane Frazier has aptly noted each person's responsibility (Frazier, 2000): 'The welfare of endurance horses depends on the knowledge and skill of their riders and is protected through evaluation of horses by veterinarians before, during, and after these events.'

A rider may be focused on taking care of their horse and negotiating the rigors of competition, such as trail, speed, and passing the veterinary checks. Sometimes, this competitive mindset creates tunnel vision. As with any learning curve, mistakes are made and horses may suffer the consequences. With more experience, riders are better able to appreciate the wisdom of all they have heard, seen, and learned from their own mistakes and successes as well as those of others.

18.6.1 Horse preparation

Performance success depends on many factors on any given day, but a critical strategy is that of conditioning preparation. Performance failure may be related to a rider's lack of commitment to a conditioning program that is appropriate to the level of anticipated competition. Conditioning of a young or novice horse new to long-distance sports is best accomplished over 3–6 months before attempting limited distance competition (25–30 miles (40–50 km)) or a slow 50-mile (80 km) ride. While undesirable, occasions do occur when a rider asks a horse to tackle a 50-mile ride, never having done more than 15 miles (25 km) in a training ride. Before attending a 50-mile event, the horse should perform occasional training distances of 20–30 miles (30–50 km). A solid foundation for a 100-mile (160 km) horse is built on two to three years of strategic training; the horse must be at least five years of age at the US national level, six years in Australia, and for FEI 100-mile (three-star and higher competition) it must be at least seven years old. A horse pays the price for riders who shortcut the conditioning process.

General fatigue may also occur for an opposite reason: over-training. Novice riders may not realize that, once a conditioning base has been achieved, it isn't necessary to demand rigorous riding four or five days a week. Current condition can be maintained with only mildly demanding exercise twice weekly. An additional weekly ride might include a light trail hack, dressage or cavaletti exercises. Training over no more than moderate mileage (70–80 miles (110–130 km) within two weeks) with sufficient rest periods improves capacity for long distances and reduces incidence of musculoskeletal injuries.

18.6.2 Ride frequency

Competition frequency and rest time between competitions impact horse welfare. Not only is a horse ridden hard at an event, but a competitor should factor in the time for transport there and back, appropriate rest time to return a horse to peak, and the effects of musculoskeletal concussion and dehydration incurred. A ride frequency that includes back-to-back rides on consecutive weekends amplifies accumulated stress.

Muscles and the cardiovascular system need time to heal and regenerate strength from a previous exertion. An ideal objective is to give a horse at least three weeks between 50-mile (80 km) events, and 5–6 weeks between 100-mile rides, with only light training in between. FEI competitions mandate specific rest time between FEI events: horses competing in distances of less than 50 miles must rest for 13 days; and those in events of more than 50 miles must rest for 20 days between competitions (FEI, 2009c).

Many horses tolerate closely spaced competitions, but eventually collective exertional demands catch up with even the most rugged horses, leading to a higher incidence of metabolic failures or lameness. Riders may not appreciate the cumulative toll that occurs on their horses and herein is the value of continuing education.

18.7 The Veterinarian's Role

The sport of endurance riding is one of the only equestrian sports to rely upon veterinarians with medical knowledge to make decisions as to the competency of a horse's 'fitness to continue' both in soundness and in metabolic capacity.

This is where the challenge lies on behalf of the endurance horse: standards and expectations should be based on what is humane and non-abusive to the horses. Many ride vets are themselves accomplished distance riders and provide an excellent resource when serving on the veterinary staff. Ideally, equality of judging across the country and around the world shares similar meaning from region to region in regard to completion and placing. Ride managers are accountable for the quality of the ride and for their selection of veterinary personnel.

18.7.1 Adherence to a standard of 'fit to continue'

An endurance horse is 'passed' through a vet check only if physical exam findings determine that he meets specified soundness and metabolic parameters sufficient to continue in competition, *ergo* he is 'fit to continue.' This tenet applies also at the finish line to qualify for completion (Figure 18.3). A thorough veterinary exam should be required at all veterinary checks, rather than abbreviated exams that provide impressions only and no objective data. A ride card accompanies the horse and rider at all times. This card includes time the horse arrived at the vet check, time to reach pulse criterion, and complete results of the veterinary exam. Graded scores (A–D) are filled in by the veterinarians at each checkpoint for every physical parameter assessed, with their signature. Notes on the card include notations about specific concerns to alert veterinarians at future checkpoints.

Following the spirit of the principle of what merits 'fitness to continue' is the responsibility of both riders and vets. Rules specify that horses that are grade 3 lame (consistent lameness at the trot on a straight line) should not be released from vet checks and should not be 'passed' for completion at the finish line check. Questionable metabolic cases are pulled in the interest of equine safety. The standard of the sport of endurance should not be sacrificed with the objective of obtaining higher completion rates.

If dissatisfied with veterinary expertise or ride organization, riders can provide feedback to ride managers and the veterinary committee. However, it is human nature for riders not to complain about inferior vetting quality that allows marginal horses through the vet gates – a rider's objective of gaining a completion often overrides the desire for more stringent veterinary controls that might preclude reaching that goal.

The challenge for both rider and veterinarian is to critically evaluate each horse as objectively as possible. If a rider feels their horse is not quite right in soundness or metabolic status, then a conscientious rider should pull their horse even if a veterinarian doesn't denote a problem. In the old days of endurance sports, some riders tried to hide problems from the veterinarians. Fortunately, this antagonistic relationship is no longer the norm; most riders are quite up-front about their concerns.

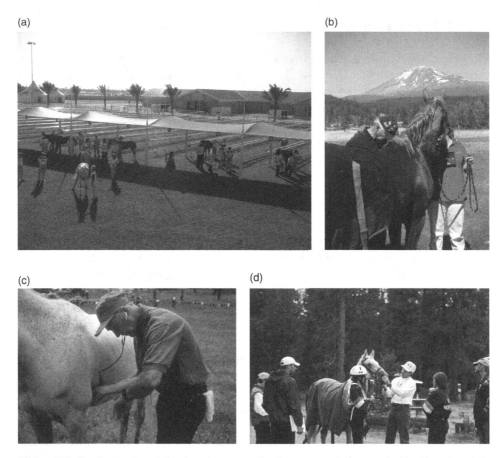

Figure 18.3 Once a horse has met the required pulse criterion to be in its hold time, it proceeds to the veterinarians for a compulsory veterinary exam of metabolic and soundness status.

They realize it is to their horse's advantage to point out issues to the vets and to approach the vet exam as a team effort in determining what is best for the horse. Good communication skills are important between vet and rider to allow open discussion without a rider being defensive or taking offense. Ride veterinarians, particularly those dedicated to the sport, are an invaluable asset to ensure equine health and well-being. Continuous monitoring of every horse during an event and in the hours following is necessary to identify problems as early as possible.

18.7.2 Cardiac recovery index (CRI) as safeguard

The cardiac recovery index (CRI) has become an important criterion for evaluation of distance horses – taken at intervals along the course, it is a measure of a horse's fitness and ability to cope with exercise demand. The CRI is evaluated throughout the event: at each vet check, at the end of the hold time at vet checks later in the ride, and at the finish exam. Once a horse's heart rate has reached pulse criterion of 64 (or 60) bpm, the horse is presented to the veterinarian, who retakes the horse's resting heart rate. Then the horse is asked to trot 250 feet (75 m) – 125 feet away and 125 feet back. Exactly one minute after initiating the measured 250-foot trot, the horse's heart rate is again counted and this value compared to the pre-trot value. (In most cases, the 250-foot trot takes less than half a minute, and the horse is allowed to stand quietly for the remainder of the minute.) The heart rate should return to the same number of beats or less than the initial resting rate. If not, this may indicate an impending metabolic problem or musculoskeletal pain – efforts are taken to corroborate other physical exam findings with a problem. Not all metabolic crises are accompanied by an elevated CRI, whereas the presence of an elevated cardiac recovery index tends to be associated with fatigue, dehydration, and other indications of exhausted horse syndrome (AERC, 2008b; Loving, 1997). To play safe, veterinarians may ask that a horse return for an additional CRI at the end of the hold time prior to leaving the vet gate – this rechecks both metabolic and soundness status to assess 'fit to continue.'

18.7.3 Veterinary staffing

While AERC only requires one veterinarian to judge a ride (AERC, 2009a), from a welfare standpoint it is more practical to hire at least two veterinarians no matter the number of entries. As a general rule, ride management may wish to hire one veterinarian per every 15 to 30 horses, depending on the intensity of the competition and difficulty of terrain and/or climate. Having two or more vets on staff ensures continuation of a ride if any horse requires veterinary attention while also ensuring availability of medical expertise to a sick or injured horse. Sufficient numbers of veterinary personnel facilitates efficient flow of horses and riders through vet checks; waiting in line otherwise wastes valuable hold time that should be directed toward care of the horse.

It is not uncommon for ride managers to seek a veterinarian at the last minute to accommodate greater than anticipated entries because not enough vets were hired in the first place or a veterinarian canceled. Staffing an inadequate number of vets has also caused veterinarian competitors to stop riding in order to attend sick horses or to help judge – a dedicated veterinarian isn't likely to turn away from helping a compromised horse.

The number of veterinarians required on-site at a competition is only one issue that affects horse welfare. AERC veterinary requirements do not stipulate which veterinarians should be employed by ride management, for example. A veterinarian with limited endurance experience may be acceptable provided s/he is working alongside a vet with extensive experience. Some individuals who have never before vetted an endurance ride may in fact be quite capable and familiar with the physiological demands of this pursuit. Yet, currently only minimal qualifications are required for a veterinarian to work local US endurance rides: the veterinarian must be an active member of AERC, pass an open book test, and acquire two hours of continuing education in sports-related topics (AERC, 2009b). In contrast, at the FEI level, veterinarians must attend specified courses every three years to ensure understanding and to acquire updates of the rules and regulations, and must judge a specified number of FEI-caliber rides within that period (FEI, 2009d). Marked interest in FEI-level competitions has produced a large pool of competent and qualified veterinarians to select from to judge FEI events.

If sufficient numbers of qualified veterinarians are not available for an event, then an improved standard suggests that a governing organization refuse to sanction that ride until certain conditions are met. There could be some form of 'accreditation' process for a governing body to verify that a national-level ride meets the standard. Most international events are scrutinized carefully, with stewards and Ground Jury present to ensure adherence to the rules and sanctioning requirements. FEI events involve a team of veterinarians to facilitate efficient control judging and regard for horse welfare (Figure 18.4). In the interest of horse safety, FEI regulations require that a veterinarian is present on the premises of the venue 24 hours a day throughout the event's duration. And FEI oversight also ensures comprehensive requirements by event organizers for risk management of controllable factors that may affect the welfare of the horses – as examples, guarantee of good-quality water available every 4.5 miles and trail design that limits use of hard-packed, vehicular roads to less than 10% of the course.

18.7.4 Meeting veterinary criteria

An endurance ride is segmented into phases, legs, or loops, each separated by a vet gate at which a horse must meet the pulse criterion and then begin a mandatory hold time. A horse typically recovers to the pulse criterion of 64 bpm within 2–3 minutes when ridden to the level of its abilities and for the conditions of the day. Upon meeting the required pulse rate as confirmed by a pulse and respiration (P&R) volunteer, the horse proceeds to a veterinarian for a compulsory physical exam (Figure 18.5). It is possible for a horse to 'pass' the required parameters of a veterinary check yet only be marginally able to continue in both mind and physical stability. Just 'hitting the numbers' does not necessarily constitute being 'fit to continue.' While not necessarily experiencing overt metabolic failure or requiring treatment, a horse may suffer discomfort and distress from the exercise demand.

Because the nature of veterinary exams relies on both objective and subjective factors, it is sometimes difficult to discern if a horse is just tired or if it is lame or experiencing more serious myositis (muscle cramps) or elements of exhausted horse syndrome related to dehydration, and energy and electrolyte depletion. An experienced practitioner is often able to recognize subtle signs of metabolic distress before a horse becomes overtly ill, based on a horse's despondent neck and/or body posture and anxious facial expressions, such as puckered lips and a glazed stare (Figures 18.6 and 18.7).

(a)

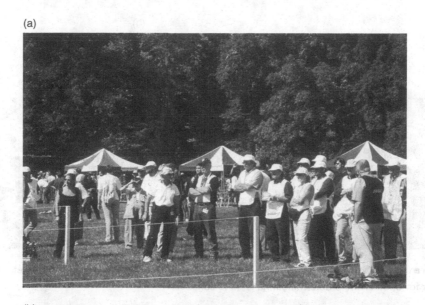

(b)

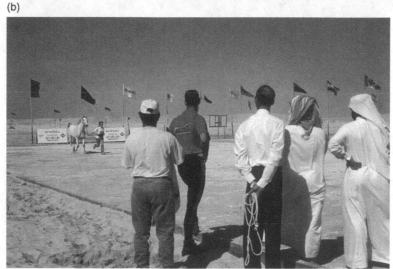

Figure 18.4 At FEI events, there is a team of veterinarians to evaluate the horses at every veterinary check.

There is not always the means to predict the outcome of releasing a horse onto the trail even with the assistance of sophisticated blood chemistry equipment. Herein lies a conundrum for veterinary personnel: conscience and science dictate doing the right thing by the horse without jeopardizing its safety and welfare while not being obstructive to the rider's objectives without just cause. Veterinary judgment relies on expertise and experience – the value of what a rider can expect

(a)   (b)

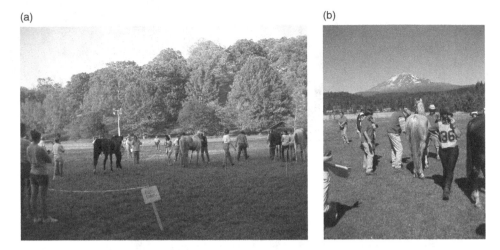

Figure 18.5   Once a horse meets the pulse criterion (64 bpm), he will proceed to the veterinary check for a full exam to determine if he is 'fit to continue.'

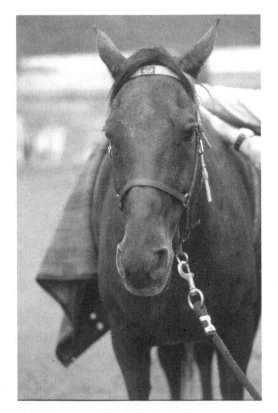

Figure 18.6   A fatigued horse will stand with a deflated posture.

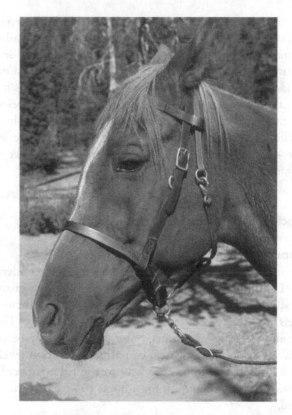

Figure 18.7 A fatigued horse and one that isn't feeling well may display anxiety by puckering his lips and/or staring with glazed eyes, not responsive to stimuli around him.

from a ride veterinarian depends on the caliber of veterinarians hired. Ultimately, though, riders have the primary responsibility for their horses (FEI, 2009e): 'Riders are challenged with regards to effective use of pace and thorough knowledge of their horses and cross country, with the emphasis on finishing in good condition rather than coming first.' An incentive to ride with this strategic approach is the goal of earning the coveted Best Condition award – one horse in the top ten finishers is judged as the most vibrant and fit to continue. This award factors in a horse's speed to finish the course, the rider's weight including tack, and veterinary scores.

18.7.5 Competent treatment veterinarians

Every ride should have on hand a veterinarian who is familiar and knowledgeable in the specific treatment of distance horse problems. Any horse can have a bad day, but no horse should suffer due to inadequate veterinary attention or due to inadequate logistics set up by ride management.

Sophisticated laboratory equipment to run serum chemistries to evaluate muscle enzymes, dehydration, and electrolyte levels is not always available but simple packed cell volume (PCV) and total protein measurements provide easily obtained information about hydration status. The most important element of efficient treatment is a veterinarian's ability to recognize a problem using his/her clinical skills based upon a wealth of experience. This skill relies not on expensive equipment, but rather on a familiarity with specialized needs of distance horses. Successful treatment also relies on implementation of appropriate and aggressive treatment in a timely manner – an experienced and competent treatment vet is invaluable to ensuring horse safety.

18.8 Risk Factors Related to Endurance Competition

18.8.1 Transport stress

Even before reaching a competition site, an endurance horse undergoes significant physical stresses. Endurance riding venues usually require long-distance hauling for most competitors. The impact of transport on a horse's performance depends upon how well it travels, and the type of trailer and driver experience. The act of balancing in the trailer and resisting vibrations, noise, and heat may be comparable to a horse having walked those miles. Season can affect hydration level through influencing how much a horse sweats on the way to the ride, particularly in hot and humid conditions. It is not uncommon for a horse to arrive at the ride site already 2–3% dehydrated.

FEI events held around the world may necessitate air travel, which is often coupled with long delays in quarantine facilities, lengthy plane transport in tight confinement, and the added stress of off-loading from the plane and overland hauling to the stabling. These factors are significant when asking a horse to perform over 50–100 miles following the intense stimulations and immune challenges that accompany travel to the venue.

18.8.2 Horse stabling

The comfort level each horse experiences at the ride site also contributes to performance. Distractions and commotion may interfere with satisfactory rest or a horse's attention to eating and drinking well. Housing is usually in small, portable corrals or stalls with little room to move, while some horses are tied to a trailer or overhead picket line for several days. A horse that is in peak athletic condition is not able to exercise at will, which affects muscle limberness and may create anxiety. Just as travel affects people, changes in routine affect a horse's circadian rhythm and mental equilibrium. Experienced campaigners do better than novice horses, but all horses are affected to some degree by changing environments, even preceding the stressors of competition.

18.8.3 Number of veterinary checks

Financial constraints and logistical issues may cause a ride to be understaffed with veterinary personnel, P&R (checkpoint) volunteers, timers, and gate control personnel such that shortcuts are taken by ride managers to make the most of available manpower. This limitation makes it tempting to design a non-FEI course with minimal veterinary checks, such as a single vet exam within a 50-mile (80 km) ride or only 3–4 vet checks in a 100-mile event. Such a budget-saving strategy is likely achieved at the expense of the horses.

Optimum design of a national-level ride is predicated on 2–3 veterinary checkpoints in a 50-mile competition for a total hold time of 1.5 to 2 hours. A 100-mile competition has 5–8 checkpoints with a total hold time of approximately 3 hours. FEI 100-mile rides are required to have at least five vet gates plus the finish line, with intervals of 12–24 miles (20–40 km) between vet gates. Although the FEI hold duration totals 2 hours 40 minutes, typical horse entries into FEI competition have demonstrated a consistent level of metabolic efficiency that enables some of them to compete at more difficult demands with success. Despite these levels of control, some horses do develop metabolic or other problems during high-caliber rides.

The sport of endurance attracts newcomers to local rides for the thrill, but these riders are not always fully aware of what is involved. The situation of a single vet check over a 50-mile course is an example of management logistics that markedly impact a horse's well-being. A single break in an entire day's effort asks a novice horse for forward movement along the trail without respite, perhaps for only an hour after completing the first 25–30 miles (40–50 km). A tough 50-mile trail through mountainous terrain takes 7–12 hours to complete. Although a crew could meet horse and rider at a trail and road junction to supply food and water for refueling and a short break, not all riders have assistants to manage these needs (Figure 18.8). Every ride should be lined out with horse safety in mind for all.

Some argue that rides with fewer veterinary checkpoints still have horses completing with few problems. In such cases, a horse relies more on the expertise and abilities of its rider, along with its inborn metabolic capacities. However, these ideal circumstances do not exist for all horses or competitors. If the goals are to protect the horses and to minimize the risk of metabolic failures, then a sufficient number of veterinary checks should be provided with sufficient duration of hold time. Then, not only do horses receive time to eat, drink, and rest, but each horse is examined at multiple checkpoints with opportunities for veterinarians to assess progressive recovery throughout the competition.

18.8.4 Vet gate timing

When a horse stops moving, adrenalin level declines and within 10–20 minutes a distressed horse may display signs that he might not otherwise demonstrate while running with the herd. It is not just novice horses that 'bottom out' – experienced

(a)   (b)

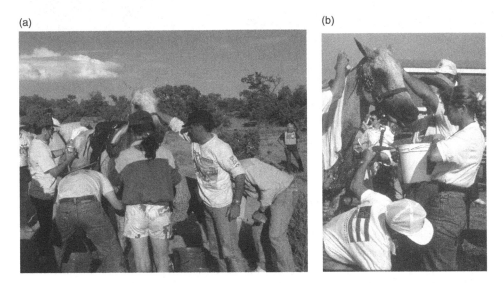

Figure 18.8 Crewing a horse at vet checks or at points along the trail provides food, water, and cooling strategies.

horses are intent on moving down the trail due to training, habit, and herd dynamics, and subtle signs may not show until there is a forced stop.

The importance of giving horses stopping time early on in an event has been suggested, particularly in light of work done on fluid and electrolyte deficits incurred within the first 20 miles (Lindinger *et al.*, 1995; McCutcheon and Geor, 1996; Ecker and Lindinger, 1995). An early vet check, in the first 12–20 miles, minimizes the number of later metabolic failures by:

- enabling refueling and rehydration to prevent the lag time for a horse's system to catch up later; and
- separating the fit horses from those pushing through on sheer adrenalin and herd instincts.

The latter is accomplished by different rates at which horses meet the required pulse criteria (heart rate usually 64 bpm) to then start the mandatory hold time. A less fit horse takes longer and so is released back on trail after more fit horses have already left the vet check.

When it is not possible to organize a full team of veterinary staff in a remote location to set up a formal vet check, rather than foregoing a check altogether, one or two veterinarians could oversee a simple 'meet pulse criteria' gate into a short hold. This strategy should not be implemented at the expense of an adequate number of veterinary checks with comprehensive veterinary exams.

(a)

(b)

(c)

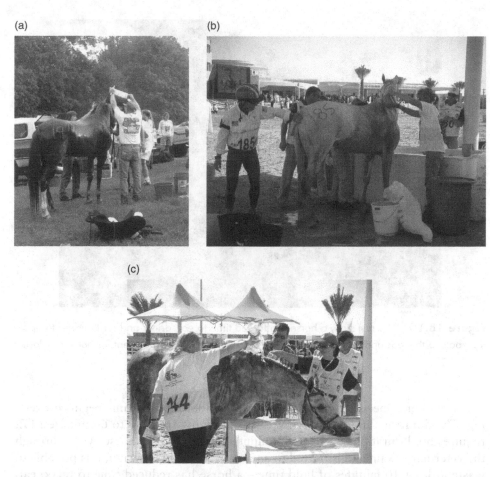

Figure 18.9 Cooling strategies are important to keep internal body temperatures within a normal range to avoid muscular fatigue; hydration is a key element to cooling and horse safety.

18.8.5 Hold time duration

The duration of each mandatory hold is subject to change relative to climate but is the same for all horses. Standing around in cold and/or wet weather may cause chilling or tight muscles whereas hot and humid environments necessitate time for adequate cooling measures (Figure 18.9), and for eating and drinking to replenish fluids, electrolytes, and energy. Pulse criteria accounts for these climatic features – a dehydrated horse takes longer to reach a pulse of 56 or 60 bpm than to reach 64 bpm. It is possible that lowering the pulse criterion may protect horse safety when weather and terrain conditions dictate more stringent controls.

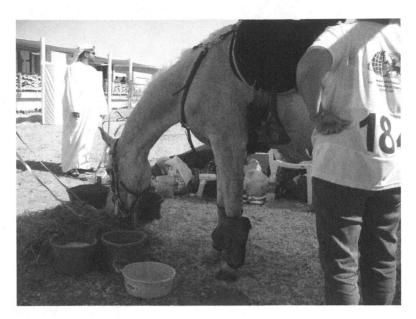

Figure 18.10   At a rest stop, a horse is afforded time to eat, drink, and for the rider to apply ice boots to the legs and attend to tack issues that might need improvement for horse comfort.

Once a horse meets the pulse criterion, a mandatory hold time begins for resting. The duration differs between vet gates, ranging from 30 to 60 minutes; FEI requires hold durations of 40 to 60 minutes. By the time a horse cycles through the veterinary exam and is moved to an area with feed and water, it is possible to waste at least 10 minutes of hold time – a horse has reduced time to relax, eat, drink, and receive electrolytes before it is tacked up and re-presented to the vets (when requested) before being let out on trail (Figure 18.10). Studies have demonstrated that it takes an hour for absorption of food and electrolytes from the gut (Clarke *et al.*, 1990; Sosa Leon *et al.*, 1997; Butudom *et al.*, 2002). Hold times should be designed to give horses a chance to utilize nutrients ingested at the rest stop.

Allowing sufficient time in the vet gates is an excellent method for screening to detect if a horse should continue on the trail. The objective is to recognize a compromised horse early, especially before it manifests a problem in a remote location out on trail, far from medical expertise.

Nothing prevents a rider from delaying departure from a rest stop past the prescribed hold time or from slowing the horse's pace along the trail. But in the spirit of competition it is human nature to want to get back into the race as quickly as possible and to ride with keen intent. While a rider's focus should be wholly on their horse, the heat of competition sometimes obscures common sense.

18.8.6 Returning eliminated horses to base camp

If a horse is disqualified at a vet gate away from base camp, trailers must be able to access the spot. Space restrictions may preclude trailer access for each rider to retrieve their eliminated horse; then it is the purview of ride management to ensure safe, sturdy trailers, and capable drivers to ferry horses back to base. When trailer safety or driver competence is in question, a competitor might decline transport of their horse, thereby delaying a horse's return to base camp and possible treatment.

18.9 Common Emergency Conditions at Endurance Events

While musculoskeletal injuries may occur at any point along an endurance ride event, the most pressing emergency situations generally involve metabolic problems. Lengthy duration of as much as 12–24 hours of protracted exercise results in depletion of body fluids and some electrolytes. Coupling this with additional demands placed on these horses from speed, challenging terrain, and possible adverse weather conditions, the most prevalent metabolic concerns fall under the umbrella of a complex known as exhausted horse syndrome, which develops due to dehydration, electrolyte imbalances, and glycogen (energy) depletion. Metabolic compromise ranges from very mild and barely detectable to extremely serious and life-threatening. A sick horse may be affected with myositis, synchronous diaphragmatic flutter (thumps), colic secondary to intestinal atony, heat stress or prostration, and also has the potential to develop laminitis.

Affected horses show clinical signs as a result of fluid, electrolyte, and energy losses, which may include: poor heart rate recovery, elevated CRI, decreased intestinal activity, reduced or absent appetite, lack of thirst, depression or disinterest in surrounding stimuli, delayed capillary refill time and/or pale or marginated mucous membrane color, delayed skin tenting, elevated rectal temperature, flaccid anal sphincter tone, synchronous diaphragmatic flutter (thumps), muscle twitching or cramps (myositis) with or without associated lameness, dark urine (myoglobinuria), increased digital pulses, recumbency, and colic.

18.9.1 Treatment and monitoring

Much of the treatment care of an endurance horse occurs in the 'field' with limited facilities, even at world-class events. The attending veterinarian should be provisioned with ample supplies to accommodate a large number of sick horses. Excellent medical care can be performed out of a well-stocked veterinary truck, but in some cases a horse must be shipped to a referral hospital for intensive and/or follow-up care or surgery. Preliminary arrangements made with the nearest referral hospital and surgical center ensure that qualified veterinarians are available for the duration of the endurance event to offer timely intervention (Figures 18.11–18.13).

Regardless of the specific metabolic crisis a horse may experience, it is necessary to replenish large volumes of isotonic fluids and to restore electrolyte balance and

(a)

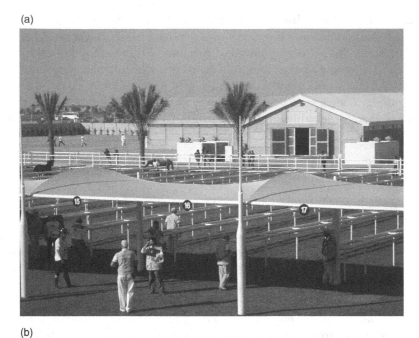

(b)

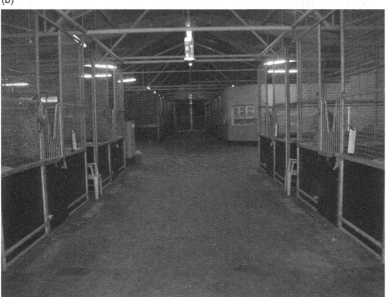

Figure 18.11 The most premier endurance events may have access to a full facility treatment hospital like this one at the Dubai Endurance village in the United Arab Emirates.

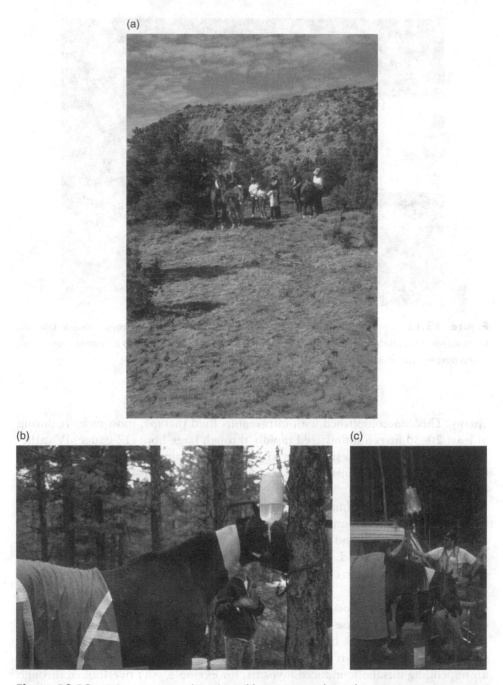

Figure 18.12 Other events conducted in wilderness areas depend on veterinary triage, using well-stocked veterinary trucks and competent treatment veterinarians. Here are examples of using trees or tree branches for hanging fluids for treatment in the field.

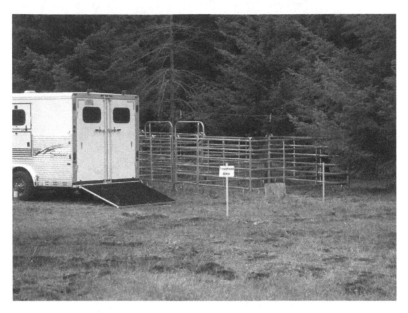

Figure 18.13 A designated treatment area may be set up to keep horses isolated from surrounding distractions and people while allowing veterinarians to continue monitoring these horses until they are well enough to be released to their owners.

energy. This is accomplished with intravenous fluid therapy, most cases requiring at least 20–30 liters administered rapidly through large-bore (12-gauge) IV catheters (Figure 18.14). For a sick horse with audible intestinal activity, electrolyte and energy-laced fluids administered by nasogastric tube also bolster quick restoration of deficits.

Competent treatment includes additional medical measures to promote intestinal motility, renal function, and neuromuscular equilibrium, to manage pain, to limit endotoxin production, and to minimize the risk of laminitis (AERC, 2008c). Often, timely restoration of fluid, electrolytes, and energy improves a horse's overall condition such that he begins to take care of himself with food and drink to further restore his losses.

Additionally, the protocol followed in most competitions encourages veterinary evaluation of every horse that is disqualified from continuing in competition, regardless of whether the horse has been eliminated due to a known metabolic or suspect lameness problem or a rider-related issue. This ensures that a horse with an impending metabolic-induced myositis, for example, isn't overlooked through an assumption that 'lameness' is caused by a musculoskeletal issue. Sufficient manpower should be available to accommodate examination and continual monitoring of all eliminated horses at regular intervals. Horses that have received

(a)

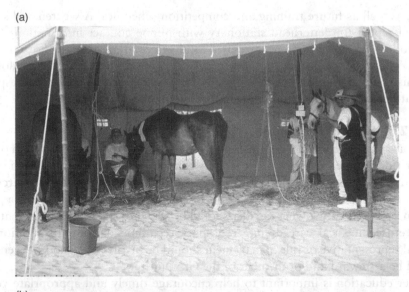

(b)

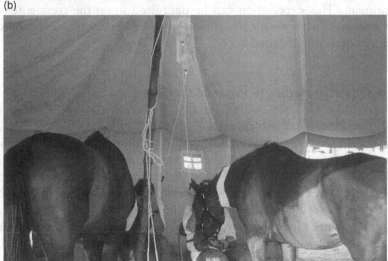

Figure 18.14 This is an example of an intravenous treatment area to get horses out of the weather, to run copious intravenous fluids, and to monitor response to therapy.

veterinary care or are in questionable medical condition should also be evaluated the following day and prior to release from the event or transport off the grounds.

The attending veterinarian contributes further to the horse's welfare by explaining to the owner and/or rider about the metabolic illness incurred by their horse during the competition, how this might affect immediate travel plans to return home, as well as future training and competition schedules. A written and signed medical report (on letterhead stationary with phone contact information) facilitates follow-up evaluation and care by a local veterinarian once the horse returns home. This report includes the presumptive diagnosis, medications and dosages administered, lab results, repetitive physical exam data tracking the horse's response to treatment, and recommendations for follow-up care (Loving, 2008).

18.9.2 Refusal of treatment

There are instances when a competition horse is in need of treatment yet an owner and/or rider refuses veterinary care despite convincing arguments on behalf of the horse. Not all owners are cooperative, due to either financial concerns, a perceived stigma to having a horse treated at a ride, or rider denial that the horse has a problem. In such cases, the owner or rider should be asked to sign a statement that they have refused medical care despite veterinary recommendations. In addition, an official representative of ride management should be involved – at an FEI event this would be a steward and/or member of the Ground Jury.

Rider education is important to help encourage timely and appropriate veterinary treatment. This expectation can be impressed upon the competitors at the pre-ride briefings, with detailed outlining of veterinarian recommendations for management of a compromised horse.

18.10 Other Strategies to Improve the Standard

18.10.1 Log books as safeguards

The Australian endurance riding community initiated a practical and safeguarding system decades ago, with the British endurance riding community and finally FEI following suit: the use of a log book or, as with FEI, a log sheet. A log book delineates a horse's complete competitive history, including the number and names of rides entered, total mileage of the horse, successful completion or elimination, and any need for treatment, with each entry signed by the ride organizer or steward. Ride officials can see a horse's ride record at a glance; this helps prevent abuse in conjunction with the rules. This written record can be a source of pride for an accomplished competitor. For other less fortunate competitors, elimination from any event is noted and the reason for elimination stated in the log book (NSWERA, 2009).

Each horse has its own number and a single log book no matter to which endurance society a horse belongs. As examples, FEI's Endurance Log Sheet must accompany a horse's passport at FEI events; all four British endurance organizations cooperate with each other, so a competitor cannot override a horse that competes in more than one organization. In countries requiring it, a log book must be presented at the start of every competition; otherwise, a horse is not allowed to start or at least not without a financial penalty. With log book in hand, vets checking in a horse with a previous metabolic incident will know how best to scrutinize the horse during competition. Historical information contained in a log book enables veterinarian and rider to formulate conscientious decisions as to the significance of a musculoskeletal injury and how that relates to participating in competition.

If a rider abuses the system and persistently presents a lame horse with a chronic injury, the horse can be banned from competing for a specified period of time – in Britain this is a four-week span. This practice has a deterrent effect, so riders are hesitant to abuse the system.

Australia and France have additionally implemented an Early Warning System (EWS) as a further protective failsafe for horses with persistent performance failure. A horse eliminated from a competition for veterinary reasons receives points appropriate to the severity of the disqualifying problem. Once allocated a specified number of points, the horse is demoted from competing in 100-mile (160 km) events to shorter distances. The EWS has provisions for an extreme case to be retired from any endurance competition for a stipulated period of rest time.

Not all countries have yet adopted the log book protocol, nor has the FEI method been used to full advantage with sufficient notes entered onto the sheet. And the value of information in keeping a log is only as good as the veterinarians making judgments on the horses and their diligent recording of the information. Even so, this strategy has the potential to go a long way toward improving equine safety.

18.10.2 Post-ride reporting

While most endurance horses that develop metabolic problems do so while on-site, there are occasions where a serious health issue doesn't arise until the horse is in transport or has reached home. Examples include colic, laminitis, and serious diarrhea (colitis, enteritis). Feedback from riders whose horses have such problems alerts the organization's governing body to the general consequences of competition and of a possible, unfortunate trend at a particular ride. This information may prove invaluable as a learning tool for vets working rides, as a means to 'grade' the safety of a ride and to consider changes to implement.

Horse safety might be improved by grading competitions much as is done in the show world. Disclosure of topographical maps denoting climbs and descents, elevation gains, along with anticipated climate conditions are helpful criteria to allow riders to judge how a ride suits their horse's ability. The number of vets planned, who they might be, veterinarian to horse ratio, number of vet checks, and hold times are relevant to a rider's decision to attend an event.

18.10.3 The cost and the value of high standards

If riders, veterinarians, and ride managers remember that the sport of endurance riding is a recreational pursuit, then it will be easier to consider not holding a ride in which welfare principles might be compromised. Raising the standard of excellence does not come without a price, such as a need to increase fees to accommodate these standards – it may be necessary to hire and fly in an experienced ride vet to help train less experienced vets. This could have a positive domino effect as more competent vets from local areas become available to the sport and each can assume the responsibility of training others new to the sport.

When all details are implemented with the welfare of the horse foremost in mind, then endurance riders will be able to proudly point to the longevity of their horses as being no longer the exception, but the rule.

References

AERC (2008a) *Ride Manager's Handbook*, Revised January 2008. American Endurance Ride Conference, Auburn, CA. Available at: http://www.aerc.org/upload/RideManager.pdf.

AERC (2008b) Guidelines for judging AERC endurance competitions. *Control Judge Handbook 3.0*, Revised November 2008, pp. 10–12. American Endurance Ride Conference, Auburn, CA. Available at: http://www.aerc.org/upload/2009ControlJudgeHB.pdf.

AERC (2008c) Guidelines for judging AERC endurance competitions. *Control Judge Handbook 3.0*, Revised November 2008, pp. 16–21. American Endurance Ride Conference, Auburn, CA. Available at: http://www.aerc.org/upload/2009ControlJudgeHB.pdf.

AERC (2009a) *Rules and Regulations*, Revised December 2009, Rule 2.1, p. 2. American Endurance Ride Conference, Auburn, CA. Available at: http://www.aerc.org/upload/Rules_Current.pdf.

AERC (2009b) *Veterinary Control/Membership Information of AERC*, May 2009. American Endurance Ride Conference, Auburn, CA. Available at: http://www.aerc.org/NewVetInfo.asp.

Butudom, P., Schott, H.C., II, Davis, M.W., Kobe, C.A., Nielsen, B.D. and Eberhart, S.W. (2002) Drinking salt water enhances rehydration in horses dehydrated by furosemide administration and endurance exercise. *Equine Veterinary Journal (Supplement)* 34(S34), 513–518.

Clarke, L.L., Roberts, M.C. and Argenzio, R.A. (1990) Feeding and digestive problems in horses. Physiologic responses to a concentrated meal. *Veterinary Clinics of North America: Equine Practice* 6(20), 433–450.

Ecker, G.L. and Lindinger, M.I. (1995) Water and ion losses during the cross-country phase of eventing. *Equine Veterinary Journal (Supplement)* 27(S20), 111–119.

FEI (2009a) *Code of Conduct for the Welfare of the Horse*. Fédération Equestre Internationale, Lausanne, Switzerland. Available at: http://www.fei.org/about-us/standards.

FEI (2009b) *Rules for Endurance Events*, 7th edn, p. 1. Fédération Equestre Internationale, Lausanne, Switzerland. Available at: http://www.fei.org/Disciplines/Endurance/Rules/Documents/Endurance_rules_2009.pdf.

FEI (2009c) *Rules for Endurance Events*, 7th edn, p. 11. Fédération Equestre Internationale, Lausanne, Switzerland. Available at: http://www.fei.org/Disciplines/Endurance/Rules/Documents/Endurance_rules_2009.pdf.

FEI (2009d) Rules For Endurance Events, 7th edn, p. 25. Fédération Equestre Internationale, Lausanne, Switzerland. Available at: http://www.fei.org/Disciplines/Endurance/Rules/Documents/Endurance_rules_2009.pdf.

FEI (2009e) *What is Endurance?* Fédération Equestre Internationale, Lausanne, Switzerland. Available at: http://www.fei.org/Disciplines/Endurance/About_Endurance/Pages/What_Is_Endurance.aspx.

Frazier, D.M. (2000) Who speaks for the horse – the sport of endurance riding and equine welfare. Animal Welfare Forum: Equine Welfare. *Journal of the American Veterinary Medical Association* **216**(8), 1260.

Lindinger, M.I., Geor, R.J., Ecker, G.L. and McCutcheon, L.J. (1995) Plasma volume and ions during exercise in cool, dry; hot, dry; and hot, humid conditions. *Equine Veterinary Journal (Supplement)* **27**(S20), 133–139.

Loving, N.S. (1997) *Go the Distance: The Complete Resource for Endurance Horses.* Trafalgar Square Publishing, Chicago, IL.

Loving, N.S. (2008) Emergency care at equine events: endurance. In *Proceedings of the 54th Annual Convention of the AAEP*, pp. 136–141.

McCutcheon, L.J. and Geor, R.J. (1996) Sweat fluid and ion losses in horses during training and competition in cool vs. hot ambient conditions: implications for ion supplementation. *Equine Veterinary Journal (Supplement)* **28**(S22), 54–62.

Nieto, J.E., Snyder, J.R., Beldomenico, P., Aleman, M., Kerr, J.W. and Spier, S.J. (2004) Prevalence of gastric ulcers in endurance horses – a preliminary report. *Veterinary Journal* **167**(1), 33–37.

NSWERA (2009) *Getting Started in Endurance Riding.* NSW Endurance Riders Association Inc., Chatham, NSW, Australia. Available at: http://www.nswera.asn.au/startingout/GETTING%20STARTED%20IN%20ENDURANCE%20RIDING.pdf.

Sosa Leon, L.A., Hodgson, D.R. and Rose, R.J. (1997) Gastric emptying of oral rehydration solutions at rest and after exercise in horses. *Research in Veterinary Science* **63**(2), 183–187.

Welfare Concerns in the Care, Training, and Competition of the Hunter–Jumper

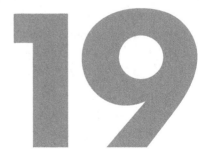

Richard D. Mitchell

19.1 Introduction

Through history, the use of the horse for military functions and cross-country hunting demanded that various obstacles encountered in the path of horse and rider had to be 'hurdled' in order to continue on course unimpeded. Such efforts required training in all but the most exceptional horses. Some horses were simply better than others for this purpose – consequently, selection and breeding arose to meet these needs. Most horses required at least some training to learn to jump with a rider, and out of this, methods were developed to consistently produce useful mounts. While training methods evolved, some were recognized as useful and productive, while others proved abusive to the horse with little long-term benefit. Since the horse was a primary mode of transportation prior to the advent of the automobile, welfare concerns arose, in part, as means to protect a valued possession.

As some horses or horse–rider combinations were perceived to perform better than others, competitions arose to recognize the best. Military and private competitions regularly matched horse–rider combinations against one another to determine

Equine Welfare, First Edition. Edited by C. Wayne McIlwraith and Bernard E. Rollin.
© 2011 by UFAW. Published 2011 by Blackwell Publishing Ltd.

the best performers. Today's equestrian jumping sport has reached an all-time level of popularity (Boswell *et al.*, 2003). As horse events have become more diverse, public concerns regarding the welfare of the horse have increased. The horse industry is learning that self-regulation of training and horse care practices may improve public perception as well as ensure the welfare of competing horses.

The horse has evolved to be a superb athlete as a matter of natural selection and survival. Being a herd animal and therefore a potential food source for carnivorous animals, the horse's ability to run away swiftly and jump obstacles in its path has historically allowed him to escape predators. While these abilities are innate, the capacity for significant repetition is limited without having physical consequences. These same traits can be enhanced in training practices to produce good performers, but improper or over-training can result in lameness, performance issues, and welfare concerns.

It is unusual to see neglect in horses of this type, but certainly issues do arise. Trainers on tight budgets may feed poorly and skimp on frequency of grooming and shoeing, but these practices have a self-limiting effect by producing poor results in the competition arena. Poor feeding and care practices are more likely to occur with the novice horse owner or in unusual instances of sudden financial hardship. Abuse is more likely to occur related to stabling, training, and medical issues.

19.2 Training the Young Jumping Horse

Jumping horses, because of the nature of their activity, must be more mature before starting jump training. A basic level of 'on the flat' training is necessary in order to have sufficient control to move on to jump training. Physical maturity will reduce the incidence of lameness issues such as physitis, bucked shins, and splints. Most breeds are three to four years of age or older before beginning jump training. Some young horses are truly gifted with the ability to jump. Such horses may be able to move along more quickly in their training, but care must be taken not to move forward to more aggressive training too quickly. Bones and ligaments need to be allowed to adjust to the activity at hand, lest injuries of these structures develop. Mild physical injuries, such as 'splints,' are common in young horses in jump training, but modification of the work schedule and appropriate medical care can often allow management of such problems (Dyson, 2003). Ignoring such issues is the simplest form of abuse and should be avoided. Young, talented horses can be moved forward in their training too quickly, producing adverse behavioral issues that may follow them throughout their careers. Patience with the talented young horse is essential for a successful outcome.

Horses that do not readily take to jumping can cause welfare concerns. Forcing such horses to jump in a round pen and through challenging gymnastic set-ups can result in injury. A modest amount of such training may bring out basic athletic ability; however, an experienced trainer can usually recognize the horse with minimal talent. The horse with poor jumping talent may be well suited for other activities such as dressage, driving, or pleasure riding, and the sooner this is recognized, the better.

Some young horses simply do not have respect for the obstacles they are asked to jump and consistently knock them down. More substantial obstacles may result in a change of attitude, but constructing unsafe and totally unyielding obstacles can be dangerous. The use of devices that inflict pain if the horse hits the jumps can be a serious welfare concern. Such devices may include jump rails with carpet tacks on the surfaces, plastic walkway runner with a tack-like underside that is wrapped around the rails underside exposed, and wires strung across the jump (sometimes electrified) that the horse cannot see. Use of such devices is unethical and abusive, yet such practices are often impossible to regulate outside of the competition venue. Some horses trained in this manner may subsequently refuse to jump. When this happens, the training may become even more abusive by forcing the horse to jump by excessive use of whip and spurs. Horses are trained by a system of reward and punishment and discipline is essential, but excessive force is a welfare concern. Creating fear in the horse is usually not a successful long-term training technique.

Poor riding technique and training by inexperienced individuals using contradictory training aids are also potential forms of abuse and may permanently affect young horses. An example would be the concurrent use of too much leg and hands sending the horse mixed signals. Training in this fashion may produce an animal that is indifferent to aids and therefore not readily trainable (Goodwin *et al.*, 2008).

How the horse is stabled and maintained on a daily basis can also lead to serious welfare concerns. Many elite performance horses live in a stall the vast majority of the time. Stabling at horse shows may be even more confining and adds the additional issues of many other horses, people, and noise. Horses evolved to be herd animals moving about and foraging 18–20 hours per day. Confinement in a small space may produce stress and alter critical physiological functions. Problems can arise related to confinement in the form of stereotypical behavior such as weaving, cribbing, and wood chewing (Hendersen, 2007). Gastric ulcers and various musculoskeletal problems may be attributable to stall confinement with little outside activity other than a training session each day (Mitchell, 2001). Dietary adjustments can be made to mimic foraging, such as multiple small meals per day. Getting out of the stall several times a day for exercise, hand walking, or walking on a mechanical walker or treadmill can be of significant benefit to minimize stress and prevent stereotypical behavior.

19.3 Travel for Training and Competition

Shipping horses has long been a very routine practice; yet numerous welfare issues may arise through ignorance or negligence. Travel itself is a stressful experience and the physical needs of the horse must be considered in shipping even modest distances. Adequate transport vehicles that provide sufficient room and safety for the horse are important. Appropriate ventilation when confined to a transport vehicle for an extended period is also important to help prevent shipping-related respiratory illness. Strict restriction of movement of the horse's head may contribute to respiratory disease. Therefore, it is often best to ship some horses in a box stall where they can put their head down if they are known to have respiratory difficulties. Periodic stops for water and rest are indicated in long-distance trips.

Horses that are constantly moving from one competition to another may begin to feel the effects of their environment. These horses may experience weight loss, stereotypical behavioral changes, and poor performance. A break from the competition schedule and stabling in a location with a more pastoral environment with occasional turnout or other similar activity may help these individuals return to normal. Certainly anti-ulcer medications and good diet can help correct these issues, and may be of benefit while the horse is 'on the road' (McClure *et al.*, 2005). The United States Equestrian Federation (USEF, 2007) and the Fédération Equestre Internationale (FEI, 2006a) allow for the use of anti-ulcer medication around and during competition due to known health and welfare issues related to gastric ulceration and traveling horses.

19.4 Schooling and Preparing for Competition

Today's equine sport is expensive and highly competitive. Many trainers are under a great deal of pressure to produce horses with near-perfect performances to achieve status and keep the horse owner happy. As a result, shortcuts are taken and unethical means of performance enhancement are sometimes utilized. These obviously can result in welfare issues. The horse show environment is stressful in many ways, from small stalls to interrupted feeding schedules, and constant noise and activity. The horse must be trained and handled in accordance with these conditions to prevent problems. The hunter is judged on jumping style, manners, and way of going. A good hunter is expected to perform in a quiet, deliberate, and obedient fashion. Any deviation from this is likely to result in penalties from the judges. This judging standard places pressure on those involved in training to get the horse 'quiet,' and a variety of methods have been used to accomplish this.

Lungeing is often used to relax the hunter before competition. A mild amount of lungeing may be beneficial for the horse in allowing a proper warm-up, but excessive lungeing to achieve fatigue is a form of abuse. Horses subjected to heavy lungeing on a frequent basis are inclined to develop soundness issues. Some horses are tied for excessive periods of time, thus preventing them from resting and possibly eating and drinking. Some trainers have actually been known to withhold water and feed intentionally prior to showing, presumably to cause dehydration and depression. These are clear abuses and against show rules but difficult to identify in the horse show environment. Various medications may be used to induce sedation or relaxation, and such practices are most often against competition rules, not only from a welfare standpoint, but also from a standpoint of concern for a level playing field with other competitors.

Preparing the jumping horse for the actual competition can bring up welfare concerns. Since it's important to have a horse jump in good form and not 'rub the jumps,' trainers will use various techniques to elicit the greatest effort from the horse. Regardless of whether the horse is a hunter or jumper, a clean performance is important. 'Rapping' or 'poling' – which is the practice of striking the horse with a rail that it is jumping over – is now forbidden at regular USEF Jumper competitions and FEI competitions (USEF, 2008; FEI, 2008), yet it may still be done by some trainers when not being watched by stewards or in private environments. This practice can result in injury to the horse, rider or the person performing the act. This practice was allowed for a period of time in the USA by the USEF with a bamboo pole only, but this has now been forbidden in regular hunter and jumper competitions. 'Rapping' can produce a profound response from the horse, but it also may instill fear and produce a reluctance to jump, especially if used too forcefully. Jumping an offset rail, which fools the horse's depth perception or doesn't allow the horse to see a rail, is still permitted at USEF Jumper competitions but has been forbidden by FEI because of safety and welfare concerns.

Occasionally owners and trainers will feel such pressure to produce a clean trip that they will resort to methods that involve sensitizing the lower legs in an effort make the horse less likely to 'rub the jumps.' Various substances that are mild to severe irritants are sometimes used to produce sensitivity, most often applied to the dorsal pastern and cannon bone regions. This process has been referred to as 'chemical rapping.' This may cause severe inflammation and 'blistering.' Use of such products is considered unethical and is a violation of rules for competition in USEF and FEI competitions. Stewards are instructed to inspect horses for the use of such substances during competitions.

The medication capsaicin has recently been cited as one that may relieve pain but at the same time may increase sensitivity in the lower leg if applied. This substance has been used by many riders for a number of years in the belief that it was not a testable substance. The drug has technically always been prohibited but until just recently was not identified in routine drug testing of performance horses. The US Horse Protection Act of 1970 made it illegal to 'sore' Tennessee Walking Horses, but this rule could be interpreted to apply to other disciplines. USEF and FEI rules do not permit horses with severe irritation on their lower limbs to compete if detected (USEF, 2008). This, of course, requires the show stewards to watch closely and identify such horses, but sensitivity to this form of abuse is sufficient at this time to insure stewardship in this area. Obviously, detection of medications or substances intended to 'sore' results in disqualification of horse and rider.

Performance-enhancing boots are sometimes applied to the hind limbs to achieve hyperflexion of the hind limbs on the jump stride. These may be weighted boots or ones applied with a greater pressure so as to reflexively produce hyperflexion.

The welfare issue with these boots is vague. The FEI has recently forbidden the use of boots weighing more than 500g (FEI, 2008); however, pressure boots are still in use. These may not be abusive, in fact, and simply may signal to the horse to flex more, but this remains unclear. Hyperflexion of the hind limbs may produce an exaggerated jumping style that can have consequences on landing and may result in the horse falling by 'tipping over' in a forward motion. These devices may likely be abusive in inexperienced hands as opposed to those of a seasoned professional (Murphy, 2008). Such boots cannot be used on hunters in the show ring as no boots of any kind are allowed, but they could be utilized in training.

In the past, electric devices such as whips and spurs have been used to elicit a greater response from the jumping horse. Again, aside from inflicting pain, these produce fear in some horses and are truly of a welfare concern. Such devices are not permitted in competition venues for training or showing. It should also be noted that excessive use of conventional whips and spurs is forbidden and may result in disqualification in both USEF and FEI competitions (USEF, 2008; FEI, 2007).

Clear infractions of rules pertaining to welfare of horses at shows carry severe penalties from governing bodies such as FEI and USEF, but enforcement of these rules still remains a problem.

19.5 Veterinary Medical and Medication Abuses

19.5.1 Current practices
The current standard for judging hunters in the USA has created a culture and need for the horse that 'never does anything wrong.' These standards will sometimes present a moral and ethical dilemma for the attending veterinarian. Playing after a jump, moving the head, and swishing the tail are all often penalized by the judges. In the jumper ring, there is a requirement for the horse to remained 'focused' on its job. As a result, trainers and owners have sought means of minimizing any undesired behavior through training means and sometimes unethical medical means. As mentioned previously, excessive lungeing prior to competition may take some of the 'play' out of a horse, but it may have long-term consequences on soundness. 'Tail blocking' is often performed on hunters to reduce movement of the tail that is considered undesirable. This practice is usually accomplished by injecting an alcohol-based substance at the base of the tail to locally paralyze the nerves. While this may be effective in stopping movement, such practice may cause more serious nerve weakness in the perineal region and affect fecal and urine retention and elimination. Severe sloughing of tissue and infection can occasionally occur, resulting in serious injury, pain, and suffering for the horse. Such practice is considered unethical by veterinary associations and is specifically prohibited by some horse show associations (AQHA, 2008).

When training alone does not accomplish the desired result, trainers, owners, and veterinarians may result to medicating the horse in an effort to influence performance. Therapeutic medication is allowed in the rule structure of a number of horse show organizations as a means for insuring the proper therapy of horses that are deemed otherwise fit to compete (USEF, 2008). In this regard such rules are beneficial to equine welfare. However, there are medications that are clearly prohibited in competition and have no place, including psychotropic medications and drugs that suppress pain such as opiates and local anesthetics.

Depending upon the organization, corticosteroids may be permissible (as in the case of the dexamethasone under USEF rules), or if the correct paperwork has been filed along with a proper withdrawal time of the horse from competition. An example of this would be the USEF rule that allows for the use of corticosteroids (other than dexamethasone) and various other medications but requires that the horse be withdrawn from competition for 24 hours and proper documentation filed with the show steward. The FEI has a strict rule structure that specifically forbids certain medications, but does allow for a limited number of therapeutic medications such as antibiotics, fluids, anti-ulcer medications, anthelmintics, anti-protozoals, and the hormone altrenogest (in mares) that are deemed not to affect performance. FEI policies require that the veterinary delegate be notified that these medications listed as 'not prohibited' will be utilized and that the appropriate paperwork be completed (FEI, 2007). Despite the prohibition of certain medications, horses may be medicated in an effort to alter behavior or mask pain.

19.5.2 Unconventional medication use

As mentioned previously, dexamethasone is permitted as a therapeutic medication at specific guideline dosages in USEF (USEF, 2007) and American Quarter Horse Association shows (AQHA, 2008). It is a popular belief, although not proven by science, that dexamethasone makes horses quiet. As a result, many hunter and jumper horses and ponies receive it ostensibly for allergies or dermatitis but are really getting it in an effort to control behavior. No medication report is necessary for the use of this medication in this fashion at the time of writing. Horses that show frequently may receive the medication several times a week, and subsequently may show several weeks in a row. The subsequent immune suppression could be a problem, allowing for severe skin and respiratory disease and possibly even laminitis. Technically, the use of the medication in this fashion is illegal by intent, but this is virtually impossible to prove. Certainly the indiscriminate use of dexamethasone poses serious welfare concerns.

Many other medications and feed additives are given in an effort to affect behavior in the show hunter and jumper. Some feed additives, such as the amino acid tryptophan, have been shown scientifically to likely not work, and others that are herbal in nature may actually contain forbidden psychotropic agents. Again, the use of herbal agents to calm the horse is illegal by intent, and using any feed additive that is not clearly labeled with ingredients poses a risk for a positive drug test and a risk to the horse's health.

Intravenous doses of thiamine are used to calm horses in the show ring. The substance itself is not prohibited, but the intent is illegal, and thiamine solutions pose a risk for serious allergic responses that can have fatal consequences.

Large doses of intravenous calcium gluconate and/or magnesium sulfate have been used to affect behavior, and these substances are not listed as prohibited in USEF and FEI rules (magnesium sulfate is on the FEI prohibited list as an 'evacuant' but reportedly difficult to detect). Certainly repeated intravenous injections of large volumes of these substances present risk for medical complications, and again the intent is illegal. Careless administration of magnesium or calcium could result in collapse of the treated horse.

Adrenocorticotropic hormone (ACTH) or synthetic analogs are frequently used in a similar fashion to dexamethasone to 'mellow' the horse that gets nervous in the show environment. Since this activates the adrenal glands, repeated use of this hormone could pose serious health concerns for the horse that may not be readily evident.

Some individuals have been known to use immune stimulants, because they will not be detected in drug testing, as quieting agents. Bacterial cell-wall derivative non-specific immune stimulants may cause brief febrile responses, and this subsequently makes the horse a little quieter. Obviously this is a form of abuse and can have serious health consequences for the horse through stress on homeostatic mechanisms.

USEF, AQHA, and the Canadian Equestrian Federation (CEF, 2008) allow for the use of specific non-steroidal anti-inflammatory drugs (NSAIDs) in horses while in competition. USEF actually allows for the use of two NSAIDs in competing horses as long as the two are not phenylbutazone and flunixin meglumine concurrently. (There is a proposal from the USEF Veterinary Committee to change this rule in 2010 and only allow one NSAID. However, this awaits the approval of the membership.) USEF, AQHA, and CEF all have lists of permitted NSAIDs, and no others are permitted for use. These are all medications that have at some time been approved for use in horses by the US Food and Drug Administration (FDA) or respective jurisdictions. These medications are again considered to be therapeutic and are intended to be used for mild problems in horses that are otherwise fit to compete. Welfare issues can arise with the use of these medications when there is a lameness for which there is no diagnosis or when horses are simply medicated 'because everyone else does it' and the trainers are seeking a more level playing field. Medicating horses unnecessarily may mask the presence of new injuries that could have serious consequences if overlooked. This becomes an even more significant issue when NSAIDs are administered by inexperienced horsemen.

When one considers that current rules in some organizations allow for more than one NSAID, and that the same rules allow for a corticosteroid to be in the horse at therapeutic levels (thereby also suppressing inflammation and pain), the potential for a significantly injured horse to compete is a real concern. Veterinarians and trainers must understand the potency of medications and make careful decisions regarding the true fitness of a horse to compete. There is the opportunity for the veterinarian to play a very important role in equine welfare in these situations.

The problem is that often the veterinarian is not made aware of the facts and often not included at all in the decision. This is a current problem in therapeutic medication rules outside of the FEI.

19.6 Future Equine Welfare Concerns

'No foreign substance' and 'prohibited substance' rules intended to prevent abuse are getting very complicated with today's advanced science of drug detection. With substances now being detected down to picograms, it becomes difficult to know when to withdraw medications given as legitimate therapy for an injury or condition so that a horse may return to competition. Rule structures need further modification to account for appropriate drug withdrawals that allow for treatment and convalescence. Horse organizations need to establish therapeutically effective levels for commonly used equine medications below which no positive call would occur. The FEI is currently working on this in a so-called 'medicine box' (FEI, 2006b). Not treating a horse with a mild problem could be considered abusive or negligent by some. Zero-tolerance rules may encourage lack of appropriate treatment or useless treatment. With zero-tolerance rules, the horseman may be encouraged to go outside of the field of known medications and experiment with newer drugs that are reportedly not detectable. This use of untested medications in the horse is yet another serious welfare concern.

Horse owners, trainers, and veterinarians have a great challenge in the future to control both physical and medication abuse in show hunters and jumpers. The temptation to lean on shortcuts and easy fixes is created in part by formidable competition and significant expense. These practices are generally not in the best interests of the welfare of the horse. Cultural changes in the past century have led to a change in the public perspective on horse competitions and what might be considered as abuse. The future of good horse sport will be dependent upon good horsemanship, an honorable sense of competition and a real concern for the welfare of the horse.

References

AQHA (2008) *American Quarter Horse Association Rule Book*, Rule 441, Prohibited Conduct, Therapeutic Medication Addendum; Rule 441(h), Show Rules and Regulations. American Quarter Horse Association, Amarillo, TX.

Boswell, R.P., Mitchell, R.D. and Dyson, S.J. (2003) Lameness in the show hunter and jumper. In *Diagnosis and Management of Lameness in the Horse*, Ross, M.W. and Dyson, S.J. (eds), pp. 965–975. Saunders, St. Louis, MO.

CEF (2008) *Equine Canada Rules*, Article 1003. Canadian Equine Federation, Ottawa, ON.

Dyson, S.J. (2003) The metacarpal region. In *Diagnosis and Management of Lameness in the Horse*, Ross, M.W. and Dyson, S.J. (eds), pp. 362–376. Saunders, St. Louis, MO.

FEI (2006a) *FEI Rules*, Annex III, Equine Prohibited List; Annex VI, Veterinary Regulations. Fédération Equestre Internationale, Lausanne, Switzerland.

FEI (2006b) *Anti-Doping and Medication Control: Reducing the Risks of Positive Drug Tests in Competition Horses*. FEI Press Release, June, 2006. Fédération Equestre Internationale, Lausanne, Switzerland.

FEI (2007) *FEI Rules*, Article 146, General Regulations, GR 143.1. Fédération Equestre Internationale, Lausanne, Switzerland.

FEI (2008) *FEI Rules, Rules for Jumping Events*, 22nd edn, Article 243.1.2, Article 257.2.3. Fédération Equestre Internationale, Lausanne, Switzerland.

Goodwin, D., McGreevy, P.D., Heleski, C., Randle, H. and Waran, N. (2008) Equitation science: the application of science in equitation. *Journal of Applied Animal Welfare Science* 11(3), 185–190.

Hendersen, A.J.Z. (2007) Don't fence me in: managing psychological well being for elite performance horses. *Journal of Applied Animal Welfare Science* 10(4), 309–329.

McClure, S.R., Carithers, D.S., Gross, S.J. and Murray, M.J. (2005) Gastric ulcer development in horses in a simulated show or training environment. *Journal of the American Veterinary Medical Association* 227(5), 775–777.

Mitchell, R.D. (2001) *Prevalence of Gastric Ulcers in Hunter/Jumper and Dressage Horses Evaluated for Poor Performance*. Association for Equine Sports Medicine, Sacramento, CA.

Murphy, J. (2008) Boots on horses: limb protection or hyperflexion training aids in the showjumping horse. *Journal of Applied Animal Welfare Science* 11(3), 223–227.

USEF (2007) *Drugs and Medications Guidelines* pamphlet. United States Equestrian Federation, Lexington, KY.

USEF (2008) *United States Equestrian Federation Rule Book*, GR410–GR412, GR839.4, GR839.4h, GR839.4j, GR843.1–3.

Welfare of Horses, Mules, and Other Equids in US Agriculture

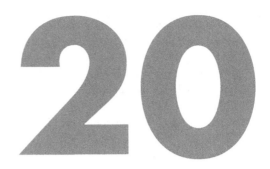

Josie L. Traub-Dargatz

20.1 Historical and Conceptual Aspects

A history of animal welfare by Baysinger (2006) suggests that, during the Industrial Revolution of the late eighteenth and early nineteenth centuries, a socio-economic revolution occurred. Both humans and animals were transitioning from rural to urban environments. The efforts to reduce child labor and abusive treatment of employees in factories ultimately extended to the bill introduced in the UK in 1822 by Richard Martin, Member of Parliament, for the protection of cattle, horses, and sheep from cruelty. In the UK, the formation in 1824 of the Society for the Prevention of Cruelty to Animals (SPCA) – later to become the Royal Society for the Prevention of Cruelty to Animals (RSPCA) – marked the beginning of the animal welfare movement. Parliament outlawed blood sports, overworking of beasts of burden, and regulated knacker yards and slaughterhouses in the late 1850s. In 1859, Darwin published *The Origin of Species* in which he proposed a new perspective on the human–animal relationship and caused society to consider that all living things might be sentient and therefore could not only suffer harm but also feel pain. In 1964, Ruth Harrison's book *Animal Machines* brought attention to agricultural animals in Europe. Subsequently the Brambell Committee was formed to investigate the state of farm animal's well-being. The Brambell Report was released in 1965 and suggested that all animals should have:

Equine Welfare, First Edition. Edited by C. Wayne McIlwraith and Bernard E. Rollin.
© 2011 by UFAW. Published 2011 by Blackwell Publishing Ltd.

(1) freedom from hunger and thirst;
(2) freedom from discomfort;
(3) freedom from pain, injury, and disease;
(4) freedom to express normal behavior; and
(5) freedom from fear and distress.

The American Society for the Prevention of Cruelty to Animals (ASPCA) was the first 'welfare' organization established in the USA, in 1866. Today, the ASPCA exists to 'promote humane principles, prevent cruelty and alleviate pain, fear and suffering in animals' (Baysinger, 2006). The Humane Society of the United States (HSUS) was formed after the ASPCA and is categorized as an animal rights organization (Baysinger, 2006). The HSUS has changed its objectives to broaden its traditional humane concerns to include a wide variety of animal and environmental issues. The HSUS concerns include research animals, companion animals, farm animals, wildlife, and State and Federal legislation. The organization People for the Ethical Treatment of Animals (PETA) was founded in 1980. PETA is dedicated to establishing and defending the rights of all animals. PETA operates under the principle that animals are not ours to eat, wear (e.g. such as leather or fur), experiment on, or use for entertainment (Baysinger, 2006).

From the brief background provided above, it is apparent there are varying perspectives regarding the welfare of animals. For this chapter, the author is assuming that the reader will accept that horses, mules, donkeys, and other domestic equids in an agricultural setting have a purpose in working with people to accomplish the goals of a ranch, farm or other agricultural pursuit. It is therefore important to consider the concept of fitness for the intended purpose of such animals, be they spelled out or inherently understood. For example, the amount of weight an animal can carry or pull is dependent on the animal's stature, confirmation, and fitness. The amount of time a horse can work in harness or under saddle depends on multiple factors including age, fitness, stature, training, behavior of the equine, the terrain, work to be done, and the existing weather conditions. Being certain that the tack or harness fits the horse and is appropriate for the intended work and that the equine has received appropriate farrier care to make the animal fit for the intended task are also important in assuring the horse's comfort while working. Thus the welfare of the animal is based on its use and general care needs.

The responsibility for assurance of the welfare of animals first falls on those who own or use them in their agricultural work. In the author's opinion, the people who are part of the agricultural setting expect of their animals what they expect of themselves. From the author's experience, farm and ranch people consistently work long hours. During a given day the people and equines working with them take periodic breaks for hydration and nutrition. Everyone, including the working equid, is expected to work until the work for the day is done.

It is logical that most of those engaged in agricultural pursuits will be good stewards of their animals, as they need them to accomplish the work that allows them to earn a living. Beyond this, many ranchers and farmers consider their horses, mules, and other equines as part of the family. These animals are given names and there is an understanding that they each have a unique personality and aptitude that needs to be taken into account in order to get the optimal performance from the animal and to make the work day go as smoothly as possible. A good example of the status some of these animals had is an account from an 85-year-old neighbor of the author's. This woman described an excerpt from a letter her father wrote to his brother, 'that come spring he hoped to have two mules and a son born.' It is interesting to note that this farmer's anticipation of the upcoming birth of the mules was mentioned, in this excerpt, ahead of, and with equal enthusiasm to, that of the upcoming birth of what would be his first son.

20.2 Demographics of Equines in the USA

A review of the demographics of equids in the USA will allow for a better understanding of the trends in the equine population in agriculture over time. Demographic changes in the equine industry in the USA occurred due to change in demand for horses and mules for farm and city work. The automobile and tractor gradually replaced the horse-drawn vehicle on city streets and roads, and the work stock on a great many farms and ranches (Sarle, 1926). According to Sarle, based on a United States Department of Agriculture (USDA) report, the decreased demand for equine stock because of mechanization of transportation and farming resulted in a 35% reduction in the value of a horse from 1918 to 1924 (Sarle, 1926). With the sharp drop in demand and falling prices for horses and mules there was a subsequent sharp drop in the number of horse and mule foals born. The Census of Agriculture for 1925 showed a 45% reduction in the number of horses and mules less than two years of age compared to the number in 1920 (Sarle, 1926).

The Census of Agriculture has collected and reported estimates of the equine inventory numbers roughly every five years since 1840 (Table 20.1). The estimate is for all places in the USA that meet the USDA's definition of a 'farm.' The current definition of a 'farm' was first used in 1974, and is defined as a place that could or did actually sell $1000.00 of agricultural products annually. In addition, as of 1987, any operation that has five or more equines (other than commercial enterprises such as racetracks) qualifies as a farm even if no other agricultural activity occurs on the operation (NAHMS, 2007).

As Table 20.1 shows, the estimated total number of equids (horses, ponies, mules, and donkeys) based on the Census of Agriculture peaked in 1920 at just over 25 million (NAHMS, 2007). The prominent role of equids in agriculture in the past is illustrated by the fact that an entire book related to diseases of horses was published by the USDA, Bureau of Animal Industry, in 1896 (Salmon, 1896). The total number of equines declined from that number to just over 4 million by 1959, further declined to 2 million by 1978, and never exceeded 2.6 million until

Table 20.1 Change in equine inventory on farms, 1850–2002.

Year/month	Horses and ponies			Mules, burros, and donkeys			Total equine inventory	Percentage of 1850
	Total inventory	Number of farms	Avg. per farm	Total inventory	Number of farms	Avg. per farm		
1850 (June 1)	4336719	N/A	N/A	559331	N/A	N/A	4896050	100.0
1860 (June 1)	6249174	N/A	N/A	1151148	N/A	N/A	7400322	151.1
1870 (June 1)	7145370	N/A	N/A	1125415	N/A	N/A	8270785	168.9
1880 (June 1)	10357488	N/A	N/A	1812808	N/A	N/A	12170296	248.6
1890 (June 1)	15266244	N/A	N/A	2251876[2]	N/A	N/A	17518120	357.8
1900 (June 1)	18267020	4530628	4.0	3264615[2]	1480652[2]	2.2	21531635[2]	439.8
1910 (Apr. 15)	19833113	4692814	4.2	4209769[2]	1869005[2]	2.3	24042882[2]	491.1
1920 (Jan. 1)	19767161	4704235	4.2	5432391[2]	2259746[2]	2.4	25199552[2]	514.7
1925 (Jan. 1)	16400623	5365513	3.1	5680897[2]	N/A	N/A	22081520[2]	451.0
1930 (Apr. 1)	13510839	5024713	2.7	5375017[2]	N/A	N/A	18885856[2]	385.7
1935 (Jan. 1)	11857850	3536597	3.4	4818160[2]	2255845[2]	2.1	16676010[2]	340.6
1940 (Apr. 1)	10086971	3148656	3.2	3844560[2]	1845517[2]	2.1	13931531[2]	284.5
1945 (Jan. 1)	8499204	2828412	3.0	3129590[2]	1486209[2]	2.1	11628794[2]	237.5
1950 (Apr. 1)	5401646	2120843	2.5	2202264[2]	1101799[2]	2.0	7603910[2]	155.3
1954 (Oct.–Nov.)	4141288[1]	1799899[1]	2.3	N/A	N/A	N/A	4141288[1]	84.6
1959 (Oct.–Nov.)	2955256[1]	1138986[1]	2.6	N/A	N/A	N/A	2955256[1]	60.4
1964 (Nov.–Dec.)	N/A	N/A	N/A	N/A	N/A	N/A	N/A	N/A
1969 (Dec. 31)	2237981	547246	4.1	66128	34309	1.9	2304109	47.1
1974 (Dec. 31)	1595640	359051	4.4	N/A	N/A	N/A	N/A	N/A
1978 (Dec. 31)	1957028	399335	4.9	56703	27631	2.1	2013731	41.1
1982 (Dec. 31)	2260791	417042	5.4	27430	10431	2.6	2288221	46.7
1987 (Dec. 31)	2456951	415565	5.9	56520	23311	2.4	2513471	51.3

Table 20.1 (Cont'd).

Year/month	Horses and ponies			Mules, burros, and donkeys			Total equine inventory	Percentage of 1850
	Total inventory	Number of farms	Avg. per farm	Total inventory	Number of farms	Avg. per farm		
1992 (Dec. 31)	2 049 522	338 346	6.1	67 692	25 589	2.6	2 117 214	43.2
1997* (Dec. 31)	3 020 117	490 517	6.2	123 211	44 096	2.8	3 143 328	64.2
2002* (Dec. 31)	3 644 278	542 223	6.7	105 358	29 936	3.5	3 749 636	76.6

Notes:

1890–1954: Number of mules on farms. Donkeys and burros were excluded.

1940: Horse and pony inventory includes only animals older than three months of age.

1954 and 1959: Horse, pony, and mule inventories reported together.

1964: No equine data.

N/A = not available.

*1997 and 2002 = Census of Agriculture adjusted for incompleteness.

Source: USDA–NASS Census of Agriculture 1997 and 2002; 1850–1992 prepared by Commerce Department US Bureau of Census.

[1] Farms reporting horses and/or mules in some States.

[2] Excludes burros and donkeys.

Source: USDA Census of Agriculture.

1997, when the total number of equines on farms in the USA was estimated at 3.1 million. The total number of equines on farms increased even further in 2002 to 3.7 million head. It is important to acknowledge that, prior to mechanization (automobile and tractor), most equines lived on farms. Since mechanization, the percentage of the equine population and the number of equines that live on premises that do not meet the Census of Agriculture's definition of a 'farm' have increased but the number is unknown. Thus it is important to acknowledge that currently the estimate from the Census of Agriculture based on their stated objective to estimate equids on 'farms' would underestimate the total equine population in the USA. The number of farms with horses peaked in 1925 at 5.3 million, while in 2002 there were estimated to be only 542 223 farms that had horses.

Based on estimates from the National Animal Health Monitoring System (NAHMS) studies conducted in 1998 and again in 2005, for operations with five or more equids, excluding racetracks, the primary use of equids for the majority of operations was pleasure followed by farm and ranch use (NAHMS, 2007). Thus, at least for places with five or more equines, farm and ranch use is one of the leading primary uses of equids in the USA.

It is doubtful that this country will ever see 20 million working horses, ponies, mules, and donkeys on its farms, ranches, or streets again, but there are thousands of working situations where horses can, do, and will perform useful work economically (Telleen, 1977). Some proposed advantages of horses over motorized equipment include (Telleen, 1977):

(1)   horses consume farm-grown feeds for their fuel;
(2)   horses return most of the fertility from their feed to the land in the form of manure; and
(3)   mares can share the work and produce foals as their replacements and for sale.

With horses, you can raise your own replacements, which appreciate in value rather than depreciate in value like tractors do. Horses in the first part of their working life appreciate in value, and with proper care can work till they are 15–20 years of age and in some instances even longer. Horses allow for the amount of power for the job to be tailored appropriately, for example, by altering the number of horses per hitch depending on the job at hand, while the use of a tractor may be an overuse of power for many jobs, thus resulting in overuse of fuel. Horses are dependable power: for example, they can work in snow and mud as well as on slopes that are either impossible or dangerous for a tractor or other motorized vehicle, such as a four-wheeler (Telleen, 1977).

Thus, despite the decline in the total number of equids from their peak in 1920, horses, ponies, mules, and donkeys are still a part of agriculture in the USA today. Therefore, a discussion of the type of uses along with the husbandry practices of such equines over time is warranted.

20.3 Agricultural Uses and Welfare of Equines in Agriculture in the USA

Agricultural uses of equines would include use as draft animals, as working cattle or other livestock, and for transportation into areas where motorized vehicles are prohibited or unable to travel on ranches, or Federal or State lands, for example in forestry for logging. There are multiple examples of the use of horses in agriculture today. A quote from Lynn Miller in his book entitled *Work Horse Handbook* (Miller, 2004) illustrates this point: 'Today in the year 2003, I work horses. In harness for field work on our ranch, for occasional logging and some highway/parade driving, I work horses. I believe in the practicality of work horses.' Miller further states his commitment to his horses by saying 'The healthier, more comfortable work horse is the more efficient and willing work horse.' He indicates there are many new aids, with more on the way, to accomplish this 'comfort' for the horse.

In general, farmers and ranchers are good stewards of the land and their animals, as they rely on both to provide sustenance for themselves and others. Using horses and mules in agriculture with respect, firm kindness, and common sense has been common place (Telleen, 1977). Per Lynn Miller, 'Although a fear-based controlling approach to horses has resulted in remarkable performance, the performance demonstrated by partnerships rooted in mutual respect and trust has won races, saved the day, plowed the fields, and protected children' (Miller, 2004).

Based on a story from *Western Horseman* magazine, Monte Jones is quoted as saying 'I came from the old school where you didn't take time to supple a horse. You just pulled him around and used him as a slave. You could get a horse broke that way, but he sure wasn't light in the bridle by today's standards and it didn't always make the horse like his job' (Denison, 2008). There is evidence in recently published articles and in practical education seminars illustrating that the methods used to train and work with horses continues to move toward a partnership between the horse and handler. In many of the horsemanship clinics today, an emphasis is placed on training the riders and handlers as opposed to training just a specific horse. The goal of these clinics is to have those participating gain new horsemanship skills that can apply to all of their horses not just the one participating in the clinic itself. The objective of many of these training clinics is to work with the natural habits of the horse in order to make this partnership easier for both the horse and the handler.

Formation of the Ranching Horse Association of America (RHAA) in 1998 attests to the current interest and popularity of horses used in ranching and performing the skills needed in ranching. The RHAA (http://www.rhaa.org) promotes the qualities and characteristics of the ultimate working ranch horse, while providing a means of competition to show these ranch horses. The RHAA sanctions local working ranch horse competitions, provides a uniform set of rules, qualifies working ranch horse competition judges, and promotes uniformity and consistency in judging. The association indicates these are their goals while maintaining traditional Western influence with historic Western sportsmanship and a cowboy ethic.

There are several components involved in providing for the welfare of equids in agriculture:

(1) providing for basic needs such as food, water, safe housing and transportation, along with farrier and veterinary care;
(2) working the equid within the limits of its ability based on its aptitude and fitness, weather conditions, and the type and level of task required; and
(3) using tack appropriate for the task which does not unduly burden or injure the equine.

Thus, when considering the welfare of equids in agriculture, there could be a negative impact if the equine were not provided the basic staples of life, if the equine is overworked, abused in order to make it work through use of severe training methods, or if it is hauled in a manner that inadequately assures the safety and reasonable comfort of the equine.

As previously mentioned, it is generally assumed the owner or their agent will provide for the welfare of the animals in their care and that the primary responsibility in providing for the welfare of equids in agriculture falls upon their owners or the person that the owner has designated to provide care.

In general, the author would suggest that farmers and ranchers are familiar with the basic needs of livestock and are likely to have access to the essentials necessary for basic care. It makes sense that horses, mules, donkeys, and other equines that are used to work in agricultural activities in developed countries live on farms or ranches where feed is abundant and there is adequate space to express normal behavior. In addition, most farmers and ranchers are experienced in the care of livestock, so they are likely to have a good understanding of the basic needs of animals in their care, including the daily provision of adequate feed, access to water, shelter, and exercise. Unlike first-time horse owners, who may fail to understand the commitment required to supply consistent provision of these staples for their animals, the farmer and/or rancher understands the commitment necessary to care for livestock and that this care is a daily, year-round job

Tim O'Bryne wrote in an article in *Western Horseman* that 'there is no official handbook outlining cowboy-horsemanship fundamentals but learning from mentors can be an important key to success as a modern working cowboy' (O'Bryne, 2005a). He indicated that the cowboy relies on good horses and is obligated to create a partnership with them in order to get the work done. He went on to say that working cowboys commit to ride and work in all weather conditions. This commitment sets them apart from the rest of the horse-loving population, leading to special requirements for the working cowboy's horsemanship profile, a profile like no other. O'Bryne (2005a) wrote of several fundamentals for the student cowboy, several of which address the welfare of the working ranch horse, including:

- tend to your horse(s) before you tend to yourself;
- do not abuse your horses;
- tend to your horse's feet; and
- work in a safe manner.

O'Bryne (2005b) gave further guidance on pacing the working ranch horse, which highlights the importance of taking into consideration:

- the age of the horse;
- the weight and ability of the rider;
- the type of work; and
- the terrain where the work is to be done.

O'Bryne went on to say that horses need to get plenty of time for recovery from long, hard days of ranch work. He notes that many ranches rotate horses several times a year, using them in a three months on and three months off work schedule. As an example, O'Bryne (2005b) suggested using more mature and capable horses for spring calving and branding and using young upcoming horses in summer and fall for moving cattle to and from grazing areas.

Guidelines related to the amount of work that equids could be expected to perform were published as recommendations for the working of cart, wagon and farm horses in 1850 in *An Encyclopedia of Agriculture* (Loudon, 1825). The recommendations for working farm horses included the recommended age at which they are put to work, the quantity of work they should perform, and their feeding and general management. This book recommends the horse be 4–5 years old when put to full work in the labors of a farm. The question of the amount of work expected depended on the circumstances, including the number of horses in the team and the type of soil to be worked. For example, this encyclopedia suggests horses may be expected to be in harness nine hours and in some situations up to 10 hours per day, with a rest to be allowed to feed for two hours in midday. The amount of weight the horse can pull depended on whether it is moving on a well-made road or pulling a plow (soil type dependent). The horse's breeding and rearing were suggested to affect when it could be put to work and how much work it could be expected to do, thus illustrating the importance of fitness for purpose when using horses in agriculture. This encyclopedia contains additional recommendations regarding housing, grooming, feeding, and the amount of land necessary for accommodating each horse.

The duration of work per day is dependent on many factors, including the fitness of the horse, the climatic conditions, and the work being done. There may be some people who consider the work done by equids on ranches and farms to be excessive based on their experiences with pleasure, show or race horses. However, horses and mules have thrived when performing these agricultural activities for decades. For example, ranch horses may be saddled in the early morning and not finish their day

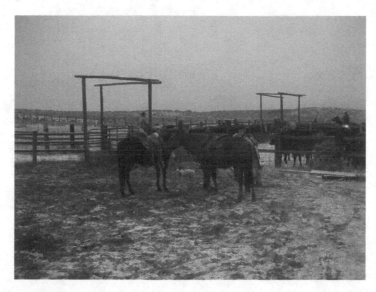

Figure 20.1   Ranch horses at pens where cattle are being sorted. Such horses may be saddled and work intermittently from dawn to dusk. Ranch horses work in all kinds of weather, such as this snowstorm in fall of the year, when cattle are typically gathered off the summer range.

until well after sundown. During this time they may be working to gather cattle, working cattle in pens (Figure 20.1), and used to move cattle back onto the range or onto trucks for transport. The horses may be transported with their saddles on between various locations in order to accomplish the gather. These horses seem to sense they have a job to do and have learned to drink when water is available at stream crossings and water tanks along the way in order to stay hydrated, and graze when allowed between tasks. Not all types of horses could be used in this manner and remain healthy. Many horses used in ranching were born and raised on a ranch, allowing them to become accustomed to the terrain and weather conditions. It takes a horse suited to its purpose to be able to maintain their weight and soundness doing this type of work, but if properly selected and cared for, some horses perform this kind of work throughout 2–3 decades of their lives. A commitment to the partnership between the rancher and horse is illustrated by a rancher in Montana who indicated to the author that he had a life insurance policy to assure the care of his horses after he died instead of the more traditional motivation, e.g., to provide for his wife in the event of his death. He went on to say that the horses that had worked with him throughout their career would have a place to live out their lives even after they could no longer work. Figure 20.2 shows three geldings that had done ranch and backcountry trail work for decades. When photographed, these horses were in retirement at a Montana ranch in a lush pasture receiving extra feed specially designed for geriatric horses in order to maintain their

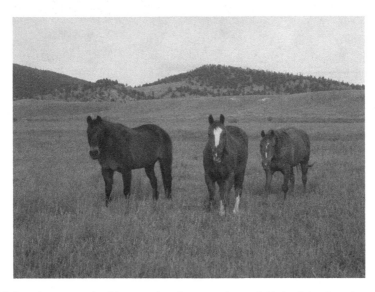

Figure 20.2   Three retired geldings in their late twenties and thirties living in retirement at their owner's ranch in Montana after having done ranch and backcountry trail work for all of their athletic years.

weight and meet their nutritional needs. They had earned their keep for life in the eyes of their owner.

Many States in the USA have provisions to assure appropriate care of horses and other domestic equids if the owner fails in their commitment to their animal's welfare. These provisions vary by State. In some States, such as Illinois, the Department of Agriculture administers a 'Humane Care for Animals Act.' While other States prohibit specific acts of cruelty, Illinois has minimum standards of treatment that must be afforded animals. Another example is Minnesota's statute[1] that defines standards for equine food, water, shelter, space and cleanliness, exercise, hoof care, and transportation requirements. In addition, specific laws have emerged in response to particular needs. A review of these laws has been published (Twyne and Stanley, 1990) and includes sections on weight-pulling contests, tail docking and setting, jumping, soring ('soring' is the intentional inflicting of pain or inflammation in the hoof area to accentuate the action in gaited horses (APHIS, 2004)), rodeos, cruelty to wild horses and burros, abandonment and sale of old horses and horses unfit for work, shelter, riding schools and hiring of horses, criteria for confiscating poorly treated and abandoned animals, dental care, transportation, possession and sale of foals, export by sea for slaughter, and horse

---

[1] Minnesota Statutes Annotated, Section 346.38, https://www.revisor.leg.state.mn.us/statutes/?id=346.38.

racing. Twyne and Stanley (1990) state that the general anti-cruelty laws of every State in the country prohibit beating, overworking, overriding, torture, torment, and neglect.

The *Legal Handbook for Inspectors* produced by the RSPCA (Flint and Pearson, 1972) points out that, while there is no legal definition of overloading, experiments carried out by experts at the request of the RSPCA found that the maximum load a horse should be required to pull on level ground is 2.5–3 times its own weight. Any pulling contest involving overloading or overdriving an equine would be in violation of the anti-cruelty laws of every State in the USA.

Regulations within the State of Pennsylvania[2] limit the hours of labor – including driving, leading, riding or working (or causing or allowing it to be done) – of horses or other animals to be not more than 15 hours in any 24-hour period or more than 90 hours in any one week. The anti-cruelty code in Washington (Section 16.52.070) states that 'whoever having charge or custody of any animal, either as owner or otherwise ... who willfully and unreasonably drives the same when unfit for labor or with yoke or harness that chafes or galls it or check rein or any part of its harness too tight for its comfort ... shall be guilty of a misdemeanor.'

Based on the National Animal Health Monitoring System equine study (NAHMS, 2006), 67.8% of equine operations with a primary function of farm or ranch administered vaccines to their equines, and this was a lesser percent than operations with a primary function of boarding and/or training, breeding farm, or 'other functions' category. Although equids on ranches and farms may lead a more isolated lifestyle and thus have less exposure to directly contagious disease agents such as viral or bacterial respiratory disease agents, equines on ranches should receive the core vaccines. The core vaccines are meant to aid in control of disease agents that have an associated high mortality rate, and exposure is possible even if the equine has limited or no exposure to equines from other operations. The core vaccines, as designated by the American Association of Equine Practitioners, include tetanus toxoid, Eastern and Western equine encephalitis vaccine, West Nile virus vaccine, and rabies vaccine. These core vaccines were the most likely type to be given other than rabies vaccine. Perhaps further education of ranchers and farmers that these core vaccines are recommended even if their equines lead a relatively isolated existence is warranted and could be accomplished through extension agent communications.

In summary, the requirements necessary to ensure the welfare of equids used for agriculture in developed countries, such as adequate housing, nutrition, and drinking water, are likely to be met, as they are readily available on ranches and farms. Ranchers and farmers generally have basic knowledge related to livestock husbandry and are committed to satisfying the basic needs of their animals. It is worth noting that written guidelines are available regarding the amount and type of work

---

[2] Pennsylvania Consolidated Statutes, Section 18-5511, http://members.aol.com/StatutesP7/18PA5511.html.

that is acceptable for equids based on their fitness for the purpose of agriculture work. However, many ranchers and farmers have inherited their knowledge of how to work effectively with equids from previous generations by word of mouth and through example. It is critical to understand there is often a partnership that exists between the animal and its owner. In the author's opinion, people unfamiliar with the use of equines in agriculture may initially think the work excessive until they understand that the amount or type of work performed by this human–equine team is acceptable if the horse or other equine is provided with appropriate care, conditioning, and selected for the intended purpose.

Acknowledgments

The author would like to acknowledge Dr. Andy Anderson for providing some of the concepts included in this text and his review of a draft of the chapter, Ms. Mary Foley and Dr. Bruce Wagner for their review of a draft of this chapter, Dr. Ralph and Candace Miller for willingness to share their Montana ranch experience and access to their ranch horses with the author over the many years of our friendship, and Ms. Verda Wilkins for sharing the content of the letter her father wrote to his brother many decades ago.

References

APHIS (2004) *The Horse Protection Act*. APHIS Animal Care Factsheet. USDA, APHIS, Animal Care, Riverdale, MD. Available at: http://www.aphis.usda.gov/publications/animal_welfare/content/printable_version/fs_awhpa.pdf.

Baysinger, A.K. (2006) Welfare: What's the consumer's perspective? A brief history of animal welfare. *Proceedings of the National American Veterinary Conference, 2006*. Available at: http://www.ivis.org/proceedings/toc3_proceedings.asp.

Denison, J. (2008) Ready to work. *Western Horseman*, July, pp. 58–66.

Flint, L.P. and Pearson, A. (1972) *A Legal Handbook for Inspectors of the Royal Society for the Prevention of Cruelty to Animals*. RSPCA, London.

Loudon, J.C. (1825) *An Encyclopedia of Agriculture; Comprising the Theory and Practice of the Valuation, Transfer, Laying Out, Improvement and Management of Landed Property; and the Cultivation and Economy of the Animal and Vegetable Production of Agriculture*, pp. 948–950. Printed for Longman, Hurst, Rees, Orme, Brown & Green, by Spottiswoode, London.

Miller, L.R. (2004) Attitude and approach – the horse as a thinking and feeling mammal. *Work Horse Handbook*, ch. 2, pp. 23–30. Small Farmer's Journal, Inc., Sisters, OR.

NAHMS (2006) *Vaccination Practices on US Equine Operations*. USDA–APHIS, National Animal Health Monitoring System, No. N454.1206.

NAHMS (2007) *Equine 2005, Part II: Changes in the US Equine Industry, 1998–2005*, pp. 2–8. USDA–APHIS, National Animal Health Monitoring System.

O'Bryne, T. (2005a) Fundamentals for the working cowboy. *Western Horseman*, July, pp. 84–93.

O'Bryne, T. (2005b) Pacing the working ranch horse. *Western Horseman*, March, pp. 68–75.

Salmon, D.E. (1896) *Special Report on Disease of the Horse.* US Department of Agriculture, Bureau of Animal Industry.

Sarle, C.F. (1926) Horse production falling fast. In *US Yearbook*, pp. 437–439. United States Department of Agriculture.

Telleen, M. (1977) The return of the draft horse. *The Draft Horse Primer: A Guide to the Care and Use of Work Horses and Mules*, pp. 1–17. Rodale Press, Emmaus, PA.

Twyne, P. and Stanley, V. (1990) Horses. *Animals and their Legal Rights: A Survey of American Laws from 1641 to 1990*, ch. VIII, pp. 126–151. Animal Welfare Institute, Washington, DC.

Welfare Issues with the Carriage Horse

Jay Baldwin

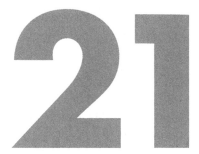

One luxury of living in a modern industrialized nation is the choice of whether or not to employ horses, and other animal companions, in for-profit businesses. In the USA, most equine enterprises are not essential for survival. Since the horses do not get to choose their own vocation, animal activists increasingly argue for the elimination of trades that involve horses working for human profit. Americans' increased appreciation of the human–animal bond has only served to highlight this discussion.

Urban carriage horses are the most visible and accessible of all horses trained to work for profit. Their nearness to large population centers, combined with their challenging work environment, has made their trade the foremost equine target of animal rights activists. Groups that have recently called for the elimination of the urban carriage horse trade include the animal rights organization People for the Ethical Treatment of Animals (PETA) and its many affiliated groups and subsidiaries, as well as more moderate groups such as the Humane Society of the United States (HSUS) and the American Society for the Prevention of Cruelty to Animals (ASPCA) (Richburg, 2007).

Horse-drawn sightseeing carriages operate in major cities in all geographic regions of the USA (Table 21.1). Of the 25 largest US cities by population, at least 17 of them host a year-round commercial carriage trade. In recent years, the commercial carriage business has diffused to many smaller cities and towns, particularly in historic districts, at least on a seasonal basis.

In spite of extensive anti-carriage horse publicity campaigns by PETA and other groups, there is no sign of the business declining. The primary reason for this is the strong public demand for horse-drawn carriage rides. Sustained public demand has created a profitable carriage trade, which often helps promote other tourist

Equine Welfare, First Edition. Edited by C. Wayne McIlwraith and Bernard E. Rollin.
© 2011 by UFAW. Published 2011 by Blackwell Publishing Ltd.

Table 21.1 A partial list of major US cities with commercial carriage horses, along with their population ranking.

City	Rank	City	Rank
New York	1	Memphis	17
Chicago	3	Baltimore	18
Houston	4	Fort Worth	19
Philadelphia	5	Milwaukee	22
San Antonio	7	Seattle	23
San Diego	8	Boston	24
Dallas	9	Denver	25
Indianapolis	12	Louisville	26
San Francisco	14	Washington DC	27
Columbus	15	Atlanta	44
Austin	16	New Orleans	47

Source: US Census Bureau (2004).

attractions in cities as diverse as New York, New Orleans, Memphis, San Antonio, Denver, and San Diego.

This chapter is intended to give a brief overview of the urban carriage horse industry of larger US cities, to describe common health problems and health regulations, and to outline some relevant welfare issues.

21.2 Common Health Problems

Despite their challenging work environment, urban carriage horses experience relatively few medical or surgical problems. The frequency or occurrence of health problems is similar to that found in most populations of pleasure (riding) horses, and it is much less than the frequency of veterinary problems in racehorses or event horses. During an intensive 18-month period of 4314 unannounced street inspections of working carriage horses in New York in 1990–1991, fewer than 20 cases of lameness or illness were found (Baldwin and Kurtz, 1992). Obviously this statistic is biased, since seriously ill or lame horses are almost never sent to work; yet this highlights the relatively low frequency of medical problems in horses performing sporadic light draft work.

21.2.1 Lameness
Continuous work on hard paved streets, along with improper or infrequent shoeing, are the major factors causing lameness in urban carriage horses. Working on pavement exacerbates any tendency toward lameness from conformational faults, and rapidly wears out all types of horseshoes. Carriage horses' frequent companions,

mounted police horses, also suffer from the constant concussion of working on pavement. In some cities, many carriage horses are retired Standardbred racehorses or retired Amish draft horses with a wide variety of healed minor injuries from their previous careers. Owing to the weight and location of the carriage hitch, hind limb soreness is most common. Because pulling a carriage represents light work for most of these horses, such defects may remain stable and painless if the horses are properly shod. Timely trimming and shoeing are essential. Proper shoeing and hoof care may be encouraged by work suspensions and fines for carriage operators who do not comply. Owners who neglect hoof care should be issued summonses until it becomes more profitable to call the farrier than to pay the fines and lose the work time.

Rubber shoes are sometimes recommended to reduce impact for horses working on pavement. Owners may refuse to use rubber shoes due to decreased wear time. Also, rubber shoes may cause slipping in wet or wintry road conditions; and rubber shoes may exacerbate conformational soreness problems in some horses. Therefore, although impact-absorbing rubber horseshoes are theoretically a good idea, they are not suitable for all horses and all weather conditions. Metal shoes with borium (tungsten carbide crystals embedded in a carrier material) caulks provide consistent traction, and require less frequent replacement. However, metal shoes provide no added cushion for the horse, and may also aggravate certain pre-existing leg problems, particularly hock problems. Rubber pads under metal shoes work well for many horses.

Leg and foot problems that all but disappeared with the draft horse, including shoe boil, quittor, and side bone, appear occasionally in city carriage horses. The diagnosis and treatment of these conditions has been well described (Adair, 1992).

21.2.2 Colic

Many urban carriage horses originate from unmechanized farms where science-based deworming is not practiced. Any newly purchased carriage horse should be suspected of carrying a large intestinal parasite load until proven otherwise. In spite of required fecal examinations, regular deworming, and conservative feeding programs, colic is still a major cause of death in carriage horses in New York City and elsewhere. It is suspected that many of these draft horses, many from agrarian origins, have an inadequate history of deworming and subsequently have resultant intestinal vascular damage. Newly purchased draft horses and mules should be aggressively dewormed. Note that most standard deworming doses are designed for a 450 kg horse and will be inadequate, for example, for a 675 kg Percheron crossbreed. Routine fecal examinations should be used to formulate a sound scientific deworming program for each individual horse. Deworming and fecal exam records should be part of each horse's individual health record.

Gastrointestinal problems may also result from lack of exercise, particularly during periods of seasonally slow tourism. Carriage horses should be turned out, or worked (even if there are no fares) during these slow periods in order to exercise the horse. Colic may result from abrupt changes in feed, poor-quality feed, or changes in feeding schedule. These problems can usually be avoided by employing experienced drivers and stable personnel.

21.2.3 Respiratory problems

Chronic obstructive pulmonary disease (COPD) or 'heaves' is the most common respiratory problem in many cities. Draft-type horses seem to be more commonly affected than Standardbreds or mules. Urban air pollution has been suggested as a contributing factor, but there is no data to confirm or deny this claim. This problem most commonly appears on hot, humid summer days. Horses with mild COPD may work humanely with good management and veterinary care. Such horses are usually worked during a night shift when it is cooler; or they may not be worked at all during humid weather. These horses should be kept near open windows, on low-dust bedding, and should be fed dust-free feed. Carriage horses with COPD that do not respond to proper management and minimal medication should be retired from urban service.

Pleuropneumonia or 'shipping fever' is not uncommon in new carriage horses that arrive from regional auctions. These horses typically become ill 24–96 hours after arrival from the sale. Obviously, immediate veterinary attention is required. Vaccination for respiratory viruses, including influenza and rhinopneumonitis, is strongly recommended for all city carriage horses to protect from viruses originating with newly arrived horses.

Activists have suggested that city living conditions – including, but not limited to, automobile exhaust – cause damage to the lungs of city carriage horses. A Tufts University study showed no significant difference in particulate matter or inflammation in airways of urban versus rural horses, although the sample size was small. The same study found that urban horses actually have less airway reactivity (a precursor to heaves or infection) than rural horses (Mazan *et al.*, 2001). Complete postmortem examinations were performed at the New York State Veterinary College at Cornell University on six New York City carriage horses that died from a variety of natural causes during the mid-1990s. Surprisingly, the postmortem examinations showed no significant chronic lung lesions in any of the horses.

21.2.4 Rhabdomyolysis

Rhabdomyolysis syndrome or 'tying up' can be a major medical problem for all carriage horses. Typically the case history includes several days of vigorous work, such as during busy holiday tourism periods, followed by a few days of stall rest without feed reduction, followed by the horse tying up in the first few hours of return to work. However, cases also may occur without any such history. Mares seem to be more commonly affected than geldings (Harris, 1997). This condition may be fatal without immediate veterinary care. Owner and caretaker education should make severe cases of rhabdomyolysis almost entirely preventable. Horses should receive regular exercise, and their feed should be reduced during times of inactivity. Horses with a history of recurrent rhabdomyolysis should be retired from city draft service.

21.2.5 Skin problems and harness sores

Open skin sores from improperly fitted harness are an obvious statement of poor horsemanship, inattention, and callousness of the carriage operator. Horses with sores under the harness must be suspended from work immediately and restricted from work by inspecting agencies. The operator should be cited with a summons and fined. Skin infections, usually *Dermatophilus* or ringworm, occur seasonally in carriage horses in the northern regions, particularly during the winter. Because sunlight may help resolve these conditions, affected horses should be allowed to work providing there is proof of veterinary care and the lesions are not underneath the harness. Harness should not be shared between horses.

21.2.6 Weather-related problems

Overheating or heat stroke is always a threat to horses working in an urban environment. Infrequent watering, poor access to electrolytes, obesity, poor conditioning, high humidity, illness, and hot pavement conditions may all be contributing factors. However, horses with none of these risk factors may be affected. Pavement temperatures usually greatly exceed ambient air temperature. Carriage horses must be watered frequently and sponged with cool water when necessary. Drivers must be trained in first aid for overheated horses. Also, stabled horses must be given free access to water and mineralized salt at all times, and stable ventilation must be adequate so that horses can replenish their fluids and electrolytes while off-duty. New York City's newest stable has installed misting fans to assist in cooling its horses. Covered outdoor misting stations would be a welcome addition to carriage routes in many cities, particularly for busy summer weekends. Most cities have extensive hot-weather regulations for carriage horses.

Few health problems have been associated with working in cold weather, primarily because most northern cities have low-temperature limits, below which horses are returned to their stables. Infrequent watering may be a problem during this time, if water sources on the carriage route are not heated. Horses that are normally housed indoors should wear blankets while standing idle at hack stands in cold weather; shivering should not be seen. It is the author's observation that horses perform well in cold weather, but drivers may not. Below 25°F (nearly –4°C), some drivers' attentions seem focused on staying warm rather than driving the carriage.

21.2.7 Trauma

The risk of accidents is a major problem for all horses working in a city environment. Horses run when frightened, and, in a confined urban environment, there is not much running room. What usually stops the runaway horse is a motor vehicle, parking meter, building, or similar large stationary object. Major accidents involving horse-drawn carriages are uncommon, particularly given the many hours that carriage horses are on the job. This is largely due to the quiet temperament of horses that are usually selected for city carriage duty. However, when a major accident occurs, the horse and passengers often sustain serious injuries, or worse. The amount of publicity associated with horse-drawn carriage accidents is major and often sensational in nature.

Pro-carriage horse groups often cite city vital statistics to promote the safety of the carriage trade. Such citations are rarely relevant or helpful. For example, during the period of growth of the New York City carriage trade from 1969 to 1989, one person died in a city carriage accident, and three died in horseback riding accidents. In contrast, in 1989 alone, 18 people died in city bicycle accidents and 635 died in motor vehicle accidents (Baldwin and Kurtz, 1992). Obviously, the death or injury rates per 'horse hour driven' need to be compared to the rates for 'automobile hours driven' to make a valid comparison; but these data are almost never available.

More common than major accidents are traumatic injuries to a horse that slips, falls, or takes a bad step on uneven pavement. In the rare instance that a fracture results, the horse may require hospitalization or euthanasia. Small cuts from horses interfering, especially on hind ankles, are seen but may be minimized by proper trimming and shoeing. Rub marks on the hips are seen in horses that are housed in traditional straight stalls. The solution is to put the horse in a larger stall, or pad the upright supports.

Emergency veterinary care is a problem for all city horses, especially in larger cities. Equine veterinarians generally do not live or work near major cities, and they also must travel through traffic to attend an emergency. Local small-animal practitioners usually are not equipped to treat horses, and often do not feel qualified.

21.3 Health Regulations

21.3.1 Identification

In many large cities, carriage horses must be identified by a city-issued registration or license number. This number indicates that the horse has been examined for fitness by a veterinarian as part of licensure by the city. The number helps with positive identification by inspection personnel and by citizens filing horse health or cruelty complaints. In New York, carriage horses must be identified by both a left-front hoof brand and a small city-issued brass number tag on the right throatlatch of the bridle. The inability to identify a suspected sick or illegally working horse is sometimes a complaint among animal activists in New York, because all these identification numbers are small in size. Some cities such as Chicago require the carriage operator's name and license number to be clearly painted on every carriage, in addition to the license plate. Most cities would benefit from larger identification numbers on carriages, to aid in following up citizen complaints. In the author's experience, more than 90% of citizen complaints about carriage horses are unfounded. Most originate from a well-intentioned complainant who is unfamiliar with horses or local rules. Therefore, easy identification of the horse and carriage works to the benefit of both the complainant and the carriage operator. A carriage driver with a well-cared-for, healthy horse should always welcome comments and questions from the public.

21.3.2 Veterinary examination

Most large cities require periodic physical examinations by a veterinarian, as part of annual licensure. New York and Atlanta, for example, require annual physical examination. Other cities require six-month exams, and a few such as Chicago laudably require veterinary examination every three months.

New York, unlike many cities, requires annual vaccinations (rabies, tetanus, Eastern and Western encephalitis) and a fecal examination as part of the annual veterinary examination. A comprehensive annual health maintenance plan has been recommended as part of the periodic veterinary examination for all carriage horses (CEN/SHARE, 1986). This proactive measure would be a very positive addition to city rules. Psychological screening has been recommended for carriage horse candidates (CEN/SHARE, 1986) and this may be a future consideration. Unscrupulous carriage horse owners have been known to illegally use two horses with the same city identification number, presumably to avoid the veterinary fees associated with the annual physical examination (Seifman, 2007).

21.3.3 Time, shift, and area restrictions

Many large cities prohibit carriage operation in congested areas during peak traffic periods. These restrictions are designed to reduce the risk of traumatic injury to horses and to eliminate traffic problems caused by slow-moving carriages. Some cities prohibit all carriage operations during peak rush-hour periods.

Most cities limit carriage horses to 8–10 hours of work during any 24-hour day. Chicago limits the carriage horse work day to 6 hours. Many cities require 10 minute rest periods each hour. New York requires 15 minutes of rest per two pulling hours. Frequent watering may be required by written regulations or by inspecting officers.

Enforcement of work day regulations is labor-intensive, and involves at least frequent spot checks and/or horse log inspections over a period of 8–12 hours. During busy holiday periods in large cities, some carriage drivers may attempt to work longer hours, illegally, by switching horse timecards or other methods – taking advantage of the fact that inspecting officers probably will not be available to watch the work area for the full 6, 8, or 10-hour day. One suggested cost-effective enforcement solution might be to implant microchip identification devices in each horse, and use microchip readers along carriage routes, to record horse work hours.

21.3.4 Weather-related rules

Most large cities require carriage horses to return to their stables when the reported temperature reaches 90°F (32°C). In New York, the temperature must be taken at an actual hack stand, because street temperatures often exceed temperatures at local weather stations. New York enforcement agencies use a sling psychrometer, a thermometer that is spun in the air to measure air temperature and humidity. The City of Charleston regulations require horse's rectal temperature to be taken after each tour, when the air temperature reaches 90°F. If any horse or mule's temperature reaches 103°F (39.5°C) thereafter, specific cooling procedures must be followed. Unlike most cities, New York has a low air temperature limit (18°F, almost −8°C) for working carriage horses. Also, all horses must be blanketed while standing at hack stands, whenever the temperature reaches 40°F (4.5°C) or lower.

Most large cities require carriage horses to stop work under adverse weather conditions, which may include snow, ice, or heavy rain or wind. Generally this regulation is enforced, so that carriage horses are returned to their stables whenever conditions become unsafe for motor vehicles. Horse-drawn carriages may be operated safely in winter conditions, but they are at high risk when cars cannot stop or steer.

21.3.5 Required reports

An unusual rule, used in New York, requires all sales, leases, retirements, removals, or deaths of carriage horses to be promptly reported to the Department of Health. Deaths must be reported within 12 business hours, and other changes must be reported within 10 calendar days. This regulation aids in tracking, and the investigation of citizen complaints and suspicious deaths of horses.

21.3.6 Records and inspections

Many large cities require logs of each horse's daily work hours, including 'trip cards' and/or daily log books. These records are accessible to inspecting agencies at all times. Time clocks may be required, to stamp trip cards with the date and time of the work period. In New York, horses, stables, and records must be accessible at all times to regulating agencies, including the ASPCA, the Departments of Health and Consumer Affairs, and the Police Department.

21.3.7 Housing

Over the last 10 years, housing for most city carriage horses has been upgraded from traditional tie (straight) stalls to box stalls. In these box stalls, the horses are generally free to turn and move around most of the day and night. In New York, stable operators have voluntarily made this change although it is not required by law. Some city regulations simply require stalls to be large enough for the horse to turn around. Others require a minimum box stall size for new stalls, such as 8 feet by 8 feet (2.4 m by 2.4 m) in Charleston or 10 feet by 10 feet (3 m by 3 m) in Chicago. Most cities require stalls to be cleaned daily, and many require minimum bedding levels such as 3 feet (0.9 m) in New York. Rodent control programs and rodent-proof grain storage are usually required. In most large cities, carriage horse stables must meet commercial building code requirements, including safe construction, hot water, adequate ventilation, cleanliness, and freedom from hazards. Annual inspection by fire inspectors is recommended. In some cities such as New York, many horses are housed on the second floor of some stable buildings, with the first floor used for carriage storage. Also, hay and straw may be housed above the horses. Both situations create higher risk in the event of a building fire. In both cases, stable buildings must be equipped with sprinkler systems.

Attendance by a stableperson 24 hours a day has been recommended for all city carriage horse stables. The advantages for horse health and fire safety are obvious. Unfortunately, this practice is employed in only about half of large city carriage stables.

Inadequate ventilation is a common problem in many horse stables in general, and likewise is a major concern in city carriage stables. Most cities require adequate ventilation, but conditions are difficult to quantify for enforcement purposes. Most laws require proper drainage in stables (no standing water) since this is a significant disease control measure. Ironically, many cities do not keep their city-owned hack stands well drained; and this is also an important public health concern. New York City also requires, by directive, that carriage horses be allowed free access to trace-mineralized salt and water, while in stalls, at all times.

21.3.8 Trimming, shoeing, and grooming

Most cities simply require that carriage horses be properly trimmed and shod. New York City requires that carriage horses be trimmed and shod every 3–6 weeks or sooner if necessary.

Many cities require daily grooming of carriage horses, whereas others require them to be clean. Seattle also requires carriage horses to be 'free from any offensive odor other than an odor normally associated with a horse that is clean, healthy, and well groomed.'

21.3.9 General working health rules

Almost all jurisdictions prohibit sick, lame, or improperly shod horses from working. When a sick or lame horse is found working, the horse must be immediately suspended from service with an order for mandatory examination by a practicing veterinarian. The driver and horse owner must be cited and fined with maximum penalties imposed.

Most cities limit the speed of carriage horses to a slow trot. Many cities also impose a passenger limit for carriages. New York enforces a limit of four adult passengers.

'Diapers' or manure-catching devices are required by most municipalities. Diaper laws are designed for general work area cleanliness, and not for horse health.

21.3.10 Carriage driver education

Driver and owner education should be a mandatory, significant part of regulation of city carriage horses. Driver apprenticeships of 1–12 weeks are required in many cities, but the apprenticeships are difficult to verify. Licensees in New York must pass both a written and practical drivers' examination, with emphasis on driving safety, city rules, and horse health guidelines. A few cities require an actual driving test, using a horse and carriage.

21.4 Welfare Issues

Historically, the partnership between humans and horses has resulted in improved survival and empowerment. Horses sacrificed their freedom, albeit unwillingly, and received protection from predation, starvation, weather, and disease. Humans received rapid transportation and mobile horsepower for doing the difficult big jobs like hauling freight and plowing fields – at the cost of considerable resources invested in feeding and caring for the horses. And a spiritual bond often developed. As Winston Churchill said 'There is something about the outside of a horse that is good for the inside of a man.' It is unknown if horses feel that there is something about the outside of a man that is good for the inside of a horse! But what is good for the inside of a horse is better, more reliable food sources, shelter for raising foals, and prompt scientific medical treatment for sickness and lameness.

In any job performed routinely by any animal (including people), there are occupational health problems associated with the repetitive nature of the job. Racehorses gradually develop osselets and suspensory ligament problems, hunter–jumpers have back problems, and office workers get carpal tunnel syndrome, for example. The key to modern humane management of domestic horses is to minimize the occupational hazards and occupational health problems for the horses, while maximizing their benefits – protection, shelter, and care. Because, unlike office workers, horses do not have any choice in their job, horse owners and caretakers must be vigilant that the benefits to the horse outweigh the liabilities as much as possible. In evaluating horse occupations, it is often useful to ask, 'What is best for the horse?' But realistically, economic realities often require that we also ask 'How will we pay for this?' or 'Who is going to pay for this?'

The crux of the urban carriage horse debate seems to be that carriage horse owners and operators are the main beneficiary of their horses' labor; and that the working and living conditions for the horses are sometimes deemed overwhelmingly difficult and negative, resulting in a poor quality of life.

To further dissect this issue, it is useful to apply the 'five freedoms of animal welfare' due to the Farm Animal Welfare Council (FAWC, 1993; see also Ewbank, 1988) to the urban carriage horse trade. Note that there is variation in the quality of horse care from city to city and, within larger cities, among different stables. However, informed generalization is still helpful.

- *Freedom from hunger and thirst* is uniformly met in the carriage industry, both by local regulations and by any owner with common sense and decency.
- *Freedom from discomfort* generally applies to adequate housing and shelter. This guideline is met, but upgrades may be needed in areas such as stall size, ventilation, and outdoor hack stand shelters.
- *Freedom from pain, injury, and disease* is generally met but is compromised when veterinary or farrier care is delayed for financial reasons, or emergency care is not readily available.
- *Freedom to express normal behavior* is limited, as with any horse not living in a group pasture setting.
- *Freedom from fear and distress* is difficult to quantify. Activists might suggest that this is never possible in conditions of congestion and traffic; others might observe that city horses, like city people, grow accustomed to city living conditions.

A more detailed summary of pertinent carriage horse welfare concerns follows. Note that carriage horse owners and operators range from callous, careless individuals who barely perform the minimum legal requirements, to compulsive overachievers who are constantly doing more for their horses. Therefore, there is some variation in horse care from city to city, and among stables within the same city. Unfortunately, in larger cities the culture of the trade tends toward the minimalists, with some exceptions.

21.4.1 Housing
Public expectations for horse care have risen over the past 20 years, and so should the carriage industry's standards for comfortable housing. It is the author's opinion that tie (straight) stalls for horses are no longer acceptable, and that box stalls should be required for all city carriage horses. Stable ventilation should be a priority for all horse owners and inspecting agencies, with experts from state agricultural colleges employed to assist as needed (it's usually free!). For safety reasons, multi-level stables and overhead hay storage should be phased out. Attendance by a stableperson 24 hours should become the industry standard.

In New York in the late 1990s, dissatisfaction with horse housing conditions and high stall rents caused a group of independent carriage horse operators to take action. They formed their own corporation, obtained a small business loan, bought a building, and opened a newer, better carriage horse stable.

Their stable features all box stalls, wash bays, good ventilation, 24-hour caretakers, and, most recently, misting fans for summer cooling. In many aspects, the stable exceeds city requirements for carriage horse housing. Less than 10 years later, the stable is the largest carriage horse facility in New York and gains new tenants every year. Moreover, their bigger, better stable has caused New York's other four carriage horse stables to upgrade their facilities. By heeding activists' criticisms and public sensitivities in their construction of a new stable, they have voluntarily raised the housing standard for all of New York's carriage horses.

21.4.2 Zone and work restrictions

Freedom from pain, injury, and discomfort for carriage horses must involve maximum prevention of trauma. Therefore, work area restrictions must constantly be reviewed to minimize horse movement in areas of heavy traffic. Ideally, carriages would work in zones where motor vehicles are prohibited. This may become less problematic in the future, as environmental 'green' restrictions result in more car-free city zones. Modern technology should be employed to enforce work hour restrictions for carriage horses. Overtime violators might be monitored by video cameras or microchip technology (something like the E-ZPass electronic toll collection system, but for carriage horses?), at considerable saving to the taxpayer.

21.4.3 Medical care

More frequent physical examinations for carriage horses might serve to ease public concerns. Chicago, for example, requires quarterly veterinary examinations. Spot checking by inspecting agencies could verify the quality of the veterinary exams. Medical records should be required for all carriage horses, to include records of all vaccinations, deworming, dentistry, and veterinary care. This is not the case in most cities. Horse medical records should be available for inspection by enforcement agencies at all times. Because city horses constantly work on pavement, standards for shoeing and frequency of shoeing must be the highest priority. Fines and work suspensions must be liberally used to ensure good shoeing practices.

Choice of horses is sometimes cited as a medical or humane issue. Retired Standardbreds are favored by some carriage owners in the East, since they are inexpensive to feed and go faster (time is money, and speed means more trips per work hour). However, Standardbreds require more of a maximum effort to pull a fully loaded carriage. Draft breeds have more power, but eat more and may be more susceptible to rhabdomyolysis and overheating. Mules seem to be heat-tolerant, but are not fast. As a result, activists have sometimes asked to restrict certain horse types in certain regions.

Emergency care for injured or critically ill horses is slow or deficient in some cities. This should be completely unacceptable to horse owners, enforcement agencies, and the public. All stable owners might be required to secure a written agreement for emergency care with a local equine practitioner, and to provide a trailer for emergency transport. Small-animal clinics located adjacent to carriage work zones might be enlisted for short-term assistance in first aid and immediate care.

Pasture or turnout facilities are absent in most cities. In some cities, turnout areas might be found in city parks with minimal disturbance to green space. In other cities, transport to rural pastures could be required by rule. Carriage horse owners might be required to exercise their horses or turn them out to pasture of their choice, during slow tourism periods to avoid illness from confinement.

21.4.4 Retirement

Both carriage horse owners and anti-carriage horse groups often advertise successful retirement placement for retired carriage horses, but documentation is purely
anecdotal. Future regulation of the carriage horse business should involve precise
documentation of average work years of carriage horses in each city, and an exact
record of where each horse goes after retirement. In order to make informed decisions about the carriage trade, the public and everyone involved in the business
must know where the horses go afterward. Many city carriage horses are obtained
inexpensively from horse sales after unsuccessful careers on unmechanized farms.
When weighing up the ethical issues to do with carriage horses, it is important to
consider what other fates might await these horses if they were not used in the carriage industry.

21.4.5 Culture of the carriage trade

Increased public awareness and concern for horse welfare dictate that carriage
horse owners and drivers must be proactively involved in supplying the best possible care for their horses. Owners and drivers must welcome public comments and
questions. Those who provide the minimum care required by law and who compromise care to reduce costs can be prompted with fines and work suspensions for
substandard care.

21.4.6 Media manipulation: the truth is out there ... somewhere

The horse lover is cautioned that both pro- and anti-carriage horse groups have a
long history of using emotional arguments and sensationalism to manipulate public
opinion. One common tactic of animal activists is the 'laundry list' technique of
listing several months, years, or decades of carriage horse illnesses, accidents, and
violations, and representing them as a day or week in the life of the carriage horse
trade. Another tactic is to involve celebrity spokespeople, usually actors or actresses
with little or no knowledge of carriage horse health or stabling. These celebrities
are then employed in place of true experts, who have medical or enforcement experience in the carriage horse trade.

A favorite technique of the carriage operators is to tell an interviewer 'If we can't
do things our way, we'll just sell the horses,' which in many regions involves a livestock or 'killer' sale. This is nothing but emotional blackmail, since the speaker is
basically saying 'Either we get to do what we want, or we kill the horse.' Fortunately,
this rarely, if ever, is carried out.

21.5 Conclusion

Highly visible and easily accessible to millions of people, urban carriage horses are
the primary equine target of animal activists. While activists employ sophisticated,
high-profile publicity campaigns to abolish the business, hundreds of thousands of

people support the trade each year by hiring horse-drawn carriages in most major cities. As in any animal industry, a variety of routine occupational health problems occur among carriage horses. Major traumatic accidents and major illnesses are uncommon but well publicized. Detailed local laws regulate horse and carriage operations in most major cities. As long as carriage horses continue to work in city environments, care of carriage horses must continually be improved to minimize health and safety hazards and to meet growing public expectations.

It is beyond the scope of one author, group of authors, chapter, or book to judge whether the urban carriage horse trade represents an acceptable life for working horses. Such determination must be made by the elected representatives of citizens in each city or state, ideally with the fact-based assistance of qualified animal health experts and experienced enforcement personnel.

References

Adair, H.S. (1992) Common lameness problems of the draft horse. In *Current Therapy in Equine Medicine*, Robinson, N.E. (ed.), vol. 3, pp. 90–91. W.B. Saunders, Philadelphia, PA.

Baldwin, J.L. and Kurtz, M.B. (1992) Health problems and health regulations of urban carriage horses. In *Proceedings of the 38th Annual Convention of the AAEP*, pp. 537–546.

CEN/SHARE (1986) *Recommended Guidelines: Urban Horse and Carriage Operations*, pp. 4–10. University of Minnesota, Minneapolis, MN.

Ewbank, R. (1988) Animal welfare. In *Management and Welfare of Farm Animals: the UFAW Handbook*, 3rd edn, pp. 1–12. Bailliere Tindall, London.

FAWC (Farm Animal Welfare Council) (1993) *Second Report on Priorities for Research and Development in Farm Animal Welfare*. Ministry of Agriculture, Fisheries and Food, Tolworth, Surrey, UK.

Harris, P. (1997) Equine rhabdomyolysis syndrome. In *Current Therapy in Equine Medicine*, Robinson, N.E. (ed.), vol. 4, pp. 115–121. W.B. Saunders, Philadelphia, PA.

Mazan, M.R., Ghio, A.J. and Hoffman, A.M. (2001) Airway reactivity, inflammation, iron, and iron-associated proteins in urban versus rural horses. In *Proceedings of the 47th Annual Convention of the AAEP*, pp. 50–52.

Richburg, K. (2007) Bill could halt New York carriage horses. *Washington Post*, December 17, p. 3.

Seifman, D. (2007) Unbridled bribery. *New York Post*, December 14, p. 3.

The Horse and its Use in Research

22

C. Wayne McIlwraith

It is the author's opinion that the critical welfare issues for horses used in research are minimization of pain and suffering, and good experimental design. These issues received attention when the author was doing PhD training, but critical oversight was relatively low compared to today. Admittedly, much of my 'learning' along the way has come from questioning of our research protocols by the Institutional Animal Care and Use Committee (IACUC), but some has also come from appropriate questions and challenges from donors to our research program, peer review of grants and manuscripts, questioning at scientific meetings, and learning from graduate students and colleagues. I am always mindful of the first clause in the American Association of Equine Practitioners (AAEP) mission statement 'To improve the health and welfare of the horse' when initiating and planning a research project involving horses. The critical aspects of this process (in my opinion) will be detailed below in this chapter.

The ethics of all animal research, including equine research, have gone through much revolution. Initial proposals from Rollin and others have become Federal law, and entrenched ideas regarding the ethics of animal research as well as animal consciousness and animal pain have changed (Rollin, 2006a). In his book on *Animal Rights and Human Morality*, Rollin (2006b) told us how his initial abstract and academic ideas became practical and immediate when he began to teach veterinary medical ethics at the Colorado State University College (CSU) of Veterinary Medicine (the first such course taught anywhere).

Equine Welfare, First Edition. Edited by C. Wayne McIlwraith and Bernard E. Rollin.
© 2011 by UFAW. Published 2011 by Blackwell Publishing Ltd.

22.2 The Ethics of Animal Research

Equine research, as with all animal research, raises complex issues that do not have simple solutions. As also pointed out by Rollin (2006a):

> Typically opponents of animal experimentation know little about research and often discredit themselves by offering wholly implausible 'alternatives' to the use of animals. By the same token some researchers considering the moral questions associated with animal experimentation discredit themselves with absurd claims that animals have no awareness, or really don't suffer, or that might makes right, or that science is value free.

I certainly was guilty of some of that in 1979, but have learned much since. I have become intolerant of research design that wastes horses and does not answer any questions. I realize intolerance is hardly a virtue, but I have heard too often, 'We had no controls because we did not have enough money,' or 'The lack of significance in our results can be attributed to too low numbers of horses, but we ran out of money' – and other unacceptable excuses.

Several years ago at the Annual Meeting of the European College of Veterinary Surgeons (ECVS) in Prague, I was the discussant on a paper in the Residents Forum. The paper described testing of an allograft osteochondral photo-oxidized implant in four sheep with no controls. When I got up to discuss the paper, I asked the resident why there were no controls and was told that 'we used controls from another study' and that study was presented at the previous year's meeting by another resident from the same institution. After, I thought, pointing out some of the errors in the design and the reasons for having no meaningful results (I thought politely), I was admonished outside the room by an equine surgeon colleague who I respect that I was too tough on the resident 'because it was the advisor's fault.' I tried to defend myself on the basis that, if these discrepancies were not pointed out, lessons would not be learned and bad examples would be perpetuated. Although my critic seemed unfazed, the current president of the ECVS came and asked me if I would be willing to come and give a presentation on research design, which I did at the Annual Meeting in Basel in 2008. There are two lessons from this:

(1) We have to stick to scientific principles and integrity rather than preserving PR by not speaking out.
(2) The majority of the veterinary profession want to do it right and are eager to do it better.

I would like to quickly point out that we still stumble toward our goal of optimal attention to equine welfare in using horses in research, but hopefully, most of the time, we learn from these unpredictable issues and continue to improve. This chapter will discuss important considerations in optimizing equine welfare when using horses for research.

22.3 Why Do We Do Research with Horses?

The first and most basic rule of medicine is, above all, do no harm, and it has been stated that this principle has been followed as a major rule of conduct of medical ethics since the code of Hammurabi was written around 1700 BC (Ramey and Rollin, 2001). Ideally, no procedure, device, or treatment should expose an animal to more risk than the risk the problem itself would pose if it were left untreated. It has also been pointed out that ethical treatment of animals is more than merely a matter of causing no harm (Ramey and Rollin, 2001). A clinician (whether it be veterinarian or physician) has moral and ethical obligation to provide treatment for which there is evidence of effectiveness, and it has been stated that society desires and expects that effective treatments be provided (Lynöe, 1992). For any given treatment, establishing proof of efficacy as well as potential risks and benefits is an ethical requirement. Part of the Veterinarian's Oath states that the taker will 'use high *scientific skills*' [emphasis added]. It has been pointed out that it is the dedication to scientific validation of treatments that sets medical professionals apart from shamans and faith healers in the eyes of society (Ramey and Rollin, 2004). It has been pointed out by physicians that science is the foundation of medical professionalism (Rothstein, 1972; Starr, 1982).

Unfortunately, not all treatments, particularly nutraceuticals, have been subjected to rigorous scientific testing. One of the factors involved in failure to test nutraceuticals, at least in the USA, is that the US Food and Drug Administration (FDA) does not require proof of efficacy for 'nutritional supplements.' Some authors have chosen to use 'alternative, complementary or integrative therapies' as the prime example of lack of scientific validation of treatments, and such authors, indeed, have much to support using these as examples (Rollin and Ramey, 2004). On the other hand, there is lack of scientific evidence for a number of 'accepted' equine therapies and treatment methods, and all treatments should be held to the same standard of providing optimal proof of efficacy. I agree with the concept of 'one medicine' – all the therapies we use need to be held accountable, but that is why we need scientifically valid equine research.

The problem of scientific validation is challenging. Some years ago the AAEP Professional Conduct and Ethics Committee perceived a need to clarify questions such as 'What are Food and Drug Administration (FDA)-licensed products and how are they scientifically validated compared with the legal medications (particularly some medications being erroneously represented as generics)?' I was requested to address current knowledge of efficacy of various nutraceuticals and the legal definitions of an approved drug, a generic drug, a device, and a feed additive (McIlwraith, 2004). As stated in that paper, getting a medication licensed is expensive and time-consuming, which is a real disincentive to corporations wishing to license medications for veterinary use. Legitimate manufacturers can be frustrated by the sale of illegal product claiming equivalence and by the sale of orally administered products that have little Federal regulation and do not require proof of efficacy. Research with horses is used to achieve a better understanding of why a disease process occurs, to improve our ability to diagnose the problem sufficiently early, or to test a putative therapy (usually one that represents a potential advance in our ability to help the horse). There are two main pathways to answering these questions through research:

(1) a clinical study with clinical cases of the disease where the new technique is evaluated in clinical studies of the disease (detailed below) or
(2) a controlled study where disease is induced in a group of horses and this is considered a basic or applied controlled research study (also discussed in detail further on).

Commonly, the animal is used as a model for human disease, and the potential benefit is only for human beings rather than for the animal itself. It has previously been argued that there is no clear-cut line between humans and animals from a moral point of view and, further, that animals have moral rights following from their nature, or *telos*, as humans do (Rollin, 2006a, b). One could, therefore, further reason that animal research should be abolished, but this is not seen as an achievable goal, primarily because most of society is not prepared to sacrifice the benefits that research brings. It has also been proposed that society is not prepared to give up faith in science as a principal way of dealing with reality, and the abolition of animal experimentation would essentially mean an end to much of science as we know it (Rollin, 2006a, b).

In some instances, the horse can be used as a model for human disease, but at the same time the research addresses a critical equine clinical problem. An example would be the use of the horse in orthopedic research to assess a punitive technique for superior repair of articular cartilage defects. Defects in the equine femorotibial joint emulate the human clinical disease and are also an important clinical problem for horses (McIlwraith and Rodkey, 2008). Such models have been used in other orthopedic research laboratories as well. While this example cannot be used as an all-encompassing argument for the use of the horse in research, it is an example of research that benefits the horse rather than being solely for human benefit.

22.4 The Basic Steps of Equine Research

In a presentation on the preparation of a scientific manuscript to ECVS in 2007, John Pascoe broke down the process of publishing a scientific manuscript into four stages:

(1) Asking the question (this causes generation of a hypothesis).
(2) Study design (represented by the materials and methods).

(3)   Results (acquisition of the data).
(4)   Interpretation (leading to discussion of the results, their relevance to the
      clinical scenario and, ultimately, telling the veterinary clinician what was
      learned and how it might change clinical practice).

The overall goal of research is to arrive at valid conclusions through scientific
inquiry. Valid conclusions can only be reached in observational or experimental
research if bias is eliminated (bias is defined as a systematic deviation from the
truth that can potentially take place in the design). Bias can be minimized by an
appropriate experimental design. Simply put, we need to ask the right question(s),
design a study to answer the question (and adequate statistical power is critical
here), analyze the results of the study, and hopefully make a worthwhile contribution to knowledge.

    There are two overall study designs: observational studies, and experimental
studies. In observational studies, the researchers observe patient groups without
allocation of the intervention. In experimental studies, researchers allocate the
treatment. Clinical studies are usually observational, but can be experimental – for
example, a randomized, controlled trial or study (RCT). Basic research studies
always have controls, whether they are *in vitro* studies or *in vivo* studies with a
disease model.

22.5 Clinical Studies and Evidence-Based Medicine

Since the term was first coined at McMaster University by G.H. Guyatt in 1991 –
with the definition 'an attitude of "enlightened skepticism" towards the application of diagnostic, therapeutic, and prognostic technologies' – *evidence-based
medicine* has permeated all fields of medicine (Bahandari and Tornetta, 2003).
It has become a common term used in both veterinary and medical practice
(Rossdale, 2003; Sackett *et al.*, 2003; Mair and Cohen, 2003; Muir, 2003; Marr,
2003). The concept is less advanced in veterinary circles compared with human
medicine, but it is important and was highlighted in a special issue of the *Equine
Veterinary Journal* in 2003 and, more recently, has been the subject of a number of
editorials in *Veterinary Surgery*. Evidence-based medicine (EBM) has been defined
by Sackett *et al.* (2003) as the conscientious, explicit, and judicious use of the current best evidence in making decisions about the care of individual patients. The
fundamental underpinning of EBM is the implication of appropriate experimental
designs and statistics (the science that deals with the collection, analysis, and interpretation of data) to medical research and medical literature (Muir, 2003).

    Evidence-based medicine involves a hierarchy of evidence, from meta-analysis
of high-quality randomized trials showing definitive results directly applicable
to an individual patient, to relying on physiologic rationale or previous experience with a small number of similar patients. The evidence-based surgeon knows

the strength of the evidence and therefore the degree of uncertainty for a particular clinical decision. These are important premises when we are discussing using the horse as a research animal and defining our data. While we need to strive for the best available evidence at all times, we should also not be judgmental of reasonable attempts at assessing data to make decisions on the best way to treat our patients. On the other hand, we must rise above the level of the anecdotal in assessing clinical data. It is tempting to use clinical data because these avoid the need to use healthy horses in research. On the other hand, the quality of clinical data needs to be considered carefully before making changes in clinical protocols.

In other words, EBM is not blanket adherence to randomized, controlled studies. It more accurately involves informed and effective use of all types of evidence (meta-analysis of randomized trials to individual case series and case reports), particularly evidence from the medical literature in patient care. In speaking of levels of evidence, the following have been established (Oxford guidelines, http//minervation.com/cebm/docs/levels html):

- *Level 1*. High-quality, randomized controlled trials/studies (RCTs), blinded with complete follow-up.
- *Level 2*. Less rigorous RCTs, cohort or observational studies.
- *Level 3*. Case-controlled studies.
- *Level 4*. Case series.
- *Level 5*. Expert opinion.

22.6 Options for Clinical Studies

The levels of evidence have been discussed previously. While high-quality RCTs are the ideal, and their use should be increased if possible, they are difficult to do and, based on experience, I feel that we usually need to fall back on using an induced model in the horse to get controlled evaluation of purported treatments. It is worth examining, however, each possible scenario of clinical studies and the relative value of them.

22.6.1 Expert opinion

This is considered level 5 evidence. Veterinarians commonly seek expert opinion, which can be very helpful in discussing the best way to handle an individual case medically or surgically, but is hard to defend in the literature.

22.6.2 Case report

This involves an uncontrolled, descriptive study design involving an intervention and outcome with a detailed profile of one patient. For any validity, this case needs to be unique and is certainly not considered a major publication or contribution to knowledge.

22.6.3 Case series

Case series are considered to be level 4 evidence and comprise an uncontrolled, retrospective review of a group of patients. No comparison is made with an untreated or alternate treatment group, and there are no controls. The results from a case series are often the first indication of a new diagnosis or treatment modality, and they can suffer from case selection bias. While ideally they are more useful as hypothesis generators, the reality with equine veterinary medicine is that many of the arthroscopic surgical techniques, for example, have data that have been validated by case series. Such studies are useful when there are sufficient case numbers and when obtaining controls is not possible. A recent paper from *The New England Journal of Medicine* comparing arthroscopic management in knee osteoarthritis to sham controls is notable as an example of the ideal, but sham surgery for an arthroscopic condition brings its own ethical compromises, and it would be very difficult to obtain an equine owner's permission for such a study (Moseley *et al.*, 2002).

On a positive note, the surgical literature most commonly presents case series, and these series are done by collecting outcome information after surgical intervention. Case series are useful for determining long-term outcomes of a given procedure, as well as for addressing complex questions influencing outcome. Typically, what we show is that the outcome with a new procedure might be better (or worse) than historical results. The critical factor in a case series is that consecutive patients are included to avoid the possibility that only patients with the best results are kept in the data set. An example would be our early efforts at reporting the results for arthroscopic surgery with carpal chip fragments in which there were large numbers and consecutive cases, a new procedure was described, and we also addressed other questions influencing outcome, including location of the fragment and the effect of articular cartilage loss (McIlwraith *et al.*, 1987).

22.6.4 Case control study

The case control study involves comparing two groups at a certain point of time (commences with subject with disease or outcome and assesses past exposure). Such a study can be used to ascertain the possible association of a potentially causative factor and a disease or outcome of interest, a group with that disease or outcome of interest or specific outcome identified (cases), and a group of subjects without the disease that become a sample for comparison. Matching can be used to assure cases and controls are similar, and an odds ratio used as an estimate of relative risk. Examples of the usefulness of these studies come from publications out of the California Horse Racing Board Post-Mortem program, where horses that have suffered catastrophic injuries are compared to horses that have not (but have been postmortemed for other reasons). From this has come good evidence for long toe grabs and a 60-day lay-up period being risk factors for fatal injury (Kane *et al.*, 1996; Hill *et al.*, 2001).

22.6.5 Cohort study

The cohort study begins with exposed and non-exposed groups, which are followed for the development of a disease or outcome. The groups are followed up to see if an outcome of interest develops. The terms 'prospective' and 'retrospective' indicate the timing of data collection (a study proposed before data collection is 'prospective'). The terms 'cohort study,' 'follow-up study,' and 'longitudinal study' have all been used where the study population is identified and followed. The strengths of a prospective cohort study are the ability of the investigator to study several outcomes with time and to ensure that data collection is relevant and accurate. The drawbacks are the expense of large numbers of subjects and the requirement for a long study period.

A retrospective cohort or historic cohort study involves identifying patients from past records and following this group backwards in time from the present to the past record. It has the advantage of being shorter in duration compared to prospective studies but lacks the ability to control selection of subjects and lacks control over outcome measurements. Cohort studies are observational in nature and subject to systematic bias. There is also no random allocation.

22.6.6 Randomized clinical trials

Randomized clinical trials are the gold standard (also called an experimental study as opposed to an observational study). Subjects are assigned to a treatment group or a control group, with control having an accepted treatment or no treatment at all, and the treatment group being assigned to the treatment of interest. Cases are randomized to eliminate selection bias and confounding. Blinding of subjects, investigators or both (double-blinded) involves concealing patient assignment so as not to influence the outcome. In equine clinical studies, the person observing the results of a punitive treatment is the one that is blinded. For example, this might be an owner or, preferably, a veterinarian doing an assessment when he/she does not know whether the horse is receiving the treatment or is receiving placebo. As mentioned previously, RCTs are the gold standard, but they are not always suitable for all research questions because of technical or ethical reasons. The present state, at least in equine veterinary medicine, is that RCTs have been rarely achieved, and questions that have not been answered by observational studies usually progress to an experimental study with horses purchased for research. Observational studies dominate the surgical literature, but we should always strive for the best level of evidence.

The author has been involved in two RCTs involving 'prophylactic' medication, and these were difficult. These studies did not require IACUC supervision, whereas if done in humans, Institutional Review Board (IRB) approval would have been required (Lubowitz et al., 2008). Recently an RCT has been performed to evaluate the value of new rehabilitation protocols following arthroscopic surgery for carpal chip fragmentation in Seattle, and this project has gone through IACUC approval at Colorado State University (CSU).

22.7 Basic Research Studies

Basic research studies have provided clinical information on pathogenesis, diagnosis, and treatments of equine musculoskeletal conditions. It is important to remember that the use of horses as experimental animals for *in vivo* research is a privilege. We justify these studies because of the benefit the research brings to the equine patients in the client-owned population. However, we also do it within the rules of the IACUC, as well as our own ethical considerations. While many animals are used as 'models' for human disease, we only do research at CSU when it is addressing an equine clinical problem.

There are some general principles with basic research studies that are critical. The research is hypothesis-based and there are controls. We require a statistical power of at least 0.8, with sufficient numbers to avoid a type II (β) error. A type II (β) error is that chance of even when a real difference associated with the treatment or some other variable exists, it is not picked up in the research study because there are insufficient numbers in each group. Many studies are flawed because of this problem. The requirement of a statistical power of at least 0.8 means that there is at least an 80% probability that, if a difference exists, it will be recognized by the experiment. I feel strongly that if you do not have controls, or the power of your study is insufficient, you are in violation of the welfare of the horses. Lack of funding or low funding is not an excuse. The design of the project will dictate significance and we need as many outcome parameters as possible in the study.

22.7.1 Hypothesis testing
The purpose of hypothesis testing is to prevent generalizations from a sample to the population. It confirms or refutes the assertion that the observed findings did not occur by chance alone, but rather occurred because of a true association between variables.

22.7.2 Controls
Positive controls are not sufficient – it is also necessary to have a negative control. We have found considerable variability between studies with our experimental osteoarthritis model. With negative controls, everything is the same except for the treatment (intervention). Historical controls have been used in observational studies, as mentioned before, but have considerable risk in an experimental study.

22.7.3 Power calculation
The purpose of power calculation is to ensure that there are sufficient numbers to decrease the likelihood of missing a significant difference when one is present. *Power* is the probability of finding a significant association if one truly exists, i.e., it is equal to one minus probability of type II (β) area. The power of 0.8 is normally accepted, and this is what is necessary at CSU for IACUC approval.

```
                    MBST power              12:26 Monday, June 11, 2007   1
                    ACS Lameness

                Two-Sample t-Test
      Group 1 Mean = 2.125   Group 2 Mean = 1.25
   Standard Deviation = .67   Alpha = 0.05   1-Sided Test

              N per
              Group    Power

               6.0     0.677
               6.1     0.684
               6.2     0.691
               6.3     0.698
               6.4     0.705
               6.5     0.712
               6.6     0.719
               6.7     0.725
               6.8     0.732
               6.9     0.738
               7.0     0.744
               7.1     0.750
               7.2     0.756
               7.3     0.762
               7.4     0.767
               7.5     0.773
               7.6     0.778
               7.7     0.783
               7.8     0.788
               7.9     0.793
               8.0     0.798
               8.1     0.803
               8.2     0.808
```

Figure 22.1 Power calculation using lameness scores from autologous conditioned serum study using CSU equine OA model. To achieve 0.8 power, the cutoff is at 8N per group.

I will use a recent request from the IACUC at CSU to reassess the statistical power with our osteochondral chip fragment model that we have used repeatedly to assess the efficacy of various treatments for osteoarthritis in horses. We selected outcome parameters that have shown significant treatment results from an (inter-leukin) IL-1ra gene therapy project and an autologous conditioned serum (IRAP™) project. We looked at print-out of results on autologous conditioned serum (ACS) for lameness (Figure 22.1), synovial fluid total protein from a triamcinolone aceto-nide study (Figure 22.2), and synovial membrane intimal hyperplasia results from the same triamcinolone study (Figure 22.3) to demonstrate that eight horses per treatment group would be needed in order to see a change in these outcome param-eters. The ideal study is typified by the gene therapy with adenoviral equine IL-1ra gene, where multiple clinical changes (Frisbie *et al.*, 2002) as well as pathologic

```
            MBST power                12:26 Monday, June 11, 2007   8
            TA Total Protein

            Two-Sample t-Test
     Group 1 Mean = 23    Group 2 Mean = 19
Standard Deviation = 2.8   Alpha = 0.05   1-Sided Test

            N per
            Group     Power

             6.0      0.744
             6.1      0.751
             6.2      0.758
             6.3      0.765
             6.4      0.772
             6.5      0.778
             6.6      0.784
             6.7      0.791
             6.8      0.797
             6.9      0.802
             7.0      0.808
             7.1      0.814
             7.2      0.819
             7.3      0.824
             7.4      0.829
             7.5      0.834
             7.6      0.839
             7.7      0.844
             7.8      0.848
             7.9      0.853
             8.0      0.857
             8.1      0.861
             8.2      0.866
             8.3      0.870
             8.4      0.873
             8.5      0.877
             8.6      0.881
             8.7      0.884
             8.8      0.888
             8.9      0.891
             9.0      0.895
             9.1      0.898
             9.2      0.901
             9.3      0.904
             9.4      0.907
             9.5      0.910
             9.6      0.912
             9.7      0.915
             9.8      0.918
             9.9      0.920
            10.0      0.923
```

Figure 22.2 Use of total protein levels from a study evaluating a second therapy, revealing that an N of 8 produces a statistical power of 0.857.

```
                    MBST power              12:26 Monday, June 11, 2007  13
              TA Synovial Membrane IH

                  Two-Sample t-Test
      Group 1 Mean = 1.58   Group 2 Mean = .67
Standard Deviation = .5    Alpha = 0.05   2-Sided Test


              N per
              Group    Power

               6.0     0.810
               6.1     0.818
               6.2     0.825
               6.3     0.833
               6.4     0.840
               6.5     0.847
               6.6     0.853
               6.7     0.860
               6.8     0.866
               6.9     0.871
               7.0     0.877
               7.1     0.882
               7.2     0.888
               7.3     0.892
               7.4     0.897
               7.5     0.902
               7.6     0.906
               7.7     0.910
               7.8     0.914
               7.9     0.918
               8.0     0.922
               8.1     0.925
               8.2     0.929
               8.3     0.932
               8.4     0.935
               8.5     0.938
               8.6     0.941
               8.7     0.944
               8.8     0.946
               8.9     0.949
               9.0     0.951
               9.1     0.953
               9.2     0.956
               9.3     0.958
               9.4     0.960
               9.5     0.961
               9.6     0.963
               9.7     0.965
               9.8     0.967
               9.9     0.968
              10.0     0.970
```

Figure 22.3 Synovial membrane histology analyzed to indicate that eight horses per group would produce a statistical power of 0.922.

changes were positively affected by this treatment regimen. In other studies, there may be only one outcome parameter showing significance (Kawcak *et al.*, 2007), but if it is a critical outcome parameter (such as reduction in articular cartilage degradation in an osteoarthritis model) this can still be useful. It is advisable to seek professional statistical advice before commencing a study.

22.8 Regulation of Animal Research, Emergence of Animal Ethics, and Origins of the IACUC

The concept of regulatory oversight as a means to facilitate the welfare of animals used in research has existed for approximately 130 years, beginning with the 1876 Cruelty to Animals Act in England (Silverman *et al.*, 2007). Modifications of this law that exist today include Home Office oversight and registration of individuals who conduct research procedures using animals in the UK. In the USA, the earliest national law addressing animal welfare was the 28-Hour Law enacted in 1887, which primarily governed animals being transported for market and did not specifically address animals for the research laboratory. The first official law addressing the care and use of laboratory animals in the USA was the Laboratory Animal Welfare Act of 1996. An amendment in 1970 changed the name to the Animal Welfare Act (AWA), by which it is known today.

By 1985, increased public concern caused two related pieces of legislation to be passed based on a model started by a Colorado group involving Bernie Rollin in 1977. One was an amendment to the Animal Welfare Act, known as the Dole–Brown Bill, that included a requirement for a IACUC as part of the USDA regulations (USDA had previously been named the responsible agency for implementing and enforcing the 1996 Laboratory Animal Welfare Act). The other bill essentially turned National Institutes of Health (NIH) policy into law and was known as the Health Research Extension Act. Since 1962, NIH had promulgated excellent guidelines for laboratory animal care, to which every research group and institution received Federal funding through NIH theoretically had to adhere (it was never enforced). In addition to establishment of a IACUC to monitor animal care and use and to inspect facilities, a 1985 amendment to the Animal Welfare Act set standards for adequate veterinary care, including use of anesthetics, analgesics, and tranquilizers, the banning of the use of paralytics without anesthetics, required consideration of alternatives to painful procedures by the investigator, and prohibition of multiple surgeries. The first US Public Health Service (PHS) policy on humane care and use of laboratory animals went into effect in 1973, was revised in 1979, and again revised in 1986. All PHS policies on this subject evolved from an NIH policy published in 1971. The 1986 PHS policy first described the IACUC in its present form and membership and, with an amendment to the AWA in 1989, USDA regulations required a similar IACUC. Most institutions now have a single committee that satisfies both PHS and USDA requirements.

IACUC-approved protocols are required for all live or dead, warm-blooded animals used in research, teaching, or testing, and registered research facilities as defined by the Animal Welfare Act regulations. The review of protocols involving the use of animals is one of the most important responsibilities of the IACUC. Particular consideration is given to animal welfare issues, such as the use of non-animal alternatives and the application of refinement techniques to reduce animal pain, discomfort, and distress. Justification of the type and number of animals must be reviewed, as must exceptions to certain specific guidelines (including multiple major survival surgery, use or non-use of pain-killing drugs, and choice of any non-standard euthanasia method). Scientific justification (or the scientific rationale for choosing a particular experimental design) is what the regulations require, but there is little regulatory guidance on the type of justification expected. The case of multiple major survival surgery is a good example in that it is acceptable for the IACUC and investigator to consider 'conservation of scare animal resources' but not 'cost-savings alone' as justification for multiple surgeries (Silverman et al., 2007).

Choosing an appropriate number of subjects is an important part of any research project, to obtain valid results and to minimize the number of individuals exposed to the potential risks and harms of research. Consequently, IACUCs are particularly interested in ensuring that a sufficient, but not an excessive, number of animals are used. If there are too few animals, there is an ethical issue because the animals are being subjected to potentially painful procedures or loss of life with relatively likely benefit in the advancement of knowledge. On the other hand, a study using more animals than are truly needed unnecessarily exposes some of them to the same harms.

Rollin (2006a) likened the history of the regulation of animal research to the history of the emergence of meaningful social ethics for animals in society. He noted that the Animal Welfare Act of 1966 represented a minimal attempt to regulate animal research and was far from morally adequate. The 1985 amendment rendered coherent the ethics for laboratory animals, but he considered the standard inadequate in many ways and enumerated these in his 2006 review (Rollin 2006a). Considerable analysis of the use and abuse of animals in research is detailed in the third edition of his text on *Animal Rights and Human Morality* (Rollin, 2006b).

In his textbook, Rollin explores moral principles for research. He discusses abolition of animal experimentation as a non-achievable moral goal, primarily because most of society is not prepared to sacrifice the benefits that research brings, especially in the area of disease control and treatment (Rollin, 2006a). On the other hand, the argument that 'the benefit to humans (or to humans and animals) clearly outweighs the pain and suffering experienced by the experimental animals' is too simple. If research is deemed justifiable, Rollin states that 'it should be conducted in such a way as to manage the animal's potential for living its life according to its nature (*telos*), and certain fundamental rights should be preserved as far as possible, given the logic of the research, regardless of considerations of cost.' Rollin calls this the 'rights principle.'

22.9 The Use of 'Alternatives' in Equine Research

In preparing a research protocol, one also should be challenged regarding alternatives to using horses in experimentation. Rollin (2006b) cites the 'three Rs' principles of Russell and Burch (1959):

(1) replacement of animals by non-animals;
(2) reduction in the number of animals; and
(3) refinement in animal use.

With regard to replacement, we use tissue and organ culture as a replacement for live animals in some instances. Our laboratory has made extensive use of an *in vitro* model system utilizing cartilage explants subjected to interleukin-1 (IL-1) treatment as a way of screening putative methods of therapy. However, alternative proof lies with *in vivo* experimentation and we have answered a number of questions on pathobiology and signaling pathways using such techniques. Two points of relevance to replacement are noted on the current IACUC form at CSU under the heading 'Living animals are required for this project' because: (a) complexity of the processes studied cannot be duplicated and/or modeled with an *in vitro* model; and (b) not enough information is known about the processes being studied to design non-living models.

Reduction can certainly be effected by attention to experimental design, power calculations, and appropriate statistical analysis. This has been discussed in detail previously.

Last, but not least, refinement in the use of the horse has certainly been an area of much progress promulgated by the IACUC and the regulations, as well as the integrity of the veterinary profession. Refinement not only includes the rules and regulations of ideal animal care, including food, water, bedding, and pain management, but also requires that consideration should be given to their *telos* or nature (Rollin, 2006a), that is, allowing horses to behave as far as possible in a natural fashion. When designing the Gail Holmes Equine Orthopaedic Research Center at CSU, attention was paid to the environment of the horse emulating the best care that horses receive in the real world. As an equine veterinary clinician and horse owner, these requirements come naturally to my colleagues and me, but may not always be considered by researchers inexperienced with a given animal (in this case the horse).

22.10 Summary

Much of our information regarding the effectiveness of treatment, as well as advances in diagnosis and understanding of disease, has been gained from case series, case control studies, and cohort studies with clinical cases. These studies spare the horse as a research animal and are the first order of priority when addressing the use of horses from a research prospective. We should always strive for the best available evidence, and randomized, controlled trials/studies are the gold standard. Because of our limitations in doing these studies, experimental studies are necessary for ongoing progress in equine welfare. However, if horses are used for such experimental studies, it is critical that they are scientifically valid and have a good chance of answering the question. In addition to paying attention to clinical relevance, issues of experimental design and statistical power, preservation of the horse's welfare, and optimal environment are also critical.

References

Bahandari, M. and Tornetta, P. (2003) Editorial Comment. Evidence-based orthopedics: a paradigm shift. *Clinical Orthopaedics and Related Research* **413**, 9–10.

Frisbie, D.D., Ghivizzani, S.C., Robbins, P.D. *et al.* (2002) Treatment of experimental equine osteoarthritis by *in vivo* delivery of equine IL-1ra receptor antagonist gene. *Gene Therapy* **9**, 12–20.

Hill, A.E., Stover, S.M., Gardner, I.A. *et al.* (2001) Risk factors and outcomes of non-catastrophic suspensory injury in Thoroughbred racehorses. *Journal of the American Veterinary Medical Association* **218**, 1136–1144.

Kane, A.J., Stover, S.M., Gardner, I.A. *et al.* (1996) Post-mortem evaluation of homotypic variation in shoe characteristic of 201 racehorses. *American Journal of Veterinary Research* **57**, 1141–1146.

Kawcak, C.E., Frisbie, D.D., McIlwraith, C.W., Werpy, N.M. and Park, R.D. (2007) Evaluation of avocado and soybean unsaponifiable extracts for treatment of horses with experimentally induced osteoarthritis using an equine model. *American Journal of Veterinary Research* **68**, 598–604.

Lynöe, N. (1992) Ethical and professional aspects of the practice of alternative medicine. *Scandinavian Journal of Social Medicine* **20**, 215–217.

Lubowitz, J., Poehling, G.G. and Burkhart, S.S. (2008) Rules of the game: institutional review boards. *Arthroscopy* **24**, 373–374.

Mair, T.S. and Cohen, N.D. (2003) A novel approach to epidemiological and evidence-based medicine studies in equine practice. *Equine Veterinary Journal* **35**, 339–340.

Marr, C.M. (2003) Defining the clinically relevant questions that lead to the best answers: What is evidence-based medicine? *Equine Veterinary Journal* **35**, 333–336.

McIlwraith, C.W. (2004) Licensed medications, 'generic' medications, compounding, and nutraceuticals – What is the scientifically validated, where do we encounter scientific mistruths, and where are we legally? *Proceedings of the 50th Annual Convention of the AAEP*, pp. 459–475.

McIlwraith, C.W. and Rodkey, W.G. (2008) The horse–human relationship: research and the future. In *The Crucial Principles in Care of the Knee*, Feagin, J.A. and Steadman, J.R. (eds), ch. 16, pp. 221–227. Lippincott Williams & Wilkins, Philadelphia, PA.

McIlwraith, C.W., Yovich, J.V. and Martin, G.S. (1987) Arthroscopic surgery for the treatment of osteochondral chip fractures in the equine carpus. *Journal of the American Veterinary Medical Association* **191**, 531–540.

Muir, W.W. (2003) Is evidence-based medicine our only choice? *Equine Veterinary Journal* **35**, 337–338.

Moseley, J.B., O'Malley, K., Petersen, N.J., Menke, T.J., Brody, B.A., Kuykendall, D.H., Hollingsworth, J.C., Ashton, C.M. and Wray, N.P. (2002) A controlled trial of arthroscopic surgery for osteoarthritis of the knee. *New England Journal of Medicine* **347**, 81–88.

Ramey, D.W. and Rollin, B.E. (2001) Ethical aspect of proof and 'alternative' therapies. *Journal of the American Veterinary Medical Association* **18**, 343–346.

Ramey, D.W. and Rollin, B.E. (2004) *Complementary and Alternative Veterinary Medicine*. Iowa State University Press, Ames, IA.

Rollin, B.E. (2006a) The regulation of animal research and the emergence of animal ethics: a conceptual history. *Theoretical Medicine and Bioethics* **27**, 285–304.

Rollin, B.E. (2006b) *Animal Rights and Human Morality*, 3rd edn. Prometheus Books, Amherst, NY.

Rossdale, P.D. (2003) Objectivity versus subjectivity in medical progress. *Equine Veterinary Journal* **35**, 331–332.

Rothstein, W.G. (1972) *American Physicians in the Nineteenth Century: From Sects to Science*. John Hopkins University Press, Baltimore, MD.

Russell, W.M.S. and Burch, R.L. (1959) *The Principles of Humane Experimental Techniques*. Methuen, London.

Sackett, D.L., Strauss, E.S., Richardson, W.S. *et al.* (2003) *Evidence-Based Medicine*, 2nd edn. Churchill Livingston, London.

Silverman, J., Suchow, M.A. and Murthy, S. (eds) (2007) *The IACUC Handbook*, 2nd edn. CRC Press, Boca Raton, FL.

Starr, P. (1982) *The Social Transformation of American Medicine*. Basic Books, New York.

The Unwanted Horse – a Major Welfare Issue

23

Tom R. Lenz

23.1 Introduction

Horses no longer wanted by their owners have been sold or discarded throughout history, but it is only in the last few years that this subset of the horse population has been designated 'unwanted.' To many, the horse is a symbol of beauty, grace, and the American West. It is a cultural icon throughout many countries of the world, but especially in the USA. A study of American attitudes toward animals in 1980 found the horse to be one of the top three most beloved animals (Kellert, 1980). This perception of the horse has greatly complicated the unwanted horse issue and the discussion of end-of-life decisions for horses. Adding to the divisiveness in the unwanted horse debate is the fact the horse industry tends to classify horses as 'livestock' whereas the public tends to classify the horse as a 'companion animal.'

23.2 The Unwanted Horse–Horse Slaughter Connection

US horse population numbers increased gradually from their introduction into North America, peaking in 1910 at 19.8 million head. That number decreased dramatically with the start of industrial mass production of motorized vehicles, and reached an all-time low of 1.6 million head in 1974 (USDA, 2008). Because most horses no longer had value as work animals and the interest in horses as recreational animals had not yet surfaced, horse surplus reduction occurred at hundreds of horse processing plants across the country where they were processed into dog food and fertilizer. Later, as the number of surplus horses dwindled and pet food manufacturers turned to cast-off products from beef and hog processing plants, the number of horse processing plants dwindled to a very few.

Equine Welfare, First Edition. Edited by C. Wayne McIlwraith and Bernard E. Rollin.
© 2011 by UFAW. Published 2011 by Blackwell Publishing Ltd.

As these events were occurring in the USA, post-World War II European populations were being encouraged to eat horsemeat, which was considered lean and a good source of iron (Reece *et al.*, 2000). The result was the development of a US horsemeat export market to European countries for human consumption. Today, over one billion people, or 16% of the world's population, eat horsemeat. According to the Statistics and Data Development Unit of the Food and Agriculture Organization of the United Nations (FAO),[1] total production of horsemeat for human consumption worldwide in 2007 was 1040450 tons (944000 tonnes), roughly five million horses. This is an increase in consumption of 27.6% since 1990. The top five leading horsemeat-producing countries in 2007 were China, Mexico, Kazakhstan, Mongolia, and Argentina. English-speaking countries such as the UK and the USA do not tend to consume horsemeat, yet often export horsemeat to non-Anglophone countries that do consume horsemeat as a protein source.

When addressing the unwanted horse problem, the issue of processing horses for human consumption has polarized the horse industry. This may be due to the change in modern American culture, which is two to three generations removed from the ranch or farm, toward animal advocacy and away from viewing animals as a food or labor source. That, coupled with increased costs in boarding, farriery, hay, fuel, and veterinary care, is making it more challenging to keep a horse until its natural death. When age, physical disability, or behavior issues decrease the horse's value below a certain point, it often ends up at a slaughter plant. And therefore, the issues of the unwanted horse and the horse processed for meat cannot be separated, as the horse sent to slaughter epitomizes the unwanted horse.

Until the bovine spongiform encephalopathy (BSE) outbreak in Europe in 2000 and the foot-and-mouth disease epidemic that occurred in the UK in 2001, Americans, both the horse-owning and non-horse-owning public, were not aware horses were being processed in the USA and their meat shipped to Europe. Both disease outbreaks were responsible for changing many European consumers' preferences from beef to horsemeat (Helm, 2000). This change drew American media attention to the fact horses were being processed in the USA and their meat exported to Europe for human consumption. Media coverage of the issue drew the attention of not only the horse-owning public, but also equine breed associations, animal rights and welfare organizations, veterinary associations, and the non-horse-owning public. Because of the resultant focused lobbying efforts, Federal legislation was introduced in Congress to prohibit processing of horses in the USA for human consumption. Knowledge that horses sent to sale barns or sold to horse dealers were being processed for meat fostered (in the horse industry) the realization there was truly an unwanted horse issue in the USA that must be addressed.

---

[1] See www.fao.org/corp/statistics/en/.

23.3 The Unwanted Horse Problem

The welfare of horses has been an issue in North American since 1641, when the Massachusetts Bay Colony included horses in legislation prohibiting cruelty to animals (Stuff, 1996). However, it was not until 2005 that the term 'unwanted horse' was first coined by the American Association of Equine Practitioners (AAEP) at a horse industry meeting in Washington DC. Unwanted horses are those no longer wanted by their current owner because they are old, injured, sick, unmanageable, or fail to meet their owner's expectations (AAEP, 2005). Generally, these are horses that are geriatric, incurably lame, have behavior problems, or are dangerous. They also include un-adoptable feral horses and horses that fail to meet their owner's expectations because they are unmarketable, unattractive, not athletic, unmanageable, have no color, are the wrong color, or cost too much to maintain. Normal healthy horses of varying ages and breeds may also become unwanted (Messer, 2004). In many cases, these animals have had multiple owners, have been shipped from one sale barn, stable or farm to another, and have ultimately been rejected.

Horses processed for meat represent the lowest economic level of the horse population and typify the unwanted horse in the USA. In 2007, approximately 58 000 horses were processed for meat in the USA, about 35 000 were exported to Canada for processing, some 45 000 were exported to Mexico for processing (T. Cordes, USDA, pers. comm.), approximately 21 000 un-adoptable feral horses were kept in Bureau of Land Management (BLM)-funded long-term sanctuaries, about 9000 feral horses were in the BLM adoption pipeline, and an undetermined number of unwanted horses were potentially abandoned, neglected or abused. Nationally, the BLM's goal is to remove roughly 4000 horses from the wild each year. Since 1971, 235 000 wild horses and burros have been removed from Federal lands and adopted by the public (Lofholm, 2008). Animals that are over 10 years of age when captured or have been put up for adoption three times and not adopted are placed in long-term BLM-funded refuges, where they live out the rest of their lives, which can be from 10 to 25 years depending on the age at which they enter. In 2007, BLM spent $21.9 million to support wild horses and burros kept in short- and long-term holding facilities (USDI, 2008). That is well over half of the BLM's 2007 fiscal budget of $38.8 million. Because feral horses have few predators, the herds double in size every four years unless animals are captured and removed. The increased cost of capturing and maintaining feral horses under the current system will inevitably cause the BLM to face difficult choices in the future management of the West's wild horse and burro program and contribute to the unwanted horse problem.

Initially, there was debate in the horse industry on what type of horses were primarily represented and who was responsible for creating the significant number of unwanted horses in the USA. However, US Department of Agriculture (USDA) export records on US horses shipped to Canadian processing plants in 2002–2005 revealed 42.8% were geldings, 52.1% were mares, 3.41% were

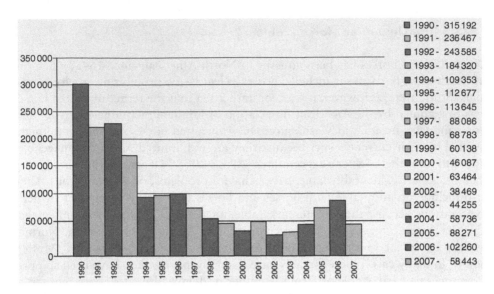

Figure 23.1 US equines processed in US plants, 1990–2007. Source: USDA, Veterinary Services.

stallions, and the gender was not recorded on 1.70%. In addition, 70% were Western-type horses, 11% were English or Thoroughbred-type horses, 3.6% were draft-type horses, and the rest included various breeds or types of horses or mules (Cordes, 2008). Observational studies conducted in 2001 reveal 'riding' horses make up 74% of the horses processed for meat as opposed to draft or other horse types (McGee *et al.*, 2001). In general, these types of horses reflect the demographics of the US horse population, with no specific type or breed of horse standing out as the quintessential unwanted horse. Therefore, the entire horse industry, all breeds and all disciplines, are responsible for the problem and must work together to find a solution. Over the past 10 years, an average of 1–2% of the 9.2 million head (75000–150000 horses) domestic equine population in the USA has been deemed unwanted and sent to processing plants (NASS, 2007; AHC, 2003). That number is down dramatically from the 339000 horses processed in 1990. See Figure 23.1 for the number of US horses and mules processed for meat from 1990 to 2007.

The question to be answered is: 'Why was there an 80% reduction between 1990 and 2007?' Was it simply a surplus reduction because of the Internal Revenue Service (IRS) tax code changes that occurred in the mid-1980s resulting in people selling off horses they were no longer able to depreciate? Was there a change in market demand or production? Or was the horse industry able to absorb this subset of the equine population through rescue and/or retirement facility efforts or by finding alternative careers for them? Some believe the

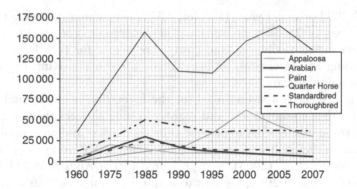

Figure 23.2   Breed registration trends.

retirement and/or rescue industry absorbed these horses and will therefore be able to absorb today's unwanted horses. It appears the reduction in unwanted horses being processed for meat followed the decrease in the number of horses bred and registered in the mid-1980s, and represented a surplus reduction as many investors left the horse industry when they were no longer able to deduct horse expenses. See Figure 23.2 for trends in horse registrations between 1960 and 2007.

According to the 2005 USDA National Animal Health Monitoring System survey, about 167000 (1.8%) horses in the USA that were 30 days of age or older were euthanized or died that year. In addition, some 112000 (1.3%) horses were processed for meat (APHIS, 2005). Therefore, the total mortality for horses in the USA in 2005 was approximately 3–4% of the horse population of 9.2 million. These percentages have varied little during the last decade (APHIS, 1999). The question facing the horse industry is this: 'If the option of annually removing unwanted horses from the general horse population via euthanasia at a processing plant is legislated out of existence, will the horse industry be able to provide adequate care and accommodations for these animals or will the industry need to absorb the cost of their euthanasia and carcass disposal?

23.4 The Retraining, Rescue, Adoption, or Retirement Option

In recent years, horse rescue, adoption, and retirement organizations have, to their credit, made a conscientious and concerted effort to provide care, funding or suitable accommodations for unwanted horses in both the private and public sectors. The number and capacity of these facilities is unknown because they function relatively independently and do not have a national organization. The AAEP estimates there are roughly 450 not-for-profit rescue and/or retirement facilities in the USA that could rescue, retire, or find alternative careers for no more than

6000 to 10 000 horses per year (D. Foley, AAEP, pers. comm.). Owing to the long natural lifespan of 25–30 years for most horses, rescue, adoption or retirement facilities face a potentially long and costly care period for each horse, and have placed funding as the critical, limiting factor for those striving to provide an adequate standard of care.

In addition, there is a strong need for the formation of a national oversight organization that could inspect and register equine shelters that meet humane husbandry standards in order to prevent animal hoarders and unscrupulous horse traders from taking in horses under false pretenses. According to a study conducted by North *et al.* (2005), and presented at the Annual World Food and Agribusiness Forum in 2005, the cost to maintain a horse until its natural death averages $2340 per year. The AAEP estimates the cost of maintaining a horse per year at $1825, not including veterinary or farrier costs (May, 2008). Based upon the North *et al.* maintenance figures, the annual maintenance cost for unwanted horses kept in rescue facilities rather than sent to processing plants in 2005 would have been $187–234 million. This annual cost, however, understates the total cost required because unwanted horses that would have been processed in previous years now remain in the horse population where they are joined by unwanted horse populations in subsequent years. For rescue, adoption, and/or retirement facilities, the financial costs can quickly exceed their capacity to meet the needs of an ever-increasing number of neglected, abandoned or unwanted horses (Ahern *et al.*, 2006).

There are a number of current options for horses that are unwanted or no longer considered useful. Some can be retrained for other uses. This is common with racehorses, which often find second careers in dressage or hunter–jumper competition, or cutting horses, which find second careers in team penning or as pleasure horses. Some are donated to university animal science departments, law enforcement agencies, veterinary teaching hospitals or therapeutic riding programs. In addition, unwanted horses can be placed in long-term rescue or retirement facilities or adopted out. As has been discussed earlier, many are simply euthanized at the request of their owners or sent to processing plants. Whenever there are large numbers of unwanted horses, there is always concern for their welfare, and the reality for many unwanted horses is that they become a burden and are potential candidates for abuse, neglect or abandonment.

23.5 The Euthanasia Option

For those responsible horse owners who do not want to burden others with the disposition of a horse that is old, lame or no longer useful, the option of euthanasia and carcass disposal is available. The term 'euthanasia' is derived from the Greek terms *eu* meaning 'good' and *thanatos* meaning 'death' (AVMA, 2001). A 'good death' occurs with minimal pain and at the appropriate time in the horse's life to prevent unnecessary pain and suffering. Traditionally, justification for euthanasia has been based primarily on medical considerations as well as future quality-of-life issues for the horse. The following medical criteria were established in 1995 by the American Association of Equine Practitioners (AAEP, 1995), and are the prime consideration in evaluating the necessity for euthanasia of a horse.

- Is the horse's condition chronic, incurable, and resulting in unnecessary pain and suffering?
- Does the horse's condition present a hopeless prognosis?
- Is the horse a hazard to itself or its handlers?
- Will the horse require continuous medications for the relief of pain and suffering for the remainder of its life?

Euthanasia at the request of the owner, because they no longer want or can care for an unwanted horse, may become a non-medical reason in the future. According to the American Veterinary Medical Association's 2000 Expert Panel on Euthanasia Report, there are three acceptable forms of euthanasia for horses: an overdose of barbiturate anesthesia, gunshot, and penetrating captive bolt (AVMA, 2001). Sodium pentobarbital is the most commonly used barbiturate for euthanasia in the horse and, when administered intravenously, depresses the central nervous system, causing loss of consciousness and deep anesthesia progressing to respiratory and cardiac arrest (Hullinger and Stull, 1999). The primary advantages of barbiturate overdose are speed of action and minimal discomfort to the animal. The major disadvantages are that the drug requires rapid, intravenous administration, which means the animal must be restrained. In addition, prolonged muscular activity, gasping, and vocalization can occur following drug administration and prior to death, which can be alarming to the owner. Because the carcass contains high levels of barbiturate and must be considered an environmental hazard to wildlife and domestic carnivores, disposal options are limited. If neuromuscular agents or potassium chloride are used in conjunction with sodium pentobarbital to prevent terminal gasping and muscle movement, they must be used after the animal is unconscious and not as a 'cocktail' with sodium pentobarbital. Unacceptable injectable agents include strychnine, nicotine, caffeine, magnesium sulfate, cleansing agents, solvents, disinfectants, other toxins and salts (AVMA, 2001).

Physical methods of euthanasia include gunshot and penetrating captive bolt. When properly applied, both cause trauma to the cerebral hemisphere and the brainstem, resulting in immediate unconsciousness and a painless, humane death. When using gunshot, the optimal site of penetration of the horse's skull is one-half inch (12–13 mm) above the intersection of a diagonal line from the base of the ear to the corner of the opposite eye (Shearer and Nicoletti, 2002). The firearm should be aimed directly down the neck, perpendicular to the front of the skull, and held at least 2–6 inches (5–15 cm) away from the point of impact. A 0.22-caliber long rifle is adequate, but 9 mm or 0.38-caliber pistols have greater penetrating potential. If a shotgun is the only available firearm, a rifled slug is preferred. Penetrating captive bolt instruments are powered by gunpowder or compressed air that provides sufficient energy to penetrate the horse's skull. Its mode of action is trauma to the cerebral hemisphere and brainstem, resulting in instantaneous brain death. Adequate restraint is important to ensure proper placement of the captive bolt, which must be held firmly against the horse's forehead. A non-penetrating captive bolt only stuns animals and should not be used for euthanasia of horses. In Europe, penetrating captive bolts are also seen as stunning rather than killing implements for livestock (although they frequently do kill), and it is a requirement that animals be bled after stunning with captive bolt (penetrating or not) to kill or to ensure death (HSA, 2001).The advantages of both gunshot and penetrating captive bolt are that they instantly render the animal unconscious, resulting in immediate brain death. In addition, the carcass is not hazardous to wildlife or domestic animals. Disadvantages include the fact that they require skill and experience, and may be esthetically displeasing for observers.

After euthanasia, it is important the horse's carcass is properly disposed of in a safe manner that does not pose a hazard to people or animals. All States, as well as many counties and municipalities, regulate the disposition of animal carcasses, and approved methods vary widely with animal species and regulatory authority. Therefore, it is important the attending veterinarian and/or owner know the specific regulations in their area regarding disposal of horse carcasses. There are a number of carcass disposal options available, including burial, composting, incineration, rendering, and biodigestion (Bagley *et al.*, 1999). Burial may be prohibited in some localities, even on the owner's own land, and therefore it is important to check with local authorities on restrictions or guidelines before beginning to bury a dead horse. Many States mandate the burial site be at least 100 yards from wells and streams. In States where individual animal burial is permitted, 3–4 feet (90–120 cm) of dirt is required to cover the carcass (Sander *et al.*, 2002). Backhoe service cost to bury a horse on the owner's property vary with the area of the country, but usually range from $250 to $500. Landfills are a reasonable alternative to burial in some States, but not all municipal landfills will accept horse carcasses, especially those that have been euthanized with barbiturate overdose. Costs, not including transportation of the carcass to the landfill, vary, but usually range from $80 to $500.

Although available in only 50% of States, rendering is an environmentally safe option for horse carcass disposal, and involves cooking the carcass to destroy pathogens and produce usable end-products such as meat, bone, and blood meal that can be used in animal feeds or fertilizers. Rendering companies will generally pick up euthanized animals and, depending upon the State, charge from $40 to $250 (Meeker, 2008). Some renderers will not accept animals euthanized with sodium pentobarbital because they market protein meals to pet food companies. Information is available on the location of rendering facilities that will pick up dead livestock.[2] Incineration or cremation is one of the most biosecure methods of carcass disposal, but is costly. Depending upon the area of the country and the local cost of propane fuel, incineration of an average-sized horse costs between $500 and $2000. To prevent air pollution, this method of carcass disposal is strictly regulated by the Federal Environmental Protection Agency (EPA) as well as State EPAs (Sander *et al.*, 2002).

A method of carcass disposal that has recently gained popularity is composting, which is defined as controlled, sanitary, aerobic decomposition of organic materials by bacteria. Composting is safe and produces an end-product that is a relatively odorless, spongy, and humus-like substance that can be used for soil supplementation. If done correctly, it takes as little as six weeks to as long as nine months to compost an intact horse carcass. During proper composting with vegetative material and moisture, the carcass tissues reach temperatures of at least 130°F (55°C) for several days or weeks. This, in turn, kills most pathogenic bacteria and viruses (Morris *et al.*, 1997). The process is usually performed in covered piles or trenches and, therefore, it is important that compost areas are placed well away from run-off and drinking water to avoid contamination. In most States, the Department of Agriculture office can provide detailed instructions for management of composters. Researchers at Texas A&M University have recently developed a low-cost, low-maintenance approach to composting individual large animals (Mukhtar *et al.*, 2003).

A relatively new method of carcass disposal is biodigestion (tissue digestion). Biodigesters are giant pressure-cooker-like machines that use alkaline hydrolysis to solubilize and hydrolyze the animal's carcass rapidly, and they have become popular with veterinary colleges and industrial research facilities. They are a less expensive, more environmentally friendly alternative to incineration and can turn a horse carcass into a pathogen-free, aqueous solution of small peptides, amino acids, sugars, soaps and powdered bone in as little as six hours. Because the carcass remains are sterile and pose no risk to the environment, they can be taken to the local landfill for disposition or used as fertilizer. Costs are about one-third that of incineration (Kuehn, 2004).

23.6 The Effect of Anti-Slaughter Legislation

A review of the unwanted horse issue would not be complete without a discussion of anti-slaughter legislation and the effect it has had on the unwanted horse issue. The term 'euthanasia' has already been defined, but because the term 'slaughter' is used frequently in the proposed legislations, it is important to understand its meaning. In North America, slaughter is used to describe the humane ending of an

---

[2] For example, see: www.nationalrenderers.org/about/directory.

animal's life under strict Federal regulations and is used only when the carcass is processed at a licensed meat plant for food purposes. In the European Union, slaughter is used by authorities to describe humane animal death, no matter the end-result of the carcass (AFAC, 2008). The 1996 Farm Bill gave the USDA's Animal and Plant Health Inspection Service (APHIS) regulatory oversight responsibility for the humane commercial transport of horses to processing plants. APHIS oversees the requirements on access to food, water, and rest during shipment, as well as defining the types of horses that cannot be shipped. These include horses unable to bear weight on all four legs, unable to walk unassisted, blind in both eyes, foals less than six months old, and pregnant mares that are near foaling. In addition, the regulations phased out the use of double-decker trailers in 2006 and require that origin/shipper certificates accompany each shipment that document identifying marks, breed, color, and gender. Falsification of any document is a criminal offense and may result in a fine of up to $10 000 or no more than five years imprisonment. The driver is not allowed to leave the processing plant until the horses have been examined by USDA representatives and horses are matched to accompanying documents (APHIS, 2002).

A major concern by proponents of the anti-slaughter legislation is that horses, despite USDA oversight, suffer during transportation to the processing facilities and many arrive injured or dead. In a study reported in 1999 and conducted at the two horse processing plants in Texas, a total of 1008 horses in 63 trailer loads were observed during unloading (Grandin et al., 1999). Conditions that were considered to be severe welfare problems in horses were: body condition scores of 1 to 2 (emaciated) in a 1–9 scale; recumbency or the inability to walk; fractured limbs; and severe wounds. It was found that 92% of the horses arrived in good condition, and 7.7% had conditions that were rated severe welfare problems; 3% of the horses had a body condition score of 1 or 2. Twelve horses had foot and limb problems other than fractures. Four horses had fractured limbs. Eighteen horses had lacerations or injuries from bites. Eight horses arrived non-ambulatory, and two had deformities. Three horses had purulent lesions, and one had a severe behavior problem. Fighting was the major cause of the injuries that occurred during transport and marketing. Abuse or neglect by the owner, not transportation, was the cause of 77% of the severe welfare problems observed (Grandin et al., 1999).

In a study conducted by Stull (1999), nine trailer loads of horses (n = 306) transported to slaughter facilities with distances ranging from 596 to 2496 km were observed to characterize the physiological responses and number of injuries due to transportation under summer conditions. The percent of horses injured was greater for double-decker 'potbelly' (29.2%) compared to straight-deck (8%) trailers; however, the stress indicators of cortisol and neutrophil/lymphocyte ratios and rectal temperature showed greater responses following straight-deck trailers. The percentage of horses injured was less in trailers with 1.14–1.31 m² of floor area than in trailers with 1.40–1.54 m² of floor area per horse. However, most physiological responses were less in horses provided more floor space (Stull, 1999).

In 2001, Congresswoman Morella of New York introduced a bill prohibiting the interstate transport of horses to slaughter. The bill was never taken up by the full House. However, it did strike an emotional chord within both the horse industry and the non-horse-owning public, and started a debate that continues today. Proponents argued the ban on slaughter would eliminate pain and suffering of those horses shipped to processing plants, and the surplus of unwanted horses that would result could easily be absorbed by the horse retirement and rescue industry. Opponents of the bill argued that banning the slaughter of unwanted horses would result in unintended consequences that would include increased neglect, abuse, and abandonment. They also argued that unwanted horses, which in the past could have been sold for a profit, would now become a cost to the horse owner to pay for care or euthanasia and carcass disposal (Ahern et al., 2006). They believed this would most severely impact the approximately 45% of US horse owners that have an annual household income below $75000 per year (AHC, 2003). They also pointed out the bill did not provide funding, an infrastructure, nor an enforcement authority to address the welfare of unwanted horses no longer processed for meat. There was also concern voiced that, if the processing plants overseen by USDA veterinarians were closed, horses would be transported longer distances without APHIS oversight and processed at foreign processing plants not under USDA's jurisdiction or US humane standards for animal treatment and handling. The bill was not passed.

However, in 2003, in the House of Representatives, Congressman Sweeney of New York introduced The American Horse Slaughter Prevention Act (H.R. 857) to prohibit the slaughter of horses for human consumption (Sweeney, 2003). A similar bill (S. 2352) was introduced in 2004 on the Senate side by Senator Ensign of Nevada (Ensign, 2004). Neither bill moved out of committee. Both bills were similar to the Morella Bill but would also limit the methods that could be used for euthanasia of horses. Under H.R. 857, injectable barbiturates would be the method of choice for euthanasia, with gunshot permitted only in cases of emergency. The bill prohibited the use of penetrating captive bolt. Captive bolt is the method that is used to euthanize horses at meat processing plants. Independent inspections of processing plants by a number of experts, including members of the AAEP's Executive Committee, verified that animals at the plants were handled properly and the use of captive bolt was an acceptable form of humane euthanasia for the horse (Grandin, 2004).

On February 1, 2005, the Horse Slaughter Prohibition Bill (H.R. 503) was introduced into the House of Representatives (Sweeney, 2005) and proposed to amend the *Horse Protection Act* by prohibiting the sale or transportation of horses to be slaughtered for human consumption or other purposes (Grandin, 2004). A similar bill, the Virgie S. Arden American Horse Slaughter Prevention Act (S. 1915), was introduced in the Senate later that year (Ensign, 2005). In 2006, H.R. 503 was passed by the House but was not taken up by the Senate. In 2007, Congressman Whitfield of Kentucky reintroduced H.R. 503 in the House and S. 311 was introduced in the Senate by Senator Landrieu of Louisiana. The bills would end slaughter of American horses for human consumption and prohibit their export for slaughter to other countries. Neither bill has moved forward.

Federal legislation to stop horse processing for human consumption became a moot point when, in 2007, a 1949 Texas law that prohibits the slaughter of horses for human consumption[3] was discovered and enforced, closing the two horse processing plants in Texas. In that same year, in Illinois, a bill was passed that amended the Illinois Horse Meat Act, thus making it unlawful for any person in Illinois to slaughter a horse if that person knows that any of the horsemeat will be used for human consumption.[4] An appeal to the US Supreme Court was unsuccessful. In 2008 The Prevention of Equine Cruelty Act of 2008 (H.R. 6598) was introduced by Congressman Conyers of Michigan and would impose a fine or prison term for possessing, shipping, transporting, etc. any horse, horse flesh, or carcass intended for human consumption (Conyers, 2008). The bill was different from previous proposed horse anti-slaughter legislation as it placed enforcement of the law under the US Attorney General rather than the Secretary of Agriculture. The primary purpose of the bill was to prevent the export of horses for slaughter. The bill has of this date not been taken up by the full House of Representatives.

23.7 The AAEP and the Unwanted Horse Coalition

Throughout the various legislative debates, the AAEP believed that horse processing was symptomatic of a much larger issue, the number of unwanted horses in the USA. In addition, their growing concern was that the extreme emotion on both sides of the debate over the legislation was driving a wedge between key groups within the horse industry, and the welfare of unwanted horses was not being addressed. To begin a dialogue to discuss the unwanted horse issue in a context outside of the legislation, the AAEP hosted a meeting in Washington, DC, in the spring of 2005 to discuss the issue and develop strategies to resolve it. Participants from breed associations, veterinary organizations, sport and discipline groups, welfare and humane groups, and rescue and retirement organizations gathered to discuss the issue of unwanted horses. The conclusions reached during the meeting included confirmation that there is an unwanted horse issue in the USA, but most of the industry was not aware of it. The group agreed that current rescue and retirement facilities were unable to accommodate all of the horses that were currently being euthanized at meat processing plants. They also

---

[3] State of Texas, The Sale of Horsemeat for Human Consumption. Texas Agriculture Code, Chapter 149.002. www.tlo2.tlc.state.tx.us/statutes/ag.toc.htm.

[4] State of Illinois, Amendment to the Illinois Horse Meat Act. Illinois Bill H.B. 1711. www.ilga. gov/legislation/fulltext.asp?DocName=09300HB17118GA.

agreed there were no large funding sources available, and the entire industry would have to take action to resolve the issue. They concluded that selectively decreasing the production of new horses was as important as dealing with discarded horses and, therefore, pre-ownership education and responsible horse ownership were key.

As a result of the meeting, the Unwanted Horse Coalition was formed, with the stated mission 'to reduce the number of unwanted horses and improve their welfare through education and the efforts of organizations committed to the health, safety and responsible care of the horse.' The coalition represents a broad alliance of equine organizations that brings together key stakeholders to develop consensus on the most effective ways to work to address the issue of America's unwanted horses. Providing a medium for the exchange of information about adoption, proper care, alternative careers, and responsible ownership is key to the coalition's mission. This is presented through a website,[5] print material, educational forums, public service announcements, and public presentations. Education of horse owners about responsible ownership, proper care, and the results of haphazard breeding are key elements of the initiative. Particular attention is given to educate potential owners on the cost of horse care, proper husbandry, training requirements, and expectations. In addition, information about life-ending decisions and the need to euthanize rather than neglect or sell is provided.

23.8 Efforts of Other Organizations

There are a number of other horse organizations working on finding solutions to the unwanted horse issue. On November 11, 2008, the Jockey Club, representing the Thoroughbred owners and breeders in North America, introduced a voluntary checkoff program that will assist two organizations that provide post-racing care for Thoroughbreds, the Thoroughbred Charities of America (TCA) and the Thoroughbred Retirement Foundation (TRF). As an incentive to encourage participation, the Jockey Club will match the checkoff on a dollar-to-dollar basis up to $200 000 in 2009. The checkoff proceeds and matching funds are to be distributed to TCA, which focuses on Thoroughbred retraining and adoption initiatives, and TRF, which focuses on retraining of Thoroughbreds at correctional facilities (Jockey Club, 2008).

On September 30, 2008, the American Quarter Horse Association (AQHA) announced plans to institute a 'Greener Pastures' program to benefit unwanted Quarter Horses. The 'Greener Pastures' logo is placed on horse registration certificates and signifies the owner of the horse has requested to be contacted in the event the horse becomes unwanted or unusable for any subsequent owners. The original owner then has the option of adopting or buying the horse back.

---

[5] The coalition's website is www.unwantedhorsecoalition.org.

In addition, an exchange forum is being placed on the association's website for the exchange of information on horses to donate, those willing to accept donated horses, and members who can help others with extra feed, hay, tack, etc. Also, a separate category for donated horses suitable for therapeutic riding programs has been established. The AQHA Professional Horseman's Council and Certified Horsemanship Association will evaluate horses for their suitability for donation to therapeutic riding centers. In the event a horse is not suitable, it will be evaluated by a veterinarian to determine if euthanasia is warranted (Barbara Linke, AQHA, pers. comm.).

The Colorado Unwanted Horse Alliance, founded in 2008 to help manage unwanted horses in Colorado, has also made a concerted effort to resolve the problem by taking a three-part approach to assess the issue and use online surveys and focus groups to determine problem awareness, source, and recommended solutions. Of the respondents, 77% were horse owners, with the remainder coming from the general public or the government. The recurring themes most commonly expressed in the focus groups were as follows (Montgomery and Fell, 2008):

(1) There is high awareness of the unwanted horse problem and a concern the problem has grown worse within the last two years.
(2) The source of the problem is closure of slaughter facilities resulting in an abundance of mid- to low-grade horses coupled with worsening economic conditions.
(3) There are mixed emotions about horses being classified as companion animals or livestock.
(4) Indiscriminate breeding is a major concern.
(5) Euthanasia options are limited and expensive.
(6) Horse rescue facilities as well as sanctuaries are full.

There was strong agreement among survey participants that horse owners are responsible for dealing with an animal they no longer want, not the government nor the horse industry. The top three identified solutions to the unwanted horse issue were these:

(1) Educate new owners regarding options and resources during economic crises and to reduce indiscriminate breeding.
(2) Provide options and resources for cost-effective euthanasia.
(3) Increase capacity and credibility for horse rescue facilities.

A reader survey conducted by *The Horse* magazine in 2008 revealed that 89% of the respondents (2370 readers) believed that low-cost euthanasia clinics should be widely available and would be a potential solution for the unwanted horse problem (Ryder, 2008).

23.9 Conclusion

The industry will never be able to completely eliminate unwanted horses. Horses will always age, sustain career-ending injuries, not perform up to owner expectations or not be attractive enough. However, the horse industry has turned its attention to the unwanted horse issue and is developing strategies to reduce the number of unwanted horses both on the front-end through responsible breeding as well as on the back-end through rescue and retirement facilities, retraining for alternative careers, and low-cost euthanasia options. It is the responsibility of all horse owners to learn the facts about the unwanted horse issue and to own responsibly. They must be aware of how their actions affect the welfare of the horses they own and consider the consequences before they breed, buy, or discard a horse at the local sale barn. It is the responsibility of veterinarians to be advocates for the health and welfare of the horse and to be a voice of reason on this emotional issue, provide factual information, and educate horse owners on the need for taking life-long responsibility for their horses. The horse industry must take responsibility for the unwanted horse, develop viable solutions, and educate the non-horse-owning public on the facts. The unwanted horse issue will not be resolved overnight. Concerted efforts to reduce the number of unwanted dogs and cats have been underway for decades, yet millions of dogs and cats are still euthanized at animal shelters and veterinary clinics each year, according to the American Humane Society.[6] However, key equine stakeholders are now working together to develop effective strategies to improve the quality of life of unwanted horses and to reduce their numbers.

References

AAEP (1995) *Euthanasia Guidelines*. American Association of Equine Practitioners, Lexington, KY.

AAEP (2005) AAEP-Hosted Unwanted Horse Summit. *The American Horse Council Annual Meeting*. American Horse Council, Washington, DC.

AFAC (2008) *The Alberta Horse Welfare Report*. Alberta Farm Animal Care, Calgary, Alberta, Canada. See: www.afac.ab.ca.

AHC (2003) *Horse Industry Statistics*. American Horse Council, Washington, DC. See: www.horsecouncil.org.

Ahern, J.J. *et al.* (2006) *The Unintended Consequences of a Ban on the Humane Slaughter (Processing) of Horses in the United States*. Animal Welfare Council, Inc., Eastwood, KY. See: www.animalwelfarecouncil.org.

APHIS (1999) *Deaths in US Horses, 1997 and Spring of 1998–Spring 1999*. National Animal Health Monitoring System's Equine 1998 Study, No. N337-0501. US Department of Agriculture, Animal and Plant Health Inspection Service.

---

[6] For animal euthanasia factsheets, see www.americanhumane.org/.

APHIS (2002) *Commercial Transportation of Equines to Slaughter*. Technical Publication. US Department of Agriculture, Animal and Plant Health Inspection Service. Available at: http://www.aphis.usda.gov/publications/animal_health/content/printable_version/pub_ahtcohorses.pdf.

APHIS (2005) *Trends in Equine Mortality, 1998–2005*. National Animal Health Monitoring System's Equine 2005 Study, No. N471-0307. US Department of Agriculture, Animal and Plant Health Inspection Service.

AVMA (2001) Report on the AVMA Panel on Euthanasia. *Journal of the American Veterinary Medical Association* **218**, 669–696.

Bagley, C.V., Kirk, J.H. and Farrel-Poe, K. (1999) *Cow Mortality Disposal*. Electronic Publication AG-507. Utah State University Extension, Logan, UT. Available at: http://extension.usu.edu/files/publications/publication/AG-507.pdf.

Conyers, J. (2008) The Prevention of Equine Cruelty Act of 2008, H.R. 6598, 110th Congress, July 24.

Cordes, T. (2008) Commercial transportation of horses to slaughter in the United States – knowns and unknowns. *The Unwanted Horse Issue: What Now? Forum, US Department of Agriculture Revised Proceedings*, June 18.

Ensign, J. (2004) The American Horse Slaughter Prevention Act of 2004. S. 2353, 108th Congress, 2nd Session, June.

Ensign, J. (2005) The Virgie S. Arden American Horse Slaughter Prevention Act, S. 1915, 109th Congress, October 25.

Grandin, T. (2004) *How to Determine Insensitivity*. See: www.grandin.com.

Grandin, T., McGee, K. and Lanier, J. (1999) Prevalence of severe welfare problems in horses that arrive at slaughter plants. *Journal of the American Veterinary Medical Association*, **214**, 1531–1533.

Helm, T. (2000) Horse meat sales soar over German BSE/Mad Cow crisis. *The Telegraph* (UK), December 19. See: www.rense.com/general6/bdse.htm; www.telegraph.co.uk/.

Hullinger, P. and Stull, C. (1999) *The Emergency Euthanasia of Horses*. University of California–Davis, Veterinary Medicine Extension, School of Veterinary Medicine. Available at: www.vetmed.ucdavis.edu/vetext/inf-an/inf-an_emergeuth-horses.html.

HSA (2001) *Captive Bolt Stunning of Livestock*, 3rd edn. Humane Slaughter Association, Wheathampstead, Herts, UK.

Jockey Club (2008) *TCA, TRF and The Jockey Club Announce Checkoff Program*. Available at: www.jockeyclub.com/mediaCenter.asp?story=354.

Kellert, S.R. (1980) American attitudes toward and knowledge of animals: an update. *International Journal of the Study of Animal Problems* 1(2), 87–119.

Kuehn, B. (2004) The breakdown on biodigesters. (News) *Journal of the American Veterinary Medical Association* **224**(7), 1060–1061.

Lofholm, N. (2008) Slaughterhouse, euthanasia possible for wild horses. *The Denver Post*, July 29. (Source: Bureau of Land Management.)

May, K. (2008) *Unwanted Horses and the AVMA's Policy on Horse Slaughter, Frequently Asked Questions*. Available at: www.avma.org/issues/animal_welfare/unwanted_horses_faq_pf.asp.

McGee, K., Lanier, J.L. and Grandin, T. (2001) *Characterizations of Horses at Auctions in Slaughter Plants*. Animal Sciences Research Report, Department of Animal Sciences, Colorado State University, Fort Collins, CO.

Meeker, D.L. (2008) Carcass disposal options. *The Unwanted Horse Issue: What Now? Forum, US Department of Agriculture Revised Proceedings*, June 18.

Messer, N.T. (2004) The plight of the unwanted horse: scope of the problem. *Proceedings of the 50th Annual Convention of the AAEP*, pp. 165–167.

Montgomery, J. and Fell, N. (2008) *Colorado Unwanted Horse Environmental Assessment Report 2008*. Animal Assistance Foundation, Denver, CO.

Morris, J. *et al.* (1997) *Composting Livestock Mortalities*. Fact Sheet. Ontario Ministry of Agriculture, Food and Rural Affairs, Ontario, Canada.

Mukhtar, S. *et al.* (2003) *A Low Maintenance Approach to Large Carcass Composting*. Society for Engineering in Agricultural, Food and Biological Systems (ASAE), Annual International Meeting, Paper No. 032263.

NASS (2007) *Livestock Slaughter Summary 2007 Report*. US Department of Agriculture, National Agriculture Statistics Service. See: http://www.nass.usda.gov/Data_and_Statistics/Quick_Stats/index.asp.

North, M.S., Bailey, D. and Ward, R.A. (2005) The potential impact of a proposed ban on the sale of U.S. horses for slaughter for human consumption. *Journal of Agribusiness* 23(1), 1–17.

Reece, V.P., Friend, T.H. and Stull, C.H. (2000) Equine slaughter transport – update on research and regulations. (Animal Welfare Forum: Equine Welfare) *Journal of the American Veterinary Medical Association* 216(8), 1231.

Ryder, E. (2008) Readers weigh in on low-cost euthanasia clinics. *The Horse*, October 30, Article No. 12990.

Sander, J., Warbington, M. and Myers, L. (2002) Selected methods of animal carcass disposal. *Journal of the American Veterinary Medical Association* 220, 1003–1005.

Shearer, J. and Nicoletti, P. (2002) *Procedures for Humane Euthanasia: Humane Euthanasia of Sick, Injured, and/or Debilitated Livestock*. Available at: http://www.vdpam.iastate.edu/HumaneEuthanasia/.

Stuff, C.L. (1996) History of U.S. equine welfare and legislation. *Pferdeheilkunde* 4, 391–392.

Stull, C.L. (1999) Responses of horses to trailer design, duration, and floor area during commercial transportation to slaughter. *Journal of Animal Science* 77, 2925–2933.

Sweeney, J. (2003) The American Horse Slaughter Prevention Act, H.R. 856, 108th Congress, 1st Session, February 13.

Sweeney, J. (2005) The Horse Slaughter Prohibition Bill, H.R. 503, 109th Congress.

USDA (2008) *Highlights of Equine 2005. Part II: Changes in the US Equine Industry, 1998–2005*. Information Sheet. US Department of Agriculture.

USDI (2008) *Challenges Facing the BLM in its Management of Wild Horses and Burros*. Fact Sheet. Bureau of Land Management, US Department of the Interior.

The Welfare of Wild Horses in the Western USA

24

Albert J. Kane[1]

24.1 Introduction

Known by many names, the wild or feral horse continues to roam millions of acres of public and Tribal land in the western USA. Paleontologists generally agree that the modern horse (*Equus caballus*) evolved in North America as well as Eurasia during the Pliocene period but ultimately disappeared from North America some time during the late Pleistocene due to climatic events as well as perhaps over-hunting by early humans. Reintroduced to North America by Spanish explorers during the 1500s, today's wild horse is a descendant of horses escaped from or turned loose by those early explorers as well as American Indians, ranchers, sheep herders, miners, and cavalry remount stations. Some of today's wild horses have stronger genetic links to the Spanish or New World Iberian lineage than others.

---

[1] Editors' Note

As a Senior Staff Veterinarian with the United States Department of Agriculture (USDA), Albert Kane manages an interagency partnership between the USDA Animal and Plant Health Inspection Service (APHIS) and the United States Department of Interior, Bureau of Land Management (BLM) Wild Horse and Burro (WH&B) Program. Dr. Kane serves as a staff veterinarian and advisor for the Program in the areas of animal health and welfare, handling, and research. Along with the several private veterinary practitioners who work for the Program, he provides veterinary consultation and support for approximately 33 000 free-roaming wild horses and burros on the range, as well as another approximately 30 000 animals in BLM preparation, holding, and adoption facilities.

This varies tremendously from herd to herd. Some have the characteristic head shape, ears, and coloration of the so-called Spanish mustang. Others, whose roots can often be traced back to particular remount stations or ranchers that managed bands of broodmares as free-roaming herds, are clearly typical of Quarter Horse, Thoroughbred or crossbred draft types of horses.

The variable ancestry of today's wild horses contributes to their symbolism, mystique, and appeal to the American public and horse lovers worldwide. It also contributes to the controversies over how to manage them on the range and even the confusion about what to call them. To most wildlife biologists and ecologists, they are *feral* animals, escaped from captivity or descendant from animals that escaped from captivity. Some argue that, because they were reintroduced following extinction, they have no place in the natural ecosystem, and because of this should take a back seat to native wildlife or be removed from the range altogether. Horses on Bureau of Land Management (BLM) and Forest Service lands were legally identified as '*wild* free-roaming horses ... living symbols of the historic and pioneer spirit of the west' by Congress in 1971. This is the term used here by this author and the BLM, which is responsible for the management of the vast majority of the free-roaming horses in the USA. Finally, there are many for whom the wild horse on Western rangelands will always be the *mustang*, with sentimental if not strong genetic ties back to horses brought to North America by the Spanish explorers.

The BLM and Forest Service have management responsibility for wild horses (and burros) on their respective lands. The BLM assists the Forest Service with roundups (called gathers) and the preparation, care, and adoption of Forest Service animals that have been removed from the range. In total, the two agencies currently manage about 33 000 horses that still roam freely on about 32 million acres of rangeland in 10 western States and another 30 000 animals that reside in BLM short-term holding corrals and long-term pasture holding facilities. These animals are the only ones afforded protection by Federal legislation.[2] The BLM's Congressional mandate is to protect, manage, and control wild horses. When Congress recognized the wild horse as a valuable cultural resource, they also gave BLM some general guidelines for management.[3] Wild horses are to be considered an integral part of the natural system of public lands and they are to be managed at a 'thriving natural ecological balance' (the Act) as 'self-sustaining populations of healthy animals in balance with other uses and the productive capacity of their habitat.' The BLM is further directed in the Act to use the 'minimum feasible level of management' that will achieve these goals.

---

[2] Public Law (PL) 86–284, the Wild Horse Annie Act, 1959; and Public Law (PL) 92–195, the Wild Free-Roaming Horses and Burros Act, 1971, as amended (the Act).
[3] Code of Federal Regulations, 2008, Part 43 CFR 4700.0-6(a), Protection, Management, and Control of Wild Free-Roaming Horses and Burros.

It seems clear that the intent of Congress was to protect and conserve wild horses but leave them on the range in a wild, free-roaming state without creating a zoo-like environment.

BLM horses are not the only wild horses in the western USA. The National Park Service manages the Theodore Roosevelt National Park in North Dakota and the US Fish and Wildlife Service has over 1000 wild horses under their management on the Sheldon National Wildlife Refuge on the Nevada–Oregon border. Under the jurisdiction of the State of Nevada Department of Agriculture are about 1000 wild horses near Virginia City, Nevada. These horses are called *estray* horses, a term that simply means they are unclaimed and considered stray feral horses. Also in the West are several populations of free-roaming wild horses on lands managed by American Indian groups such as the Yakama, Colville, Warm Springs, Paiute, Apache, Navajo, and Ute Tribes. Other herds of wild horses live in scattered areas across the USA. The National Park Service manages about 200 animals on the Assateague Island National Seashore in Maryland. On the southern end of Assateague Island, separated by a boundary fence, live about 150 privately owned feral ponies of the Chincoteague Volunteer Fire Department. Small groups of free-roaming wild horses also live on military installations, private, County, and State lands in Missouri, Louisiana, Georgia, and North Carolina (mid-Atlantic coastal barrier islands), Arizona, New Mexico, and California. There is no organized reporting of the sizes of these populations, but it seems likely there are another 20 000 wild horses in the USA on lands not managed by the BLM or Forest Service. Each management agency may have different objectives and parameters within which the horses are managed. Some regard them as a cultural resource to be preserved or conserved. Others view them as a source of commercial revenue, and others an invader or pest that competes with native wildlife but whose presence is often tolerated due to public interest. While none of these non-BLM horses are protected by the same Federal laws applicable to BLM and Forest Service horses, most are protected in some manner from unauthorized capture, branding, harassment, and destruction.

As varied an appearance and uncertain an origin as any wild horse might have, one thing is certain. They are remarkable animals deserving of humane treatment and proper management. Whether our responsibility comes to us by Congressional assignment, moral obligations due to the feral horses' domestic origins, or an enthusiasm and respect for all wild or domestic animals including the horse, we must endeavor to protect their well-being and provide for their welfare. For wild horses, this invariably means managing the animals and, more importantly, their environment so they remain healthy and have the opportunity to thrive. Given their wild nature, the practicality of individualized animal care often needs to be weighed against the problems that can be created when trying to capture or restrain an animal for treatment on the range or in a facility. Stress levels can be high in the wild, during capture operations, and while animals are adjusting to captivity. To avoid all stress seems unrealistic in any management scenario. The responsible goal therefore is to minimize the animals' stress levels whenever possible. This can be done by creating the best environment possible, avoiding unnecessary handling, and handling the animals in a quiet, efficient manner when necessary. Signs of distress should be uncommon and generally indicate a problem with the animal's condition, the environment or the handling procedures.

24.2 Horses on the Range

Protecting the welfare of wild horses on the range is largely about protecting the well-being of the herd through good range management and crisis prevention more than addressing problems with individual animals. This is mostly accomplished by keeping the size of the populations in balance with the water and forage resources available so that the animals can naturally maintain their body condition and good health. The saying 'healthy rangelands and healthy horses' is more than just a catchphrase. If water and forage resources are in good condition, which generally means that feed and water are relatively abundant and evenly distributed throughout a herd management area, then wild horses generally remain in good body condition and good health.

The most common welfare problems on the range are related to limited feed and water availability. Some seasonal variation in body condition is expected. Mares in particular will decline in condition when nursing a foal or when forage may be limited due to drought or snow cover. The Henneke et al. (1983), body condition scoring system (1 = extremely emaciated to 9 = extremely fat, Henneke et al. 1983) has proven to be a useful method of describing the body condition of wild horses. A body condition score of 4 might be good for younger (three-year-old) or older (15-year-old or older) lactating mares coming out of winter. A score of 3 might not be alarming for the same mares in the early spring. Heading into winter, however, condition scores of 3 should probably be reason for concern. If a small percentage of mares, say 2–5%, are affected, it is probably an indication that individual animals have problems, such as advanced age, severe dental abnormalities, lameness or other health problems. If a moderate percentage of mares are affected, say 20–30%, that likely suggests an imbalance between grazing pressures and the available resources. When 50% or more are in poor condition, this is likely a sign of a serious mismatch between grazing pressures and forage availability, with a potential crisis on the horizon. There are no good natural mechanisms that will decrease foaling and population growth rates until the animals are clearly suffering from starvation and there is severe overgrazing damage to the rangeland resource. Conception rates might decline a little, but conception occurs in a previous growing season. Wild horse mares will continue to foal until body condition affects their overall stamina and well-being, typically Henneke scores of 1 or 2, or they are much older (more than 20 years old). In some areas it is not uncommon for thin mares over 20 years old to still be foaling, and it is a myth that population growth rates will naturally match forage availability. Before the horses show signs of starvation, the range will typically be severely overgrazed, with resource damage that may take many years or even decades to recover.

In herd areas where water is a limiting resource, the amount as well as the distribution of available water is important. If horses can drink their fill when they go to water, they will readily travel 10, 20 or even more miles (15–30 km or more) each day to areas with good forage, returning to water on a daily basis or even every other day. If they cannot drink their fill or 'tank up' in a relaxed non-competitive manner, they cannot travel as far to graze and will overgraze areas near water sources to a greater degree. Under these conditions, horses will eventually reduce the area within a mile or so of a water source to bare dirt. Under these conditions, there may be adequate forage several miles away but horses will still face starvation if they cannot or will not travel to those areas. In challenging desert range conditions, there is also some herd-level memory that can play an important role in making efficient use of the available forage. This is akin to an institutional memory, where over many years the herd has learned to travel long distances to areas with good forage. Some groups of animals regularly follow rainstorms to areas that historically have produced good forage when seasonal rains come to the desert. Relying on small dams and puddles for water when it is available, horses will then return if necessary to their original, permanent water sources maybe 20 or 30 miles (30–45 km) away when water resources again run low.

Regardless of whether the limiting resource is forage or water, it is the range that must be monitored first to prevent starvation problems. The utilization of available forage will suggest an imminent animal problem before the grazing animal's body condition reveals there is a problem. By the time a majority of the animals are thin, the range will have suffered long-lasting or permanent damage and an emergency situation will already be at hand. It is before these emergencies that measures should be taken to safeguard the well-being of the animals. If domestic livestock are present, grazing competition can be reduced by removing them earlier than scheduled. Ultimately gather and removal actions (roundups) may be necessary to ensure the well-being of the animals. Normally, this means that only a percentage of the animals are removed from the range. A core breeding population, large enough to ensure the viability of the herd but small enough to be sustained by the remaining natural resources, is usually left on the range. Exceptions might include areas affected by wildfires that destroy all the available forage at one time. In these areas or areas that have been affected by severely limited resources on a reoccurring basis, a temporary or indefinite complete removal of all animals from that herd area may be warranted to prevent future animal welfare crises.

Often it is suggested that artificial water sources such as wells or pipelines be developed or that animals be fed hay to get them through bad times or a harsh winter. While this may seem like a good short-term solution to prevent a catastrophic die-off, for example, it can also cause long-term problems. Water wells are subject to mechanical breakdowns and pipelines break or can be turned off even by well-intentioned people. On large low-pressure pipeline systems, opening a valve at one trough to help horses that may be looking for more water can inadvertently dry up a second trough a few miles away and put other horses in danger. Given the vast areas where wild horses live, hundreds of thousands or even millions of acres in a single herd management area, few management agencies would have the manpower to visit every critical well or water tank daily or every other day. Horses can learn to adapt to natural variations in water availability that occur slowly over time, but they are unlikely to learn how to adapt to a water tank suddenly going dry because of an unforeseen mechanical failure or sick caretaker. There may be a place for manmade water developments to improve the distribution of available water, but relying heavily on artificial water sources without adequate redundancy seems to be asking for trouble in the long run.

Winter or drought feeding grounds have been established to provide for some wild-life species such as elk outside Jackson, Wyoming, or deer along the Continental Divide in Colorado. However, these unnatural provisions can also create problems and may not be an option if the legal mandate is to manage for a 'thriving *natural* ecological balance' at a 'minimum feasible level of management' as in the BLM's case. Feed grounds create an unnatural congregation of animals that will affect the spread of infectious or contagious diseases and parasitism in the population. Over the long term, this usually creates an even greater set of problems for the wild animal population as well as domestic animals that may be trying to share the available resources.

Free-roaming horses on the range rarely have health problems that aren't related to poor condition or very old age. Horses generally live in small social groups or bands that range in size from three or four animals to perhaps 10 or 15 in a band. Interactions that take place between bands depend largely on the time of year and the distribution of water and forage. For the most part wild horses and burros try to avoid confrontation with animals outside their social group by avoiding contact with other groups. However, during the breeding season in particular, there may be mingling or transfer of individuals between bands, and in areas with limited water resources many bands may congregate near water sources during different times of day. In some herd areas it is not uncommon to see bands keeping distances of a mile or more between them. In other areas, particularly where there are few water sources, multiple bands may congregate in the same area at the same time, forming large groups of 50, 60 even 100 horses within a square mile (260 ha).

When horses are widely dispersed over an arid landscape, the spread of infectious or contagious diseases, such as bacterial or viral respiratory diseases or internal parasitism, is much less likely. When they congregate in large groups, it may be more common. Infectious upper respiratory disease caused by *Streptococcus zooep-idemicus* and *Streptococcus equi* have been documented in free-roaming wild horse herds; however, they are rarely a problem with horses on the range. Often herds that are known to have endemic bacterial respiratory infection also have a history of some animals from the herd having been gathered and confined in a facility for a period of time then later released back to the range.

With the exception of a few small herds along the mid-Atlantic coast, most wild horse herds are not vaccinated on the range. For the BLM, vaccinations and individual medical treatments of horses on the range seem contrary to the 'minimum feasible level of management' mandate. Horses on the mid-Atlantic Barrier Islands have on occasion been affected by Eastern equine encephalitis virus, but overall this or clinical problems associated with West Nile virus infection seem rare. Similarly, the equine infectious anemia (EIA) virus has infected some horses on the East Coast Barrier Islands as well as a BLM herd and an American Indian herd in the Uintah Basin of Utah and an American Indian herd in Oregon. During gathering operations, BLM animals in the area affected by EIA are quarantined on-site in temporary corrals until they test negative and can be shipped outside the herd management area. Thankfully, these infections are also very rare overall. Surprisingly, no clinical signs associated with the West Nile virus have been noted in the 179 BLM herds throughout the West.

One important aspect of protecting animal health and welfare on the range involves ensuring sufficient genetic diversity to avoid inbreeding depression. Small herds and those that may have experienced a population bottleneck in the past are at risk for excessive inbreeding, leading to insufficient genetic diversity. The herd size necessary to avoid problems isn't exactly known for wild horses, but it is thought to be about 50 effective breeding age animals or 150 total animals in the population (Singer et al., 2000). While many wild horse herds are smaller than this, ongoing genetic testing of BLM herds has not yet identified any herds in imminent danger of having a critical problem. When inbreeding depression is a concern, it is relatively easy to address by introducing one or two young mares from another wild horse herd every 10 years or so. If young wild horse mares living in a similar environment are used for relocation, they usually assimilate well into existing herds. Trying to introduce domestic stock, older mares or stallions is usually problematic. These classes of horses may travel back to their original range, fail to assimilate into the breeding population, or may not survive the transition.

Welfare and health concerns of individual animals on the range are usually related to debilitation from old age and acquired or congenital physical defects. Although rare overall, naturally occurring injuries such as lower limb fractures that heal poorly and severe angular and flexural deformities are most common. In most cases horses with these deformities are not seen during the acute stage of the injury but after they have adapted to the problem on the range. Under this circumstance many will get along surprisingly well as long as there is adequate forage and water and they aren't traveling long distances, 20 miles or more, every day. Although they may have a severe gait abnormality or lameness consistently observable at a trot, for example, they may be in good body condition and keep up and interact with their peers in a normal manner. Horses that do have crippling injuries or injuries that are affecting their overall condition are suffering and may need to be destroyed on the range in the quickest and most humane manner possible.

In some herds physical problems with a clear genetic link such as the club foot deformity, dwarfism or blindness associated with cataract formation have occurred.

These conditions affect not only the well-being of the individual animal but also the viability of the herd. Other conditions with a genetic link such as ventral abdominal hernias and cryptorchidism may not affect animal well-being but can create a management problem and are considered a serious physical defect or unsoundness in the domestic horse world. These situations can usually be addressed during a roundup. At the least these animals should not be allowed to return to the range. If the condition cannot be corrected or causes lameness or other health problems, euthanasia should be considered. At these times it is helpful to have a clearly written and agreed-upon policy for euthanasia in place before the need arises. Some personnel will still be reluctant to follow these policies. A veterinary consultation early in the process can be very helpful to ensure an accurate assessment of the animal's condition and increase the confidence and comfort level of field personnel and management with these decisions.

24.3 Population Control

Wild horses are remarkably adaptable animals that can maintain population growth rates of 20% or more per year, doubling herd sizes every four or five years, even under adverse conditions. It is unlikely that wild horse mares are inherently more fertile than their domestic counterparts, but the natural breeding model that includes true seasonal breeding, live cover, breeding several times a day, and often by more than one stallion is an effective one. While the age structure of the herds varies depending on the climate, terrain, and type of horses present, most horses live and reproduce well into their teens. In some herd areas it is not uncommon to see mares foal up to or beyond 20 years of age. Forage, drought, and other weather and environmental conditions have a large impact on foal survival. Pregnancy and foaling rates however don't seem to be easily affected by environmental conditions or the body condition of the mare. It is not uncommon to see thin mares with a Henneke body condition score of 2 or 3 nursing a foal, maybe also nursing their yearling colt, and being successfully rebred all at the same time. Short of catastrophic die-offs of a large proportion of the adult population, as sometimes occurs with severe winter weather or drought, it is a myth that population growth somehow balances out with the available forage.

Horses will reduce standing vegetation of all types to dirt and starve to death in large numbers before foaling rates and the resultant population growth rates will be reduced. Some advocate letting nature take its course in these conditions, but this is a cruel and miserable death. When the grasses and edible forbs are gone, horses will eat brush and trees. When consumed in large quantities by starving horses, sagebrush, greasewood, and other woody plants are toxic and cause physical as well as physiological problems in the gastrointestinal tract and nervous system. When the grass is gone, horses will brush away dirt and sand with their noses to eat the roots of the grass. This along with drinking out of puddles and even hoof prints leads to sand accumulation in the colon and causes acute and chronic gastrointestinal problems. When death comes, it is slow and insidious, often occurring over the course of several days. Starving horses will spend more and more time recumbent, eventually working a hole into the ground under their nose when they are unable to get up. Scavengers that normally feed on carcasses do not always wait until an animal has passed. Birds and coyotes will begin to feed on an animal's hindquarters or head before it has died. Maybe this was understandable before the turn of the last century, when animals could potentially migrate over hundreds of miles, but in the twenty-first century – with interstates and development limiting most herd areas to tens or hundreds of thousands of acres instead of tens or hundreds of millions of acres – this doesn't seem at all like a responsible course of action.

Apart from occasional winter die-off, usually due to sudden blizzards, effective natural population control seems limited to the few areas where mountain lion predation of foals and debilitated older horses balances with the foal survival rates. It is unusual to record successful lion attacks on strong, healthy adult horses; but in a few BLM herd management areas lion predation seems to keep population numbers stable. So responsible herd management means responsible population control, and, where possible, responsible suppression of population growth rates.

Periodic roundups, called gathers by the BLM, and removal of a proportion of animals from the range are the most common approach used for population control. When done in a responsible manner, gathers can be done humanely and efficiently with no detrimental, long-term effects on the horses. Most herds are gathered about every five years, depending on population growth rates. Helicopter drive trapping is the most common method used. With this approach, a small helicopter maneuvers much a like a border collie herding sheep to push horses toward and ultimately into a corral. Using natural trails, travel corridors, and terrain to locate the site, small corrals called traps are constructed of 6–7 feet (2 m) tall portable steel panels. These are similar to the panels used for round pens or arenas but made of slightly heavier tubing. At the entrance to the trap is a pair of 'wings.' The wings are usually made of rolls of burlap hung on metal T-posts temporarily driven into the ground. These temporary, solid-looking fences form a type of funnel, which serves to direct horses into the trap. When the horses are brought in quietly by a skilled pilot, these wings only need to be about 4–5 feet (1.5 m) tall and perhaps 100–400 feet (30–120 m) long. Horses enter a trap at the back end where most of the panels in the first pen are uncovered so as not to look too much like a solid wall or enclosure. This first pen leads to a second pen and often into a third smaller pen that feeds a short alley for loading horses onto stock trailers. A typical trap may only be about 20–30 feet (6–9 m) wide at the widest point and 60–100 feet (18–30 m) long, to accommodate a typical run of 20 or so horses. A small colt pen is often added on the side of the trap so small foals can be temporarily sorted away from the adults before shipping to a nearby holding corral.

Other traps, depending on the terrain and horse density, may be attached to a much larger temporary holding corral that includes alleyways and a working chute and can hold 200 or more horses separated into half a dozen separate pens. The corrals should always be designed to minimize the risk of injury. Plastic snow fence or burlap is used to cover most of the panels and gates to create more of a visual barrier than the panels alone. Wild horses will often challenge or crash into fences and gates where they first enter a pen if they don't appear to be almost solid. The trade-off is if panels were completely solid it would be more difficult to get the animals to enter the pens. Corrals constructed from panels may be anchored to the ground in a few key locations but the fact that the panels are relatively lightweight and have some give where each hinges to the next helps prevent injuries when a horse challenges the enclosure or tries to jump out.

Helicopter-assisted roping is another technique used to capture some horses. With this method a helicopter brings horses toward a team of three or four cowboys mounted on fast, sure-footed horses. The pilot directs the ropers to an area free from hazardous terrain and brush, and they usually stay somewhat concealed, behind a hill, for example. When the helicopter brings the wild horses past the riders, they have an advantage, and can usually catch a horse or two without incident. Unassisted ropers are rarely able to capture free-roaming wild horses. The saddle horses simply could not catch up to most wild horses, and the danger to the horses and riders would be too great. Even with the advantage of the helicopter hazing the horses toward the saddle horses, it takes a very skilled and experienced roper to catch an adult wild horse or foal and slowly bring it to a stop without injury to the horses or riders.

Under BLM contracts, only dally roping, where the rope is held in the roper's hands and not tied hard and fast to the saddle horn, is allowed, and captured horses are never intentionally tripped or tipped over as part of the capture. Usually roping is reserved for small groups of horses or horses that cannot be brought to a trap. The single horse here or there that will not enter a trap is usually allowed to get away. Under some situations, such as horses that are outside the herd management area boundaries and must be captured for removal, every horse must be captured if possible.

Helicopter-assisted roping is also an advantage for the safe capture of very young colts, and old, injured or debilitated animals that cannot be brought safely to a trap. In these cases the pilot will usually allow the animal to fall back away from the larger group of horses, make a note of the location, put the main group into a trap and return minutes later with a ground crew to capture the horse left behind and load it onto a trailer for the trip to the trap. Extra effort is also put toward capturing every mare in a band that has very young colts. This makes it less likely that a colt will be captured while its mother runs off and remains on the range.

With the assistance of a helicopter, many horses can be safely, humanely, and efficiently captured with these methods. A skilled and patient pilot can safely bring even newborn foals and debilitated animals into or near a trap using these techniques.

Ground pursuit by horseback over any significant distance is usually much more stressful to the animals and will often result in more injuries and foals separated from the herd. The wings of a trap typically need to be 6–7 feet (2 m) tall when using mounted riders to haze horses into a trap because the animals are more panicked and running harder when brought in by these methods. The use of planes and ground vehicles such as motorcycles or all-terrain vehicles for herding and capture are prohibited by Federal law for BLM and Forest Service horses and are not used by these agencies. Typically horses are brought to a trap by a helicopter from distances of less than 10 miles (15–16 km). They may run at a gallop when first located and when very close to the trap, but usually travel most of this way at a slow lope, trot or even a walk. Horses should arrive at a trap only slightly winded, not blowing hard or lathered in sweat. It should be comparable to an endurance horse coming into a checkpoint, not a Thoroughbred after finishing a race. Animals should recover to a normal respiratory rate for an excited or nervous horse but not be blowing within 5–10 minutes. At no time should they display signs of exhaustion or metabolic distress. In the summer, accommodations must be made for the heat. Trapping and sorting should not be done during the very hottest part of the day. As long as temperatures are above 0°F (–18°C), winter is a good time to capture wild horses. A small amount of snow cover makes horses easier to spot and prevents dust problems. Deep snow can be a problem as it tires the horses more quickly and can lead to signs of exhaustion or distress. Experience, monitoring the condition of the animals as they are captured, and knowing when to adjust the methods are essential to ensure safe gather operations.

Bait or water trapping are also routinely used to capture wild horses. With this technique, a trap similar to the one described earlier, but without the wings, is built near an area frequented by the horses. Often they are built around an existing water source. The horses are lured into the trap with feed, water, salt or a mineral block as a lure. A gate is then closed by a trip rope, electronic trigger or person hiding nearby. Usually this technique is reserved for capturing small groups of horses that might frequent a certain area. Under drought conditions, when alternative water sources are limited or non-existent, however, over 100 horses a day can be captured using this technique. Many assume this is a kinder, gentler technique compared to helicopter drive trapping, but this is not necessarily the case. Except for those already debilitated by drought, the horses are usually fresh when the gates are closed and seem more likely to crash into panels and gates when surprised by the presence of humans. Water trapping the second half of a population can be a slow process and there is a tradeoff between coaxing the animals into the trap and holding them off water. Traps must be designed to allow wildlife such as antelope a chance to drink, and every second or third day the horses must be allowed to drink or some would die from thirst rather than enter the trap.

It is difficult to emphasize enough how important the skills of the pilot and crew are for a safe, humane, and efficient gather operation. Usually 30 to 50 horses are captured in a single day, but it is not uncommon to capture 100 horses in a day using helicopter drive trapping. While it doesn't pay to be in a great hurry, time and money are usually limiting resources when managing wild horses, and an efficient operation is usually in the best interests of the horses and the management program. There are many subtleties to trap location and design, hazing by helicopter, roping and working horses in a corral. Bystanders, camera crews, and extra vehicles in the area can easily spook wild horses and make it more difficult to bring them into a trap or work them through the pens. Most injuries that occur are minor scrapes and cuts. This author has participated in the capture of 10 797 horses, with an accidental death loss attributable to gather activities, which includes sorting and temporarily holding the horses on the range, of just 55 animals – or about 0.5%. While every death is an unfortunate and regrettable event, that they are extremely rare and lower than one might expect given the wild nature of the horses is some comfort.

Alternative capture techniques such as darting with chemical immobilization agents and aerial net-gunning (using a helicopter to shoot nets over a running animal from a sort of cannon) have been tried over the years but almost always lead to higher injury and death rates. These techniques are extremely dangerous for the personnel involved, and it is difficult to imagine how they could be applied efficiently when thousands of animals need to be captured each year. These techniques should not be used for routine or large-scale capture activities.

The most common welfare concern encountered during gather activities is how to handle horses that are found to have serious pre-existing injuries or physical problems. Although rare, when limb deformities and problems such as club feet do occur, they tend to be severe because of the demands of traveling long distances on the range. These conditions along with old fractures or injuries that heal poorly and severe arthritis can cause crippling lameness and eventually starvation in the older horse. Some would have managers release these animals to let nature take her course. How this can be considered humane, to make a crippled horse travel for miles each day in search of feed and water, is difficult to understand. To compound the problem, conditions such as club feet have a genetic component and herds with a management history that includes turning these animals back onto the range quickly see an increasing incidence of the problem. The most humane course of action in most of these situations is to euthanize the animal in a timely manner.

Another challenge is how to handle large numbers of horses that are in very poor condition. The occasional young or middle-aged horse that is very thin will likely do fine when removed from the range and placed on feed in a facility or an adoptive home. Often these are mares nursing foals that simply need a chance to catch up to the demands of lactation with a more readily available source of feed. Older animals, particularly those with severe dental abnormalities, may not be able to recover their condition and adapt to new surroundings after being placed in captivity. Is it humane to expect a 20-year-old stallion with worn teeth, arthritis, and the other perhaps minor infirmities associated with old age to adjust to captivity, castration, and domestic life? The vast majority do survive and make the adjustment, but is it always in the horse's best interest to put them through that process?

A greater challenge is how to handle large numbers of horses that have been facing starvation and must be removed from the range. Invariably these horses have turned to eating brush and other plants that may have toxic side-effects. This can cause damage to their digestive system, and they can have difficulty getting back on feed. These horses can put others at risk in facilities if they develop problems such as infectious diarrhea. In extreme cases, to protect the health and welfare of the larger population in a facility, it may be necessary to euthanize some animals in the field that have a poor prognosis for recovery, even if that recovery may be possible.

There is no single solution for these problems. They must be addressed on a case-by-case basis by experienced managers and veterinarians who are on-site. The goal of a good management plan is to prevent these large-scale problems. Thankfully, with careful management, they rarely occur.

24.4 Fertility Control

A safe, effective, and affordable alternative to gather and removal strategies for controlling population numbers would be a welcome tool for wild horse managers. Fertility control or contraception has the potential to provide the alternative, but it has been a difficult and slow process to produce a practical and long-lasting agent. Early research in the 1970s and 1980s focused on using hormones in stallions and mares to control the reproductive cycle. Although this approach reduced fertility, these methods proved inefficient, dangerous for the animals, and threatened the natural food chain. Although many still ask why you can't simply castrate the stallions or perform vasectomies on them, the focus has shifted away from the stallion, as one missed stallion can impregnate many mares. Research has shown that under normal conditions 15–33% of foals are sired by non-harem stallions (Bowling and Touchberry, 1990; Kaseda and Khalil, 1996; Asa, 1999). With mares continuing to cycle for extended periods of time, providing ongoing opportunities for secondary stallions to get mares bred, it seems unlikely that fertility control focused on males would be an effective or efficient method of slowing population growth rates. Wild horse mares are difficult to spay under field conditions, so this option is not appealing. Intrauterine devices that prevent pregnancy have been tried, but they typically fall out of horse mares in the course of natural breeding. Each of these techniques also requires the mare be open when treated, and wild horse mares of breeding age are generally pregnant for most of the year.

In 1990 a breakthrough was achieved when a previously tested but unproven immunocontraceptive agent using a porcine zona pellucida (PZP) antigen was used to suppress fertility of wild horse mares on the Assateague Island National Seashore (Kirkpatrick et al., 1990). Although this agent is not approved by the Food and Drug Administration, it has been under development since the late 1980s (Liu et al., 1989) and is available for investigational use. The liquid form used on Assateague Island National Seashore has been shown to stabilize population growth when given by remote delivery (darting) on an annual basis (Kirkpatrick and Turner, 2002). After 11 years of annual treatments, the population size decreased by natural mortality by 23% from 175 animals to 135 animals (Kirkpatrick and Turner, 2008). This works well on the Island and in other areas where animals can be approached within 50 yards or so for darting. Unfortunately, on most Western ranges, wild horses are usually difficult to approach to within less than a half of a mile. So while annual darting is being used in a few BLM herds, its widespread practicality remains uncertain.

Between 1992 and 2003, 11 studies of PZP immunocontraceptives were performed on BLM herd management areas (Kirkpatrick, 2005). Long-term stabilization of population growth has not been demonstrated in any of these areas. One of these studies included novel timed-release PZP pellets designed to last for two years (PZP-22). This application was reported to reduce foaling rates from 54% in untreated mares to just 6%, 14%, and 32% in years one, two, and three, respectively, following treatment (Turner *et al.*, 2007). Since 2004 the BLM has administered 2200 doses of this agent and the original liquid PZP in ongoing field trials in 56 of their 179 herd management areas. These trials conducted by the BLM and the Department of Interior's US Geological Survey are trying to demonstrate a long-term suppression of population growth rates, and some are examining the effects of immunocontraception on behavior. Stabilization of population growth rates over several years has not yet been demonstrated, but the work is ongoing. It is the policy of the BLM to analyze use of the PZP vaccine in every gather plan and use it if feasible. The vaccine causes no harm to unborn foals. However, to maximize the effectiveness and longevity of the vaccine, it must be given 3–4 months prior to breeding. Also, to effectively reduce population growth rates, it is believed that a vaccine that is highly effective must be administered to 70–90% of the breeding-age mares. This means capturing 80–100% of the actual population, which is often not possible. The BLM has considered gathering some herds more frequently, every two years, to apply fertility control without removing horses. In some areas this may work, but in most it is feared that it would get harder and harder to safely capture the animals, as they do catch-on to the process and over time become more and more resistant to being hazed into a trap.

Research aimed at producing a longer-lasting PZP agent has been funded by the BLM for the past several years, and this work continues today. Developing a safe, highly effective, single-shot, long-lasting but reversible contraceptive is a tall order to fill. This has never been done for any other species, including man. There are no products of this type available anywhere in the world today. Research on long-acting products where it is important to demonstrate reversibility is by nature a slow process, often taking five years or more to do one study of a three-year agent. If the agent doesn't work as planned, it is back to the laboratory and another wait of five or more years to see if the second attempt works better. The cost of the pelleted PZP agent is about $250 per dose, which is high for a vaccine but seems more reasonable compared to the costs of gathering and caring for unadopted animals.

The biggest limitations remain the impracticality of darting horses every year on most Western rangelands, and that, although they can clearly reduce foaling rates in treated mares, these relatively short-acting agents have not been demonstrated to slow population growth rates over several years without annual darting of the liquid agent.

Two other fertility control agents, SpayVac™, which is a novel liposome vaccine using a PZP antigen, and GonaCon™, which is a gonadotropin-releasing hormone (GnRH) vaccine, have also shown promise for use in wild horses (Killian et al., 2008). It is disappointing that after over 30 years of work there are still no approved or long-lasting products available for fertility control in wild horses. However, there has been progress, and research with all these agents continues in the effort to produce a safe, effective, and practical management tool for use on a wide variety of Western wild horse herds.

24.5 Preparation for Adoption, Holding, and Shipping

Following capture, wild horses are taken either to a nearby temporary holding corral set up on the range or to a nearby permanent facility. On arrival, every horse, except perhaps the youngest foals, are put through an alley that includes a padded chute. The stallions are separated from mares, mares are examined to see if they are nursing, and mares and foals are marked with chalk to facilitate keeping track of which foals are nursing which mares and keeping the pairs together. Weanlings and yearlings are separated from the adults. Often the animals are aged by examining their teeth at this time, samples may be taken for genetic testing, and veterinary care is provided if necessary. The sooner this sorting can be accomplished, the less fighting and fewer injuries will occur. When separated from mares by even a narrow double fence, such as an alleyway, stallions will get along and fight less than if mares are in an adjacent pen. It is a rare event that a particularly aggressive and dominant stallion or pair of stallions need to be separated. Mares tend to kick and bite each other much more than stallions. They need adequate pen space to keep some distance between them. Once a group is somewhat stable, removing the more aggressive animals only serves to re-stir the dominance hierarchy and start the process over again.

Some have advocated trying to keep family groups together throughout the gather and removal process. This is rarely a good idea. Many bands will be mixed together before they even arrive at a trap and even regular observers of a herd have difficulty identifying the horses from a particular band when they are mixed together. Many bands have more than one stallion as a member. When mares are allowed to stay with stallions there is invariably a lot more fighting, and just placing one young stud or mare in the wrong group could have terrible consequences. The injury rate for foals is also much higher if the mare–foal pairs are not separated from the stallions. Early and efficient sorting is one of the best ways to reduce fighting and injury rates among the horses following capture. Hay and water are provided upon settling the horses into the corrals. Dust control throughout this time is an important part of preventing future problems with pneumonia. Little can be done about the miles of dirt roads that are traveled in the desert range, but trap sites, temporary holding corrals, and roads next to the corrals can be watered down repeatedly to minimize dust exposure and the risk of dust pneumonia.

Some management agencies hold adoptions or sales of newly captured animals at or near the capture site. The BLM occasionally holds a small local adoption soon after a gather, but most often horses are first shipped to what BLM calls Preparation (for adoption) and Short-Term Holding facilities. This first journey should be short, preferably less than eight hours in length. Later, BLM shipping policies limit travel to less than 24 hours, with offloading and 12 hours of water, feed, and rest required before animals can resume a long journey if needed. Foals and weanlings should be separated from the adults for shipping, with nursing foals paired back with their dams following arrival. All BLM shipping is done either in stock trailers pulled by pickup trucks or straight, single-deck semi-trailers bedded with wood shavings. Wild horses should never be transported in double-deck or pot-belly trailers.

Upon arrival at a preparation facility, horses are separated by gender but kept in groups with their herd mates. They are given hay and water and allowed a period of time to adjust to captivity. All horses are examined by a veterinarian following their arrival. Most horses adjust to captivity without serious problems. There is a period, however, about 3–5 days following capture, when fatigue and the stress of the new environment seem to set in. Horses may go off feed, be reluctant to move about freely, and generally act depressed. Even horses that come off the range in poor condition will actually lose weight and condition for several days before they start gaining and improving in condition. A good wrangler or manager will anticipate this, recognize the signs, and allow time for each group of horses to adjust at their own pace. It may take a week or it may take three weeks or longer depending on the conditions that existed on the range, the horses' condition when captured, and the general temperament of the particular herd. Each situation can be different and should be addressed on a case-by-case basis.

Prior to adoption or sale, every wild horse should be tested for exposure to the EIA virus. The BLM also vaccinates and deworms every horse removed from the range, records its age, and applies a permanent freeze mark number to the left side of the animal's neck. This mark identifies it as a BLM horse and contains the animal's year of birth and a unique identifying number as well. Booster vaccines are administered about a month later, and after that time stallions are gelded prior to adoption or sale. All gelding is done by a veterinarian using anesthetic protocols similar to those used for domestic horses. Hoof trimming is done as needed in padded chutes that lift the animals and lay them on their side. Wild horses typically have strong well-shaped feet, but with the change to the domestic environment they need hoof care similar to a domestic horse.

During this period of preparing the horses for adoption and holding, the biggest welfare concerns are related to helping horses regain body condition if they come off the range starved or in poor condition, and keeping them healthy as they make the transition to domestic life. Managing the health of large numbers of newly captured wild horses in a facility is a lot like managing a daycare center during the cold and flu season. Stress levels are higher than normal, living conditions are crowded compared to conditions on the range, and most horses will be immunologically naive to common infectious respiratory conditions in particular. Aggressive vaccination programs are used to try to lessen the severity of illness, but many infections agents such as equine rhinovirus, *S. equi* (the bacteria species that causes strangles) and *S. zooepidemicus* may simply need to run their course so the animals develop their own natural immunity. An emphasis is placed on keeping groups of animals together as much as possible to limit the spread and explosive nature of an outbreak that may occur, and allowing animals to recover before shipping them to other facilities or adoptions to prevent the spread of infectious diseases outside a facility. Thankfully, most of these conditions are self-limiting and horses usually recover uneventfully with no individual treatment needed.

24.6 Adoption, Compliance, and Care of Unadopted Animals

Most wild horse management programs offer horses removed from the range for adoption or sale. Some place no restrictions or limitations on who adopts or buys the horses or what the new owner does with the horse, but most, including the BLM, have contracts that limit what can be done with newly adopted or purchased animals. Animals removed from BLM and Forest Service lands are the only ones protected by Federal laws. These laws and a well-established set of regulations and policies currently prevent the BLM and new adopters from sending horses to slaughter and require humane treatment of the animals. They also prevent the commercial exploitation of the wild nature of the animals, such as using them for wild horse races. Until the animals are gentled and accustomed to fences, the facilities of BLM adopters must meet certain requirements for space (at least 400 square feet (36 m²) per animal) and be constructed appropriately for safety (6 feet (1.8 m) tall, heavy plank, pipe or panel construction). Adopters are required to demonstrate they can provide adequate shelter, feed, and care to safeguard the well-being of the animals. Persons with convictions for inhumane treatment of animals are not allowed to adopt.

Animals adopted from the BLM are randomly selected for compliance inspections during the year following adoption. If problems or complaints do arise, the BLM, sometimes assisted by veterinarians or technicians with the United States Department of Agriculture or volunteers trained by BLM, step in to investigate and if necessary correct the situation. The BLM retains ownership of the animals it places through adoption until the adopter applies for and receives title to the animal. There is a one-year waiting period before an adopter can apply for title, and a statement on the application that confirms the animal has been cared for humanely must be signed by a veterinarian, extension agent or animal control or humane society official before title will be granted. Every effort is made to educate new adopters and create a win–win situation for the adopter and the horse, but if necessary, animals that are not being cared for properly can be taken back into BLM custody if they are untitled. These safeguards cannot prevent all problems that can arise following adoption, but they foster responsible animal care and help create good homes for the horses. Titled animals are legally private property, outside of BLM jurisdiction.

Welfare concerns with titled animals must be handled by State or local authorities just like for any other horse. Since 1973 the BLM has placed over 220 000 wild horses into good homes by adoptions and sales. On average about 5500 compliance checks are performed each year to check on the well-being of these animals following adoption. This arguably makes the BLM 'Adopt a Horse or Burro' Program the largest and most successful equine adoption program in the world. While not perfect, the vast majority of these placements are successful. There are many examples of BLM wild horses going on to great success as pleasure and performance horses. Palominos in the Marine Corps Color Guard, horses serving in the Caisson Platoon at Arlington National Cemetery, dozens of horses used by the US Border Patrol, and various champions in dressage, reining, and endurance riding are only a few of the examples that come to mind.

The success of wild horse adoption programs notwithstanding, there is still a major problem in that the supply of available animals greatly exceeds the demand. Although the Act that protects BLM horses directs the Agency to 'humanely destroy excess animals for which an adoption demand does not exist,' the BLM has been reluctant to do so. Public sentiment opposes the idea, and until recently Congressional appropriations law superseded the Act and prohibited this approach. After more than 30 years of protecting these horses, there is also strong resistance to destroying healthy animals within the BLM itself. A 2004 amendment to the Act caused controversy, requiring certain animals to be sold, such as to the highest bidder at livestock sale barns. BLM implemented a sale program, but currently sells horses only under contract. At this time, the BLM contract requirements specify that animals only go to good homes, and buyers must promise not to send or sell purchased horses to slaughter. Further confusing the issue, in 2008, the Government Accountability Office (GAO) found that BLM was not in compliance with the Act because the Agency was not euthanizing or selling excess horses without limitations. The GAO recommended that the agency discuss with Congress and other stakeholders how best to comply with the Act or amend it so that BLM would be able to comply (GAO, 2008).

Although the BLM does not identify animals as unadoptable, it has moved over 20 000 horses that remain unadopted and for which the supply exceeds the demand into long-term holding on an extensive collection of pastures spanning tens of thousands of acres in the tall grass prairies of the Midwest. Here the animals live out their natural lives waiting, in theory at least, for the opportunity for adoption or sale into private homes. In the management of unwanted dogs and cats, the euthanasia of excess, unadopted animals has become an unfortunate and regrettable reality for most animal shelter and rescue organizations. For horses, however, it seems the public, the politicians, and the largest Agencies in charge of wild horse management are not yet ready to follow this paradigm.

24.7 Conclusion

Wild horses provide some unique challenges – from their management on the range, to controlling population numbers in balance with available forage resources, to capture and removal operations, adoption, and gentling into the domestic world. Myths, misconceptions, and historical prejudices run strong. It is difficult to describe their character even to knowledgeable horse people. They aren't simply like poorly behaved or unbroken domestic horses. They are truly wild animals, more akin to a 1000-pound (450 kg) whitetail deer than a domestic horse in some ways. Yet, in other ways, they are simply horses, just like other horses, simply amazing and simply magnificent. They are not one type of horse. They are Spanish and cobs and Quarter Horse and Thoroughbred types. They are drafts and even ponies in some herds. They are ultimately from the same genetic seed stock as domestic horses with the same physiology and mostly the same nutritional and animal care needs. Theirs is a rough-and-tumble world where natural selection constantly challenges the weak and rewards the strong. The emphasis in their management and care is about preventing problems rather than treating the individual. We are bound by the law and our ethical obligation to them as animals placed in our care to protect their well-being and provide for their welfare. As a veterinarian, my highest priority is to prevent their suffering, cure it if I can, and end it if I must. But we all share a larger ethical dilemma with the Agencies responsible for their care, and it is a dilemma that has no easy solution.

Tens of millions of dollars are spent feeding and caring for animals removed from the range to prevent the destruction of rangeland resources and their ultimate starvation. Would the horses as a whole be better off if these funds were spent instead on range management or fertility control research? Some will argue if we removed all the cattle and sheep from the public lands more horses could live there. Yes, that would be true for a time, but what would happen in 20 years after their numbers doubled, tripled or quadrupled. Would we then allow them to starve by the tens of thousands or remove the deer and elk to provide still more forage for the horses? The superhighways will never be plowed up and replaced with migration routes for the large ungulates across North America. So we are left with our dilemma. Remove wild horses from the range when we must to protect the rangeland resources and the horses themselves; push fertility control use as far as the science will allow while working to produce more effective and practical contraceptive agents; feed the ones in captivity for now or forever? All of this must be done while we strive to prevent the exploitation of wild horses and provide for their welfare.

Acknowledgements

The information, ideas, and opinions expressed are those of the author and do not necessarily represent those of the United States Department of Agriculture or the United States Department of Interior. The author would like to thank the many wild horse and burro specialists, wranglers and facility managers of the BLM Wild Horse and Burro Program, the owners and crews of the Cattoor Livestock Roundup Service and K&G Livestock, and the private veterinary practitioners who work with the BLM for sharing their knowledge of wild horses over the past ten years.

References

Asa, C.S. (1999) Male reproductive success in free-ranging feral horses. *Behavioral Ecology and Sociobiology* 47, 89–93.

Bowling, A.T. and Touchberry, R.W. (1990) Parentage of Great Basin feral horses. *Journal of Wildlife Management* 54(3), 424–429.

GAO (2008) *Bureau of Land Management: Effective Long-Term Options Needed to Manage Unadoptable Wild Horses.* GAO-09-77, October, Government Accountability Office, Washington, DC. Available at: www.gao.gov/new.items/d0977.pdf.

Henneke, D.R., Potter, G.D., Kreider, J.L. and Yeates, B.F. (1983) Relationship between condition score, physical measurements and body fat percentage in mares. *Equine Veterinary Journal* 15, 371–372.

Kaseda, Y. and Khalil, A.M. (1996) Harem size and reproductive success of stallions in Misaki feral horses. *Applied Animal Behaviour Science* 47, 163–173.

Killian, G., Thain, D., Diehl, N.K., Rhyan, J. and Miller, L. (2008) Four-year contraception rates of mares treated with single-injection porcine zona pellucida and GnRH vaccines and intrauterine devices. *Wildlife Research* 35(6), 531–539.

Kirkpatrick, J.F. (2005) The wild horse fertility control program. In *Humane Wildlife Solutions, The Role of Immunocontraception*, Rutberg, A.T. (ed.), pp. 63–75. Humane Society Press, Washington, DC.

Kirkpatrick, J.F. and Turner, A. (2002) Reversibility of action and safety during pregnancy of immunization against porcine zona pellucida in wild mares (*Equus caballus*). *Reproduction Supplement* 60, 197–202.

Kirkpatrick, J.F. and Turner, A. (2008) Achieving population goals in a long-lived wildlife species (*Equus caballus*) with contraception. *Wildlife Research* 35(6), 513–519.

Kirkpatrick, J.F., Liu, I.K.M. and Turner, J.W. (1990) Remotely-delivered immunocontraception in feral horses. *Wildlife Society Bulletin* 18, 326–330.

Liu, I.K.M., Bernoco, M. and Feldman, M. (1989) Contraception in mares heteroimmunized with porcine zona pellucida. *Journal of Reproduction and Fertility* 85, 19–29.

Singer, F.J., Zeigenfuss, L. Coates-Markle, L. and Schwieger, F. (2000) A demographic analysis, group dynamics, and genetic effective number in the Pryor Mountain wild horse population. In *Managers' Summary – Ecological Studies of the Pryor Mountain Wild Horse Range, 1992–1997*, Singer, F.J. and Schoenecker, K.A. (eds), pp. 73–89. US Geological Survey, Midcontinent Ecological Science Center, Fort Collins, CO.

Turner, J.W., Liu, I.K.M., Flanagan, D.R., Rutberg, A.T. and Kirkpatrick, J.F. (2007) Immunocontraception in wild horses: one inoculation provides two years of infertility. *Journal of Wildlife Management* 71(2), 662–667.

Welfare Issues in the Event Horse

25

Kent Allen

25.1 Introduction

Each discipline in equestrian sport has its own set of welfare concerns. Eventing challenges the equine athlete to compete in dressage, show jumping, and cross-country jumping phases of an equine triathlon. These horses must be fit enough for the cross-country jumping demands, and disciplined and athletic enough to perform in dressage and stadium jumping. Welfare concerns of the event horse are often related to the cross-country phase of the competition. During this phase, the horse is negotiating a technically difficult course on turf with solid jumping obstacles while at speed. The national and international organizations that regulate the sport of eventing have welfare codes and rules to assure that all horses and riders are capable of such a competition. The Fédération Equestre Internationale (FEI, International Equestrian Federation) addresses equine welfare by stating the following:[1]

> The Fédération Equestre Internationale (FEI) requires all those involved in the international equestrian sport to adhere to the FEI's Code of Conduct and to acknowledge and accept that at all times the welfare of the horse must be paramount and must never to subordinated to competitive or commercial influences.

(1) At all stages during the preparation and training of competition horses, welfare must take precedence over all other demands. This includes good horse management, training methods, farriery, tack, and transportation.

[1] FEI Code of Conduct, Fédération Equestre Internationale, Avenue de Rumine 37, CH-1005 Lausanne, Switzerland. Statement reproduced courtesy of the Fédération Equestre International (FEI) website.

Equine Welfare, First Edition. Edited by C. Wayne McIlwraith and Bernard E. Rollin.
© 2011 by UFAW. Published 2011 by Blackwell Publishing Ltd.

(2) Horses and competitors must be fit, competent and in good health before they are allowed to compete. This encompasses medication use, surgical procedures that threaten welfare or safety, pregnancy in mares and the misuse of aids.

(3) Events must not prejudice horse welfare. This involves paying careful attention to the competition areas, ground surfaces, weather conditions, stabling, site safety, and fitness of the horse for onward travel after the event.

(4) Every effort must be made to ensure that horses receive proper attention after they have competed and that they are treated humanely when their competition careers are over. This covers proper veterinary care, competition injuries, euthanasia, and retirement.

The FEI is also engaged with World Horse Welfare (www.worldhorsewelfare.org), which is a leading international equestrian welfare organization. In addition FEI is committed to continued consultation with riders, trainers, officials, and veterinarians to thoroughly research the welfare issues. Also, further education of stewards will also continue to ensure that welfare issues at FEI events are dealt with promptly and professionally.

FEI and national federations, especially the United States Equestrian Federation (USEF), participate in international and national education and exchange programs for stewards. Stewards have education requirements that must be met to qualify and maintain their national and international steward levels. The stewards and technical delegates are the monitoring arm of the regulatory bodies and as such are critical to welfare and rules enforcement. In the FEI system, the Ground Jury and Veterinary Delegates are in place at the competition for additional welfare and rule enforcement and immediate enforcement of the rules and common sense competition welfare issues.

While FEI codes and guidelines of welfare govern eventing at international venues, these recommendations should apply to all levels of the sport. Domestically, the United States Equestrian Federation (USEF) and United States Eventing Association (USEA) have their own welfare codes and committees. These organizations reflect the views of the FEI on animal welfare and provide these guidelines to all levels of the sport.

25.2 Competition and Equine Welfare

Equine welfare is the primary priority during competition. The process begins with proper identification, vaccination, and quarantine, which are followed and enforced by the selected Veterinary Delegate at all FEI competitions. The purpose of this process is to prevent the spread of disease and to protect the health of all competition horses. Additionally, facility layout, course design, and footing choices are all planned and continually monitored in the interest of animal welfare.

The cross-country course designer is a critical aspect of eventing. There is a national and international course designer consultant who evaluates newly designed cross-country courses. The technical delegate also evaluates the courses for consistency with the rules and whether the heights and spreads are correct and the course construction is of a safe nature. The Ground Jury then evaluates the course for rida-bility and suitability. Then finally a rider representative is nominated and can bring any specific rider concerns to the Ground Jury and the technical delegate.

Experience has shown that the consideration of environmental conditions is par-amount. Both the Atlanta Olympics in 1996 and Beijing Olympics in 2008 were in hot, humid environments. Prior to these competitions, extensive research was con-ducted regarding the effects of heat and humidity in the exercising three-day event horse, and these data were utilized during the Olympic Games with success (Jeffcott and Kohn, 1999; Bradbury and Allen, 1994; Jeffcott et al., 2009). Pertinent changes included a cooling stop during phase C (following the steeplechase portion) and a shortened portion of the cross-country course. Better cooling processes were also researched and instituted. Pressurized micro-nozzle misting fans were used to cool the areas horses frequented. Additionally, the riders and grooms were educated on proper use of ice and water to cool their horses. Horses were allowed intravenous fluids if needed, similar to many human athletic events. These adaptations by the FEI and USEF were the most significant accommodations and rule changes relating to the welfare of the three-day event horse at the time.

25.3 Injuries

This discipline requires strength, stamina, and speed. Fitness- and exhaustion-related injuries include exercise-induced pulmonary hemorrhage (EIPH), tendon and ligament injury, rhabdomyolysis, and trauma from hitting obstacles. During training and at a three-day event, competitor's soundness, fitness level, exhaustion, musculoskeletal heat load, and trauma should be addressed and considered. Soundness is evaluated at the jog-up prior to the start of competition and again after the cross-country phase, just prior to the show-jumping phase. This helps to ensure that the horse is fit to compete. Competing with an unsound horse can have devastating consequences for both horse and rider. The horse may be unable to adequately perform due to pain, resulting in breakdown injuries, falls or crashes, and possibly death. Fitness and exhaustion play a large role in the welfare of the event horse. Soft tissue injuries typically occur when supporting musculature becomes exhausted and tendons and ligaments are subjected to abnormal forces. Speed also plays a role in EIPH, as the majority of horses running at speed will have some degree of clinical or non-clinical bleeding (Allen, 2008). Many different inju-ries may be sustained by the event horse. They can be categorized as lacerations and abrasions, speed-related injuries, and jump-related injuries.

25.3.1 Lacerations
Lacerations of the distal limb are common due the horse jumping over fixed fences and varied terrain. Overreach wounds of the heel and stud-related punctures are quite common and can be painful to the horse. Because of the water jumps these

wounds are often contaminated and will require antibiotic therapy as well as a drawing poultice and tetanus prophylaxis if needed. Abrasions of the carpus are associated with water jump falls and a too deep or a rough gravel surface. These can be significant injuries and, if several of them are seen at the same event, they should be pointed out to the technical delegate and/or organizer, who may not be aware of the deteriorating surface under the water. If any of the wounds are near or are suspected to be penetrating injuries of a synovial structure, they should be carefully examined and possibly sent to a referral center for a more detailed assessment than may be available at the competition.

25.3.2 Speed-related injuries

Speed-related injuries can be many and varied. These will often be similar to injuries of the Thoroughbred racehorse.

Bleeding or exercise-induced pulmonary hemorrhage (EIPH) can be quite mild with a trickle of blood seen and not clinically relevant or can be more severe and require rest and a significant workup to determine the underlying cause. The worst expression of this is rupture of an aortic or pulmonary vessel and often presents as sudden death during exercise.

Running at speed can result in a variety of tendon and ligament injuries. These may present with obvious swelling and pain, with lameness in the affected area. They may also present as lameness with no apparent swelling (some superficial digital flexor core injuries and origin of the suspensory) and the swelling may develop later. The most common injury is tendonitis of the superficial digital flexor (SDFT), with desmitis of the suspensory ligament being the second most common. Injuries to the inferior check ligament, suspensory branches, origin of the suspensory, and collateral ligaments of the coffin joint are next most significant injuries. These injuries almost without exception will require withdrawing the horse from the competition once they are detected. Anti-inflammatory therapy, cold therapy, and support wraps as well as ultrasound diagnostics to determine the degree of the injury are indicated as soon as possible. However, it is rare that it is necessary to medicate the horse on the field of play, and it is safer and more prudent to transport the horse back to veterinary care in the barns and do a more detailed assessment. Severe manifestations of SDFT and suspensory injury may require the use of a Kimzey splint or a Robert Jones type bandage to appropriately support the non-weight-bearing leg and allow the horse to be loaded in a trailer and be taken to its stall or a pre-designated surgical referral center for further evaluation.

Exertional rhabdomyolysis (ER) or tying-up is common in the event horse and may be seen even at lower-level events. It may present as a horse that has stiffness in the hind limbs or it can present as a horse that is unable to walk. In its extreme form ER can present as a recumbent horse who may need fluids to rise, and it can present as a unilateral shortness of stride in the front or hind limbs. The significant factor is that it is recognized for what it is, and the horse is transported off the course and examined in more detail. Sometimes it presents as a horse reluctant to leave the stall, and stiff and short after the competition, with stiff and hard muscle mass most commonly in the area of the middle gluteal muscle group. A mild case may require nothing more than an anti-inflammatory injection and the horse is usually withdrawn from competition. For a moderate to severe case, the treating veterinarian should have a large-bore 14-gauge intravenous catheter to insert in the jugular and have a large-bore intravenous fluid administration set with the ability to run 20, 40 or more liters of a balanced electrolyte solution rapidly. Obviously poor conditioning, pressing an exhausted horse, or adverse environmental conditions can increase the chance for ER.

25.3.3 Jump-related injuries

Impacting a solid fence is a common scenario in the cross-country phase of the event horse. It may have no injury associated with it; however, the fall of the horse (hip and shoulder striking the ground) would normally eliminate the horse and rider combination. It also can result in a wide variety of injuries, with the most common being trauma to the stifle area and shoulder, carpus, pelvis, and neck. The mild versions of these injuries are ones that surface as abrasion, stiffness, and swelling after the cross-country phase, and the horse should be examined to see if the injury is mild and the horse can continue in the competition with icing and minor treatment. Some trauma is minor, such as foot bruising and lacerations. Some injuries are more major: patellar fractures and soft tissue stifle injuries occur when horses hang their hind legs over solid obstacles. The more significant injuries are those where the horse has gone acutely lame and requires transportation off the field of play.

25.3.4 Change in format – has it made a difference?

The original long format of eventing containing steeplechase and roads and tracks certainly tested the endurance and speed of the horses. The recent change to the short format was done in an effort to reduce the amount of fatigue-related injuries. As a consequence of the shortened format, course designers have designed more technically challenging courses. In response, riders rode their horses slower at the more technical aspects of the course and faster between the jump elements. This type of riding may result in greater fatigue in contrast to the steady pace once seen on the long-format courses (Murray *et al.*, 2006).

25.3.5 Effects of heat

Heat and exercise are major concerns in event horses. Musculoskeletal fatigue and heat load may therefore lead to further injury. Severe hyperthermia alone can result in collapse and brain damage in affected individuals (Sharma and Hoopes, 2003). Muscles, tendons, and ligaments generate an incredible amount of heat during exercise. This heat must be dissipated through sweating and evaporation. Any remaining heat can result in degeneration at the cellular level in soft tissue structures (Birch *et al.*, 1994). FEI, USEF, and USEA rules provide for modifying courses in extreme heat. Leg boots and wraps should all adhere to USEF/FEI regulations. Leg boots and wraps[2] must be carefully chosen in order to provide protection and adequate cooling, thus preventing significant tissue damage (Yamasaki *et al.*, 2001).

25.3.6 Falls

There has been a recent rise in dramatic rotational falls, which has greatly increased the risk to both horse and rider. In response, the USEA, USEF, and FEI technical committee assembled a forum to study horse falls in three-day eventing. The development of this group has led to the recent use of frangible (meant to break on impact) pins and deformable jump materials in competitions. Research into these and other safety options is ongoing.

25.3.7 Cardiovascular and respiratory problems

The role that the cardiovascular and respiratory systems play in event horse welfare has become of recent concern. Several horses have collapsed on course or had falls at obstacles directly related to exercise-induced pulmonary hemorrhage (EIPH), aortic rupture, or other unknown cardiac events. Studies relating age, physical condition, illness of the cardiovascular and respiratory tracts, as well as fitness are ongoing by the USEA Equine Safety Task Force (C. Kohn, Columbus, OH, pers. comm.). These studies hope to gain insight into how to prevent these catastrophic events. The USEA has also offered to provide necropsies for horses that die on course at eventing competitions. These research efforts should improve the understanding of why horses die on course and help prevent tragic accidents in the future.

25.4 Medication

Medication and anti-doping regulations also play a major role in eventing welfare. Recent changes to the FEI drug and medication rules mirror the welfare concerns of the sport. International (FEI) medication rules have an effect on welfare during competition and allow horses to compete on a level playing field. Additionally, these rules help ensure horses are free from pain and illness during competition. The purpose of this rule is that horses competing with an injury or unsoundness may increase the likelihood of a catastrophic event for both horse and rider.

Internationally, the FEI medication rules limit the number of medications a horse may receive before or during the time of competition. The FEI also provides a list of prohibited medications that cannot be given to the horse at any time. Additionally, there is a sub-list called the FEI list of detection times. This list includes drugs that

---

[2] Marlin, D. (2009) Leg protection for the event horse. Presentation at the USEA Annual Meeting and Convention, New Orleans, LA.

may be given within a certain time frame before the start of competition. All pharmaceuticals on the list are well researched, and the FEI provides accurate acceptable dosages and detection times.

25.4.1 Testing

The FEI has standardized all competition laboratories worldwide for accurate testing of some of these substances. They also have recently proposed changes in their medication rules that have provoked much discussion in 2009 and 2010. In early 2009, the FEI updated their approach regarding medication rules, in order to bring themselves more in line with the World Anti-Doping Agency (WADA). This is the agency that governs drug rules for human athletes. This new approach by the FEI is helpful because, when a challenge occurs with an FEI medication ruling, the issue is managed with WADA-like principles by the Court of Arbitration for Sport in Switzerland.

Part of these new changes consisted of compiling an extensive list of drugs and medications (similar to WADA) and then deciding which pharmaceuticals were and were not allowed during FEI competitions. The FEI produced a final list of pharmaceuticals, with yearly modifications, known as the Equine Prohibited Substance List. This list is split into two parts: prohibited medications and controlled medications. The controlled medications are substances that are regularly and legitimately used in equine veterinary medicine but are not allowed during FEI competitions.

25.4.2 Medication – the rules and why we have them

Most of the controlled medications are commonly used in veterinary medicine, such as acepromazine, detomidine, lidocaine, and flunixin meglumine. Nevertheless, any controlled drugs found in the horse at detectable levels under FEI rules carry the possibility of a six-month to two-year suspension. Possible shorter suspension times may apply depending on individual mitigating circumstances. This controlled medications list contains the sub-list of researched drug detection times (FEI List of Detection Times) to assist treating veterinarians with pharmaceutical administration prior to competition. Prohibited medications are pharmaceuticals used in human or veterinary medicine that are strictly banned for use in competition horses at any time.[3] If a veterinarian is going to administer a medication close to an FEI event, they should select a controlled medication within the acceptable detection time if at all possible.

Antibiotics, anti-ulcer medications, anti-EPM medications, vitamins, fluids, and progesterone supplementation for mares are allowed for use under FEI regulations. There are obvious restrictions as to how, when, and under what supervision they can be administered to a horse in an FEI compound. Owing to integrity concerns

---

[3] See FEICleanSport.org.

brought forward by national federations after controversy about unapproved treatments provided to horses at the Olympic Games in China, an FEI Commission
chaired by Lord Stevens was instituted. The commission made several recommendations that resulted in increased stewarding and preventive injections able to be given
in a designated treatment stall under steward supervision. Forms will have to be filled
out for this and any other permission to medicate. Competitors should check with
their veterinarian or FEI Veterinary Delegate for the forms or for further details.

New in 2010, Legend®, Adequan®, and Pentosan Equine Injection® will be
allowed for administration to horses in the FEI compound under FEI Veterinary
Delegate or competition steward supervision.[4] Allowing these treatments reflects
the FEI's attitude towards preventive maintenance joint therapy that doesn't have
potent performance-enhancing properties.

Also in the new FEI Veterinary Rules will be a requirement for exhibitors to keep
a medication log book on each individual horse. There will be some guidelines
available to download a template log, or exhibitors may create a log book themselves. Each FEI horse should have their own log that lists the date of treatment, the
name and dose of the medication, how the medication was administrated, and who
administered the drug to the horse.

Nationally, USEF and USEA medication rules have also changed recently. USEF
medication rules in the past have allowed for the use of up to two non-steroidal
anti-inflammatory drugs (NSAIDs) at restricted levels. Over a two-year period of
time there has been discussion about reducing this to a single NSAID with a
restricted level. The discussion in the end focused on horse welfare in all equine
disciplines. It was decided that more than one NSAID in the horse may be additive,
can cover up a significant lameness, and may have detrimental side-effects to the
gastrointestinal tract, urinary tract, and joints. The discussion then changed to the
time of when the switch to a single NSAID rule should occur. Some disciplines
within the USEF became very concerned that the proposed implementation date of
December 1, 2010, was too soon and their members couldn't comply. A compromise was reached that delayed rule implementation but gave a start date for the
single NSAID rule. Beginning April 1, 2010, USEF members will need to file a form
prior to competing declaring the use of two NSAIDs. The implementation date for
reducing NSAID usage to one at a time was pushed back until December 1, 2011.

To use two NSAIDs between April 1, 2010, and December 1, 2011, a rider must
go to the show office and pick up and fill out and then turn back in a NSAID
Disclosure Form. This form will list the two NSAIDs that are being used, the dose
and the time, and the diagnosis of the problem, as well as the veterinarian prescribing them. Normal prohibitions such as the use of phenylbutazone and flunixin
meglumine together will still apply.

[4] Legend®, Bayer Animal Health, Bayer, KS 66201, USA. Adequan®, Luitpold Pharmaceuticals,
Inc., New York, NY 11967, USA. Pentosan Equine Injection®, Nature Vet, Glenorie, New South
Wales, Australia.

Shauna Spurlock states in the United States Hunter Jumper Association (USHJA) Resource guide, 'The potential for the NSAIDs to affect normal physiology in the joints, intestinal and bone healing, in addition to the increased risk of gastrointestinal ulceration and kidney damage, has led to the rules that limit this practice and limit the risk for the horse. Even when using two NSAIDs in accordance with the existing rules, it should be done understanding the real risk as well as the potential benefits.' Based on USEF Drug and Medication program statistics, a large number of trainers, owners, and amateurs understand the danger associated with administering two NSAIDs. Since the program started discussing this problem in 2007, the use of double NSAIDs in horses tested has dropped from 4.8% in 2008 to 3.1% in 2009 (S. Schumacher, Staff Veterinarian, USEF Equine Drug and Medication Program, Hilliard, OH, pers. comm.). This is a reduction of thousands (extrapolated from number of horses tested to number of horses competing) of horses being administered two NSAIDs and shows a significant concern for horse welfare at the national level. The final implementation of the single NSAID rule by the end of 2011 will further demonstrate this commitment to equine welfare. Often changes in Drug and Medication rules mirror public and veterinary concern for horse welfare. Such rule modifications demonstrate the concerns of the individual competition disciplines, the governing federations, and equine sport as a whole.

25.5 Challenges of Eventing and Response of the Industry

The sport of eventing has had a challenging decade, with some highly publicized casualties to both horses and riders. The sport has responded with new and more stringent rules as well as new research into jump materials. The sport is also pursuing new avenues of equine research, including the cardiovascular system. Eventing has risen to equine welfare challenges such as coping with heat and humidity issues at the Atlanta 1996 Olympic Games. The sport is continuing to work to reduce rotational falls, study cardiovascular issues, and change drug and medication regulations for the good of the equine eventing athlete.

References

Allen, A.K. (2008) Emergency preparedness for eventing. In *Proceedings of the 54th Annual Convention of the AAEP*, pp. 149–152.

Birch, H.L., Wilson, A.M. and Goodship, A.E. (1994) The effect of exercise-induced localized hyperthermia on tendon cell survival. *Journal of Biomechanics* 27, 899–905.

Bradbury, E. and Allen, A.K. (1994) Equi-mist fan/mist system evaluation. In *On to Atlanta '96*, Clarke, A.F. and Jeffcott, L.B. (eds), pp. 75–78. Equine Research Center, University of Guelph, Ontario.

Jeffcott, L.B. and Kohn, C.W. (1999) Contributions of exercise physiology research to the success of the 1996 Equestrian Olympic Games. *Equine Veterinary Journal (Supplement)* 31(S30), 347–355.

Jeffcott, L., Leung, W.M. and Riggs, C. (2009) Managing the effects of the weather on the equestrian events of the 2008 Beijing Olympic Games. *Veterinary Journal* 182, 412–429.

Murray, J.K., Senior, J.M. and Singer, E.R. (2006) A comparison of cross-country recovery rates at CCI 2* with and without steeplechase competitions. *Equine Veterinary Journal (Supplement)* 38(S36), 133–138.

Sharma, H.S. and Hoopes, P.J. (2003) Hyperthermia induced pathophysiology of the central nervous system. *International Journal of Hyperthermia* 19, 325–354.

Yamasaki, H., Goto, M., Yoshihara, T. *et al.* (2001) Exercise-induced superficial digital flexor tendon hyperthermia and the effect of cooling sheets on Thoroughbreds. *Journal of Equine Science* 12, 85–91.

Index

Page numbers in *italics* denote figures and tables.

Equine Welfare, First Edition. Edited by C. Wayne McIlwraith and Bernard E. Rollin.
© 2011 by UFAW. Published 2011 by Blackwell Publishing Ltd.

Printed in the United States
By Bookmasters